CORONARY CIRCULATION

DEVELOPMENTS IN
CARDIOVASCULAR MEDICINE

CORONARY CIRCULATION

From basic mechanisms to clinical implications

edited by

JOS A.E. SPAAN
Department of Medical Physics, Faculty of Medicine,
University of Amsterdam, The Netherlands

ALBERT V.G. BRUSCHKE
Department of Cardiology, University Hospital,
Leiden, The Netherlands

and

ADRIANA C. GITTENBERGER-DE GROOT
Laboratory for Anatomy and Embryology, Faculty of Medicine,
University of Leiden, The Netherlands

1987 **MARTINUS NIJHOFF PUBLISHERS**
a member of the KLUWER ACADEMIC PUBLISHERS GROUP
DORDRECHT / BOSTON / LANCASTER

Distributors

for the United States and Canada: Kluwer Academic Publishers, P.O. Box 358, Accord Station, Hingham, MA 02018-0358, USA
for the UK and Ireland: Kluwer Academic Publishers, MTP Press Limited, Falcon House, Queen Square, Lancaster LA1 1RN, UK
for all other countries: Kluwer Academic Publishers Group, Distribution Center, P.O. Box 322, 3300 AH Dordrecht, The Netherlands

Library of Congress Cataloging in Publication Data

```
Coronary circulation.

  (Developments in cardiovascular medicine)
  Based on a Boerhaave course organized by the Faculty
of Medicine, University of Leiden, the Netherlands, Apr.
9-10, 1987.
  Includes index.
  1. Coronary circulation--Congresses.  I. Spaan, Jos
A. E.   II. Bruschke, Albert Vincent Godefridus.
III. Gittenberger-de Groot, Adriana C.   IV. Rijksuniver-
siteit te Leiden.  Faculteit der Geneeskunde.
V. Series.  [DNLM: 1. Coronary Circulation--congresses.
W1 DE997VME / WG 300 C8216 1987]
QP108.C67  1987      612'.17      87-19614
```

ISBN-13: 978-94-010-8013-2   e-ISBN-13: 978-94-009-3369-9
DOI: 10.1007/978-94-009-3369-9

Book information

This publication is based upon a Boerhaave course organized by the Faculty of Medicine, University of Leiden, The Netherlands

Copyright

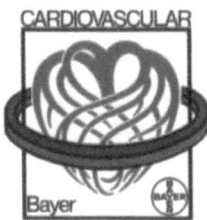

Acknowledgement

The organizers of the symposium "Coronary Circulation" on which this publication is based, gratefully acknowledge the support of Bayer Nederland B.V.

C O N T E N T S

VIII

FOREWORD

Few diagnostic methods in Cardiology have heralded such revolutionary developments as the introduction of coronary arteriography. When, in the early 1960's, Dr. F. Mason Sones demonstrated that visualization of the coronary anatomy in living humans was not only feasible but sufficiently safe and reliable to be used as a clinical tool in the evaluation of patients with known or suspected ischemic heart disease, the thusfar somewhat neglected area of coronary circulation became the focus of interest. Naturally, for a considerable period of time a great deal of emphasis was placed upon coronary anatomy. Simple relations between narrowing lesions, impediment to flow, and prognosis were assumed to exist. Spectacular results of surgical coronary revascularization seemed to confirm this concept.

Gradually it has become evident that the pathophysiology of coronary artery disease is considerably more complex. Diagnostic methods were introduced to assess and quantify exercise-induced myocardial ischemia. At first, these tests were used mainly to achieve a more discriminative selection of candidates for coronary arteriography and the coronary arteriogram remained the gold standard. Currently, these techniques have evolved to the point where they provide valuable functional and metabolic information. They have become powerful independent tools in clinical investigations and evaluation of individual patients.

At the same time major advances have been made in basic research on the coronary circulation and its interaction with myocardial contraction and metabolism. New techniques, which include the use of computer models, radioisotope labelling of natural substrates of myocardial metabolism, and nuclear magnetic resonance spectroscopy, have opened up unforeseen possibilities to explore myocardial physiology and metabolism under a variety of conditions. Studies of the micro-anatomy and embryologic development of the coronary arterial system have further broadened our understanding of coronary circulation.

However, despite the great strides made in both clinical and basic research, until recently, there has been too little acknowledgement of the benefits to be gained from a multidisciplinary approach, in which scientist and clinicians work closely together. Such an approach is mandatory to effectively study the intricate problems related to coronary circulation and to ensure optimal treatment of pathological conditions.

We compiled this volume which brings together the results of research and clinical investigations. We trust that this endeavor will set a precedent for the future, resulting in better mutual understanding. The impact of multidisciplinary studies on clinical decision making will continue to be felt in increasing proportions as new diagnostic possibilities and methods to restore coronary flow become available.

The papers presented are of interest to anyone involved in the management of patients with coronary artery disease or to anyone conducting research related to one of the many aspects of coronary circulation.

We are grateful to the authors, whose great expertise and didactic skill resulted in this presentation of the state of the art.

The Editors

L I S T   O F   C O N T R I B U T O R S

- Bruschke, A.V.G.
Department of Cardiology, University Hospital, Rijnsbugerweg
10-C5-P, 2333 AA   Leiden, the Netherlands
Co-author: B. Buis

- Downey, J.M.
Department of Physiology, University of South Alabama, Mobile
AL 36688, U.S.A.

- Gittenberger-de Groot, A.C.
Laboratory for Anatomy and Embryology, State University
Leiden, Wassenaarseweg 62, 2333 AA   Leiden, the Netherlands
Co-authors: A.J.J.C. Bogers, M.M. Bartelings

- James, T.N.
University of Alabama, University Station, Birmingham, Alabama
35294, U.S.A.

- Karp, R.B.
University of Chicago Hospital, 5841 South Merryland Avenue,
P.O. Box 152, Chicago, Illinois 60637, U.S.A.

- Kramer, J.R.
Department of Cardiology, Cleveland Clinic Foundation, 9500
Euclid Avenue, Cleveland, Ohio 44106, U.S.A.
Co-authors: S. Strikwerda, C. Kittrell, M.S. Feld

- Krauss, X.H.
Co-authors: A. de Roos, S. Postema, J. Doornbos, E.E. van der
Wall, A.E. van Voorthuisen, A.V.G. Bruschke
Department of Cardiology, University Hospital, Rijnsburgerweg
10-C5-P, 2333 AA   Leiden, the Netherlands
Present address of X.H. Krauss: Department of Cardiology,
Zuiderziekenhuis, Groen Hilledijk 315, 3075 EA   Rotterdam, the
Netherlands

- Laarse, A. van der
Department of Cardiobiochemistry, University Hospital,
Rijsburgerweg 10-C5-P, 2333 AA   Leiden, the Netherlands

- Reiber, J.H.C.
Thoracic Centre, Erasmus University, Dr. Molewaterplein 50,
3000 DR   Rotterdam, the Netherlands
Co-authors: C.J. Kooyman, C.J. Slager, J.J. Gerbrands*, A. den
Boer, J. van Ommeren, F. Zijlstra, P. Serruys
*Information theory group, Delft University of Technology,
Delft, the Netherlands

- Reneman, R.S.
Department of Physiology, Biomedical Centre, State University
Limburg, P.O. Box 616, 6200 MD   Maastricht, the Netherlands
Co-authors: Th. Arts, C.H. Augustijn, F.W. Prinzen, G.J. Vusse

- Ruigrok, T.J.C.
    Department of Cardiology, University Hospital,
    Catharijnesingel 101, 3511 GV Utrecht, the Netherlands and
    Interuniversity Cardiology Institute, the Netherlands
    Co-author: J.H. Kirkels*
    *Interuniversity Cardiology Institute, and department of
    Cardiology, University Hospital, Catharijnesingel 101, 3511 GV
    Utrecht, the Netherlands

- Sauer, U.
    Deutsches Herzcentrum, Lothstrasse 11, 8000 Muenchen, B.R.D.
    Co-authors: A.C. Gittenberger-de Groot*, K. Buehlmeyer, F.
    Sebening, J. Apitz, I. Hammerer, W. Hoffmann, M. Wimmer
    *State University Leiden, Leiden, the Netherlands

- Sibley, D.H.
    Department of Cardiology, University of Alabama, Birmingham,
    35294 Alabama, U.S.A.

- Simoons, M.L.
    Thoracic Centre, University Hospital Dijkzigt, Dr.
    Molewaterplein 40, 3015 GD Rotterdam, the Netherlands

- Spaan, J.A.E.
    Department of Medical Physics, University of Amsterdam,
    Meibergdreef 15, 1105 AZ Amsterdam, the Netherlands
    Co-authors: I. Vergroesen, J. Dankelman, H. Stassen

- Steendijk, P.
    Department of Paediatrics, University Hospital, Rijnsburgerweg
    10, 2333 AA Leiden, the Netherlands
    Co-authors: A.D. van Dijk, J. Baan

- Tillmanns, H.
    Abteilung Innere Medizin III, Medizinische Universitaets
    Klinik, Bergheimerstrasse 58, D-6900 Heidelberg, B.R.D.
    Co-authors: H. Leinberger, F.J. Neumann, M. Steinhausen
    N. Parekh, R. Zimmermann, R. Dussel, W. Kuebler

- Tomanek, R.J.
    Department of Anatomy, College of Medicin, University of Iowa,
    Iowa City IA 52242, U.S.A.

- Wall, E.E. van der
    Department of Cardiology, University Hospital, Rijnsburgerweg
    10-C5-P, 2333 AA Leiden, the Netherlands
    Co-authors: E.K.J. Pauwels, A.V.G. Bruschke

- Wieringa, P.A.
    Department of Physiology and Physiological Physics, State
    University Leiden, Wassenaarseweg 62, 2333 AL Leiden, the
    Netherlands

I
Coronary anatomy

MICROANATOMY OF THE CORONARY CIRCULATION

Robert J. Tomanek

INTRODUCTION

Myocardial O_2 supply is dependent upon a variety of factors. Since oxygen extraction is high in the myocardium, blood flow and $\dot{V}O_2$ are tightly coupled. Thus, increases in cardiac work require increases in flow which are commensurate with the enhanced O_2 demand. In addition to its dependency on flow, O_2 supply to the cardiocyte is also linked to the density and arrangement of capillaries. Therefore, the distribution of flow, a function of the microcirculation, is dependent upon 1) flow through the arterioles and 2) the numbers and spacing patterns of capillaries. This statement suggests that architectural and anatomical considerations are important in the various adaptations of the coronary circulation. Moreover, anatomical changes often underlie decrements in perfusion and O_2 delivery.

These anatomical changes can involve either precapillary or capillary vessels. Atherosclerosis occurs primarily in the large epicardial arteries, while arteriosclerosis may involve the general population of coronary arteries. Cardiomyopathies and cardiac hypertrophy in response to hypertension are characterized by an inadequate growth of the microvascular bed. While these diseases may not affect myocardial perfusion at rest they usually are accompanied by a decrement in coronary reserve. In addition, anatomical changes in the walls of resistance vessels, such as fibrosis or medial reorganization, might limit the vasodilator capacity of the vessel. Thus, the nutrition of the myocardial cell can be compromised by 1) limitations of flow through precapillary vessels or 2) reductions in capillary density or enhanced heterogeneity of capillary spacing. This communication focuses on three topics. First, the anatomical characteristics of the microvessels and their functional correlates are described. Second, experimental data on the consequences of hypertension and left ventricular hypertrophy on the coronary vasculature are presented. Third, evidence for angiogenesis during long-term hypertension and LVH is documented.

HISTOLOGICAL CHARACTERISTICS OF CORONARY VESSELS

Coronary arteries and arterioles are quite similar to their counterparts in other vascular beds. Endothelial cells together with the subendothelium and internal elastic membrane (which is absent in the smallest arterioles) comprise the intima. The major difference between arterioles, small arteries and large arteries is the number of layers of smooth muscle in the tunica media. As lumen diameter decreases so does the number of smooth muscle layers. However, the medial thickness does not decrease in proportion to luminal diameter and, therefore, wall thickness/lumen diameter ratio is largest in the smallest (terminal) arterioles (Figure 1).

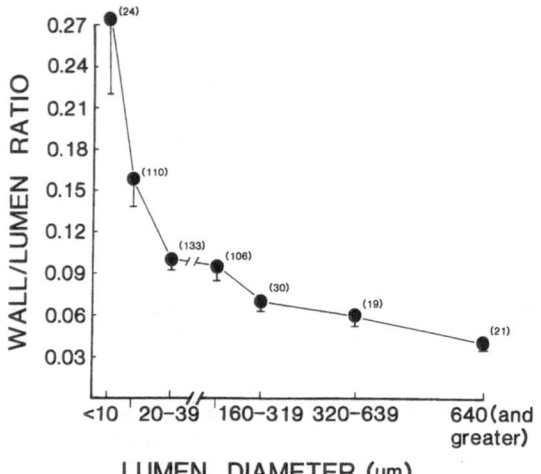

FIGURE 1. Wall/lumen ratios of coronary arteries and arterioles with various lumen diameters are illustrated. The values are means ± SEM based on 8 dogs; the number of vessels measured is indicated in parentheses.

The microvascular bed is numerically dominated by capillaries which have densities of 3,000-4,000/mm^2 and indent into adjacent cardiocytes (Figure 2).

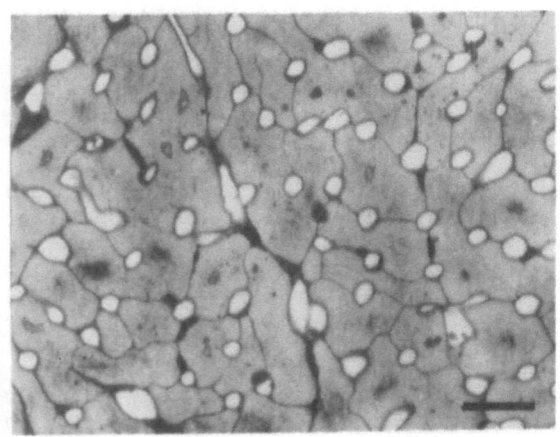

FIGURE 2. Cardiocytes cut in cross-section to illustrate capillary profiles (round-oval translucent areas. The bar represents 20 μm.

Arterioles, defined here as precapillary vessels with lumen diameters of 200 μm or less, usually have one or two layers of smooth muscle in their media (the largest have up to three). In data obtained from dog left ventricle we noted that over 50% of arterioles are less than 30 μm in diameter and generally constitute terminal arterioles. Whether precapillary sphincters occur with consistency in the coronary vasculature is uncertain, although they have been described in man (12) and dog (11). Such structures are important in the regulation of flow to a given capil-

lary bed.   Recent work on the left ventricles of rabbits indicates that
under resting conditions approximately one-half of the total number of
arterioles and capillaries are perfused at any given point in time (21).
This finding is consistent with the concept of capillary recruitment,
which suggests that progressively greater numbers of capillaries become
perfused as O_2 demand increases.

Myocardial capillaries are characterized by a continuous endothelium
which is about 0.2-0.3 μm thick and contains numerous plasmalemmal
vesicles.   Intercellular clefts, about 10-20 nm wide, occur between
adjacent endothelial cells.   These clefts are periodically interrupted
by occluding (tight) junctions.   Passage of small molecules occurs via
the clefts, which appear to represent the small pore system elaborated
through the use of molecules of graded size.   Larger molecules, experimentally represented by electron-dense tracers, e.g., horseradish perox-
idase (MW = 40,000), have been used to demonstrate transcapillary exchange via plasmalemmal vesicles.   However, utilizing three-dimensional
reconstructions of ultrathin serial sections and electron microscopy it
has recently been demonstrated that myocardial endothelial "plasmalemmal
vesicles" are actually components of more complex channels which allow
communication between the capillary lumen and extracellular compartment
(1).   Such a system of channels probably allows for the passage of macro-
molecules.

DISTRIBUTION OF CORONARY ARTERIOLES

To appreciate the three-dimensional structure of the coronary vasculature we arrested rabbit hearts in diastole with procaine, which also
serves to maximally vasodilate the coronary vessels, and then introduced
a plastic compound (Batson's) into the coronary arteries. By using a
fairly viscous mixture and injecting a limited amount of the compound we
were able to fill most parts of the left ventricle as far as the terminal
arterioles and parts of the capillary bed.   Subsequently, the heart tissue was digested by a saturated KOH solution (60°C).   Figure 3 illustrates the branching patterns of arterioles and arteries as observed via
scanning electron microscopy.   We followed the branches of the left
anterior   descending   artery   (LAD).   Our   observations   warrant   several
conclusions.   First, an artery may have branches which vary greatly in
size, i.e. from arteries with diameters close to the parent artery to
small arterioles.   Such variation is seen in Figure 3A.   Second, the
number of generations of arteries and arterioles preceding the capillary
bed is extremely variable as is their size distribution.   In Figure 3B a
third order artery (i.e. with reference to the LAD which is considered
the primary vessel) is parent to an arteriole (100 μm diameter, 4th order
vessel).   The branching of successive arterioles ends in a terminal
arteriole which in this case is a seventh order vessel.   In contrast, the
260 μm diameter artery (second order) seen in Figure 3A has a terminal
arteriole arising directly from it (arrow). Figure 4 summarizes some of
the variations in the origins of terminal arterioles.   In this illustration terminal arterioles are seen to range from third to fifth order, and
vary in diameter from 12 to 30 μm.   However, it should be noted that
these vessels, as measured in histological sections, may have luminal
diameters smaller than 10 μm (Figure 1).   Finally, it is obvious that
terminal arterioles are extremely short, usually about 100 μm, compared

6

to capillaries which often extend for one millimeter before reaching a venule.

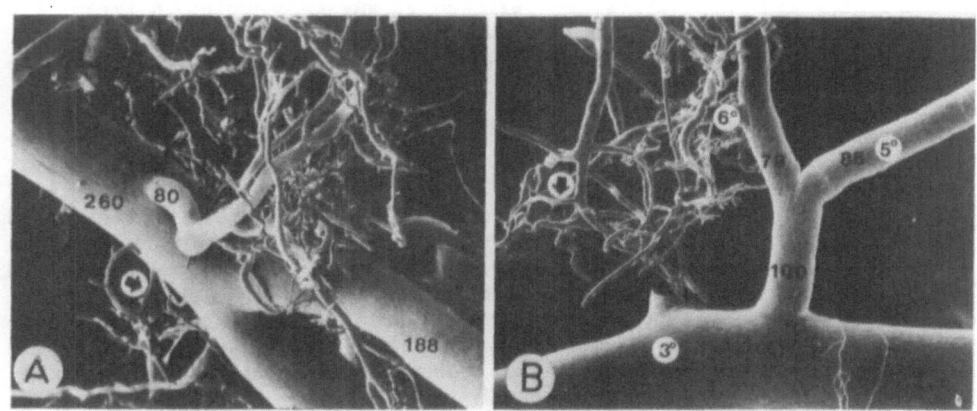

FIGURE 3. Coronary casts of rabbit LV. Arterial and arteriolar diameters are given; terminal arterioles are indicated by arrows. In B the generation or order of vessel is given in some cases (LAD = 1°). These vessels were obtained from the epicardial half of the myocardium.

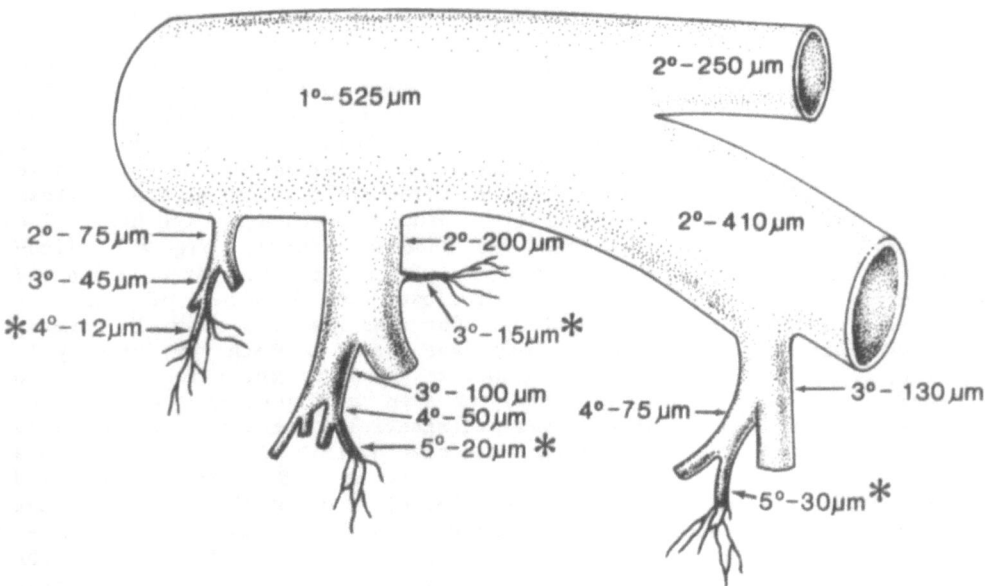

FIGURE 4. Illustration representing a summary of origins, branching patterns and diameters of arterioles. Terminal arterioles are indicated by asterisks. The generation or order of arteries and arterioles is indicated (LAD = 1°).

ARTERIOLAR CONTRIBUTIONS TO VASCULAR RESISTANCE

Resistance to flow in a vascular bed is primarily a function of a vessel's luminal radius as indicated by Poiseuille's Law which relates flow (Q) in cylindrical tubes to the pressure gradient (ΔP), the radius of the tube's lumen to be 4th power (r^4), the viscosity of blood (η), and the tube's length (l) in the equation: $Q = \Delta P \pi r^4/8\eta l$. Resistance (R) can readily be calculated from the equation: $R = \Delta P/Q$. One can easily appreciate that even a very modest change in arteriolar radius has a marked effect on blood flow, e.g. if radius decreases by 50% and ΔP remains constant, flow decreases 16 fold. During maximal pharmacolog-ically-induced dilatation, coronary flow can increase five fold over resting flow (4). A number of functional alterations can contribute to an increase in vascular resistance as evidenced in hypertensive states. These include 1) altered sensitivity to vasoactive substances, 2) increased myogenic activity, 3) increased sympathetic activity and 4) increased plasma renin levels.

To specify the distribution of resistance in the coronary vascula-ture, a recent study measured microvascular pressures and vessel diameters in beating cat hearts (2). Figure 5 illustrates the pressure drop in coronary vessels in these experiments.

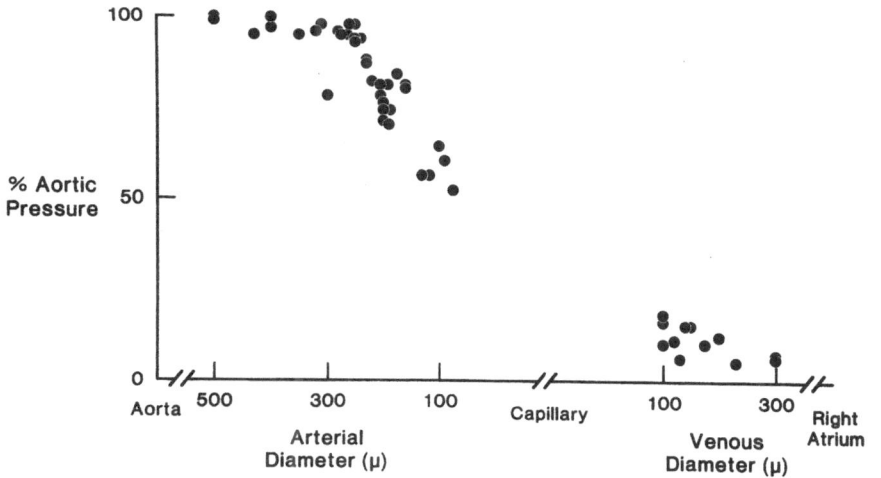

FIGURE 5. Coronary microvascular pressure distribution in anesthetized, open-chest cats. Data courtesy of W.M. Chilian; see reference 2 for further details of this study.

These data suggest that there is a negligible drop in pressure from the aorta to 300 µm arteries. However, as diameter decreases from 300-200 µm pressure clearly begins to fall in the coronary circuit. In summary a noteworthy 25% of the coronary resistance resides in vessels above arterioles with 200 µm diameters, 20% in 100-200 µm arterioles and 55% distal to 100 µm arterioles. During maximal vasodilation the distribu-tion of resistance shifts so that 90% resides in arterioles <200 µm in diameter, a finding which indicates that a substantial dilation occurs in vessels proximal to 200 μm arterioles. Thus, it is suggested that a wide size range of arterioles may contribute to the regulation of coronary flow.

MICROVASCULATURE IN HYPERTENSION AND LVH

One of the major liabilities of LVH during hypertension is a decrement in coronary reserve (3). This decrement can be demonstrated by a reduction in peak/resting flow velocity during reactive hyperemia (9), or by an increase in minimal coronary vascular resistance (MCVR) calculated from maximal myocardial perfusion measured with radioactive microspheres (8). An increased MCVR/unit mass could be due to any of several anatomic variables. These include: 1) failure of vascular growth to match the magnitude of LVH, 2) a decrease in lumen radius of resistance vessels due to medial hypertrophy, 3) a decrease in vasodilatory capacity due to medial fibrosis, and 4) arteriolar rarefaction, i.e. absolute decrease in the number of arterioles - as demonstrated in other vascular beds, e.g. skeletal muscle (7,10) - due to systemic hypertension. If lumen diameter decreases or arteriolar rarefaction occurs then one would expect total MCVR to increase. Such a trend was observed in our study on six month old spontaneously hypertensive rats (18). When the SHR were treated from the time of weaning with hydralazine, hypertension was completely prevented while LVH was not significantly attenuated. Under these conditions both total and per unit mass MCVR was reduced, suggesting that hypertension plays a direct role in modifying the coronary vasculature. This conclusion is consistent with data on the right ventricle of SHR which experiences the same pressure in its coronary vasculature as the left ventricle, but does not exhibit myocardial hypertrophy. Yet MCVR/unit mass in the right ventricle is significantly elevated in SHR (18, 20).

Subsequently, we studied dogs with renovascular hypertension of six weeks duration (16). MCVR per unit mass was elevated by 67% although LV/body weight ratio was only 27% above controls. Yet we found no evidence of an increased wall/lumen ratio of any size class of arterioles or arteries. Since total MCVR was not significantly altered, it would appear that most of the increase in MCVR/unit mass was due to a decrease in arteriolar density. A similar situation may occur in humans who presumably have normal coronary arteries but severe left ventricular hypertrophy secondary to valvular aortic stenosis. When the reactive hyperemic response was evaluated with a Doppler probe (flow velocity in the LAD was measured before and after a 20 second occlusion) it was found to be severely impaired (8). In contrast reactive hyperemia in the right coronary artery was nearly normal. These data on humans suggest that the substantial increase in LV mass has a marked effect on coronary reserve. Taken together the data from these studies suggest that both the increase in LV mass and the presence or persistence of hypertension may contribute to a decrease in coronary vasodilator reserve.

At the present time, it is not possible to adequately define the vascular alterations, particularly those in arterioles, which might explain the decrements in coronary vasodilator reserve which occur with the development of LVH in response to hypertension. However, it is obvious that a number of factors influence the response of the coronary vessels during LVH, e.g. 1) the stimulus for the LVH, 2) the duration of the LVH, 3) the age of the animal when LVH is induced, and 4) the species studied. These points have been addressed in a recent review (3).

While little information concerning the major resistance vessels, the arterioles, in LVH is available, considerable data have been generated on myocardial capillaries. A reduction in capillary density is a consistent finding during the development of LVH in various animal models of hypertension (13). Thus, the development of LVH in hypertensive states is characterized by at least a limited growth response (proliferation) of the capillary bed. Depending on the extent of the decrement in capillarity, the potential for cardiocyte hypoxia may be increased. Henquell et al. (5) noted that a 30-40% increase in LV mass in hypertension led to a 2.4 μm increase in minimal (anatomical) intercapillary distance, which could limit the diffusion distance for oxygen to the cardiocytes. Such a change may not be significant under resting conditions, but could be most important during periods of high oxygen demand.

In addition to numerical density, the heterogeneity of capillary spacing is important in oxygen supply to the myocardial cell (14,19). Estimates of myocardial oxygenation for tissue cylinder radii 8 to 18 μm indicate that the percentage of anoxic tissue increases with increasing heterogeneity of capillary spacing (14). Such data indicate that the heterogeneity factor is an important determinant of tissue oxygenation irrespective of the mean values for PO_2. This variability of intercapillary distance can be estimated from histological sections. A recent method is that of utilizing a computerized digitizer to prescribe capillary domains (Figure 6), and derive the log SD which represents an index of variability. It can be seen that the individual capillary domains (perfusion field of a single capillary) vary. An increased log SD has been demonstrated in spontaneously hypertensive rats (6), suggesting that the heterogeneity of capillary spacing is increased in this model of LVH. This change could presumably render certain cells more vulnerable to hypoxia during high O_2 demand.

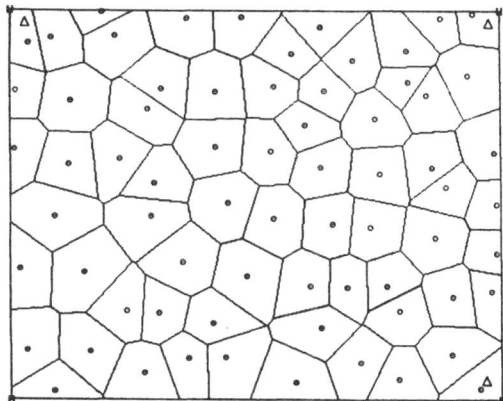

FIGURE 6. Capillary domains as generated by computer-assisted digitization from Turek et al. (19) with permission. Each capillary (small circles) has demarcated around it a "domain" established by analysis of intercapillary distances.

ANGIOGENESIS AND LVH DURING HYPERTENSION

The above discussion pointing out decrements in vasodilator reserve and capillarity would imply that the appropriate stimulus or growth factor for vascular growth is unavailable or inadequate. However, a variable angiogenesis may occur as evidenced by recent experiments. In SHR myocardial capillary numerical surface and volume densities become normalized (comparable to normotensive controls) between seven and 15 months of age, a time interval which corresponds to stabilized LVH (17). Autoradiographic experiments on 12 month old rats in this study demonstrated that thymidine incorporation into endothelial nuclei of SHR, an index of DNA synthesis, was more than twice that of the WKY. Moreover, coronary reserve measured with microspheres (20) or by determining peak resting flow velocity with a pulsed Doppler (9), is similar in SHR and normotensive WKY after this period of stabilized blood pressure and left ventricular growth. These lines of evidence would tend to support the idea that angiogenesis involving arterioles and capillaries occurs after a long period of hypertension and corresponds to the period of stabilized LVH.

Most recently we examined the effects of long-term (seven months) renovascular hypertension on the microvascular bed in dogs. In contrast to a six week period of hypertension (16) MCVR/unit mass was not significantly increased despite a large increase in LVW/body weight (46%). Arteriolar profile density was similar in the dogs with LVH and the controls, suggesting arteriolar growth which is consistent with the MCVR data. We also examined, morphometrically, a number of capillary parameters summarized in table 1. While capillary numerical density tended to be lower in the dogs with LVH the difference between the groups was not significant. If no capillary growth had occurred the density of

TABLE 1. Effects of 7 mo. renovascular hypertension and LVH in dogs.

Parameter	EPI	MID	ENDO
	(percent increase: LVH group vs. control group)		
Cardiocyte cross-sectional area	45	55	48
Capillary numerical density	NS	NS	NS
Capillary domain: mean area	NS	17	22
Capillary domain: log S.D.	NS	NS	NS

EPI = epimyocardium, MID = midmyocardium, ENDO = endomyocardium these vessels would be about 46% less than the controls; the actual, non-significant, decrement ranged from 5% in the epimyocardium to 14% in the endomyocardium. Therefore, a rather marked capillary growth occurred in these hypertensive dogs which nearly compensated for the increased LV mass.

In order to evaluate the degree of heterogeneity of capillary distribution we utilized the method employing capillary domains described in the previous section. A comparison of the log SD's of the control and LVH group indicated no significant difference in any of the three layers of the free LV wall analyzed. These data led to the conclusion that capillary growth during LVH is similar to that occurring during normal growth.

CONCLUSIONS

The hierarchy of the coronary vasculature is specialized in conductance, capacitance, and regulation of flow as well as exchange between the cardiocyte and the vascular compartment. Both flow, per se, and its distribution are important in maintaining the functional integrity of the cardiocyte. Thus, diseases which reduce flow in the arteries, decrease arteriolar or capillary density, or increase the hypertrophy of capillary spacing may effect O_2 delivery to the myocardium, especially when O_2 demand is high. During the development of hypertension and LVH, coronary reserve is usually reduced, capillary density decreased and heterogeneity of capillary spacing increased. However, there is evidence that a significant angiogenesis occurs with long-term hypertension which normalizes coronary reserve and capillary parameters. The search for angiogenic factors is an important research direction which may lead to interventions which minimize myocardial ischemia in certain clinical entities.

REFERENCES

1. Bundgaard M., Hagman P., and Crone C.: The three-dimensional organization of plasmalemmal vesicular profiles in the endothelium of rat heart capillaries. Microvas. Res. 25:358-368, 1983.
2. Chilian W.M., Eastham C.L., and Marcus M.L.: Microvascular distribution of coronary vascular resistance in beating left ventricle. Am. J. Physiol. 251:H779-H788, 1986.
3. Chilian W.M., Tomanek R.J., and Marcus M.L.: The coronary vasculature during myocardial hypertrophy. in The Stressed Heart, M.J. Legato, ed. pp. 87-105. Boston. Martinus Nijhoff.
4. Folkow B., and Neil E. Circulation. New York: Oxford Univ. Press, 1971.
5. Henquell L., Odoroff C.L., and Honig C.R.: Intercapillary distance and capillary reserve in hypertrophied rat hearts beating in situ. Circ. Res. 41:400-408, 1977.
6. Hoofd L., Turek Z., Kubat K., Ringnalda B.E.M., and Kazda S.: Variability estimated on histological sections of rat heart. in Oxygen Transport to Tissue. VII. F. Kreuzer, S.M. Cain, Z. Turek, T.K. Goldstick, eds., New York, Plenum Press, 1985, pp. 239-247.
7. Hutchins P.M., and Darneel A.E.: Observation of a decreased number of small arterioles in spontaneously hypertensive rats. Circ. Res. 32/33 (Suppl. 1):150-161, 1974.

8. Marcus M.L.: The Coronary Circulation. McGraw-Hill, New York, 1983.
9. Peters K.G., Wangler R.D., Tomanek R.J., and Marcus M.L.: Effects of long-term cardiac hypertrophy on coronary vasodilator reserve in SHR rats. Am. J. Cardiol. 54:1342-1348, 1984.
10. Prewitt R.L., Chen I.I.H., and Dowell R.: Development of micro-vascular rarefaction in the spontaneously hypertensive rat. Am. J. Physiol. 243:H243-H251, 1982.
11. Provenza D.V., and Scherlis S.: Coronary circulation in dog hearts. Demonstration of muscle sphincters in capillaries. Circ. Res. 7:318-324, 1959.
12. Provenza D.V., and Scherlis S.: Demonstration of muscle sphincters as a capillary component in the human heart. Circulation 20:35-41, 1959.
13. Rakusan K.: Microcirculation in the stressed heart in The Stressed Heart, M.J. Legato, ed., pp. 107-123. Boston. Martinus Nijhoff, 1987.
14. Rakusan K., and Turek Z.: The effect of heterogeneity of capillary spacing and O_2 consumption - blood flow mismatching on myocardial oxygenation in Oxygen Transport to Tissue. VII. F. Kreuzer, S.M. Cain, Z. Turek and T.K. Goldstick, eds., pp. 257-262, New York, Plenum, 1985.
15. Rose C.P., Goresky C.A., Belanger P., and Chen M.J. Effect of vaso-dilation and flow rate on capillary permeability surface product and interstitial space size in the coronary circulation. A frequency domain technique for modeling multiple dilution data with Laguerre functions. Circ. Res. 47:312-328, 1980.
16. Tomanek R.J., Palmer P.J., Pieffer G.W., Schrieber K., Eastham C.L., and Marcus M.L.: Morphometry of canine coronary arteries, arterioles and capillaries during hypertension and left ventricular hyper-trophy. Circ. Res. 58:38-46, 1986.
17. Tomanek R.J., Searls J.C., and Lachenbruch P.A.: Quantitative changes in the capillary bed during developing, peak, and stabilized cardiac hypertrophy in the spontaneously hypertensive rat. Circ. Res. 51:295-304, 1982.
18. Tomanek R.J., Wangler R.D., Bauer C.A.: Prevention of coronary vasodilator reserve decrement in spontaneously hypertensive rats. Hypertension 7:533-540, 1985.
19. Turek Z., Hoofd L., Rakusan K.: Myocardial capillaries and tissue oxygenation. Can. J. Cardiol. 2:98-103, 1986.
20. Wangler R.D., Peters K.G., Marcus M.L., and Tomanek R.J.: Effects of duration and severity of arterial hypertension and cardiac hyper-trophy on coronary vasodilator reserve. Circ. Res. 51:10-18, 1982.
21. Weiss H.R., and Conway R.S.: Morphometric study of the total and perfused arteriolar and capillary network of the rabbit left ventricle. Cardiovas. Res. 19:343-354, 1985.

ANATOMY AND PATHOLOGY OF SMALL CORONARY ARTERIES

Thomas N. James, M.D.

All normal arterial blood flow in the myocardium passes through the small coronary arteries. In addition to being this essential conduit they also serve as the principal site of flow regulation by virtue of their vasoreactivity. To discuss these clearly important vessels this presentation will deal first with their normal anatomy and then with the nature of pathological changes in them, concluding with a section on functional interpretation.

ANATOMY

Small coronary arteries are arbitrarily defined as those with external diameters of 0.1 to 1.0 mm. Such vessels are normally abundant throughout the myocardium but are most numerous in the left ventricle, proportional to the dominant mass of myocardium there. The course of small coronary arteries is generally parallel to the epicardium of the two atria and the right ventricle but is much different in the thicker walls of the left ventricle. There, small arteries may follow a brief epicardial course but more often penetrate at right angles to the surface of the heart and usually pass to the endocardial surface. These small left ventricular arteries may branch either in the epicardium or during their intramural course, but they often branch little or not at all before they reach the endocardium only to turn again at right angles to distribute terminal branches in a plane parallel to the endocardium (Figure 1). The length of small coronary arteries varies greatly and is not always in proportion to their diameter. Among arteries of the caliber being considered, it is unusual to find them to be less than one centimeter in length, and an average length is about 2 or 3 cm. Within the interventricular septum and certain other regions of the left ventricle one often finds small coronary arteries which are 5 or more centimeters long.

In every human heart there are certain special small coronary arteries which deserve particular comment. For example, all normal intercoronary anastomoses belong in the category of small coronary arteries (1,2). Thus, those diseases affecting small coronary arteries which provide primary blood supply to the myocardium will also at least randomly affect the source of collateral circulation. When any such disease also affects large coronary arteries (e.g. diabetes mellitus or amyloidosis), the cumulative effect upon the coronary circulation can be devastating.

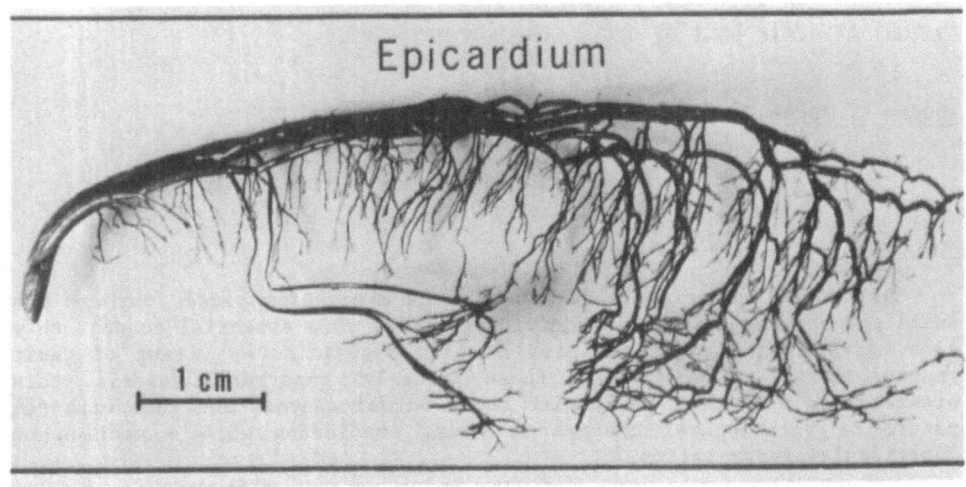

FIGURE 1.   Vinylite cast of human left ventricular coronary artery
branches.

Other special small coronary arteries include those supplying the
cardiac conduction system (1) and those normally perfusing a coronary
chemoreceptor (3,4). Attention to these two groups is important not only
because the structures being supplied have a unique purpose but also
because the anatomical course and location of these vessels is
predictable. They can therefore be compared from one heart to another in a
way which is more difficult for less predictably located small arteries.

PATHOLOGY

One useful way to consider structural abnormalities of small coronary
arteries is in two categories: those changes which reduce the lumen of
the vessel (Figures 2 and 3), and those which damage the tunica media and
thereby impair its vasoreactivity (Figures 4 and 5). Of course, some
diseases cause both problems, not only in the same vessel at different
sites but even at the same site. In that context it is important to keep
in mind the focal nature of virtually every structural abnormality of a
small coronary artery. Most lesions are relatively short in length even
if they completely occlude the small artery, and there may be normal
segments of the same vessel in between two such lesions. Since flow in
the vessel is linear, any obstruction will preclude flow, although the
more proximal the location of the obstruction within the overall length of
the vessel, the more functionally significant it will be since a larger
volume of subtended myocardium will be jeopardized.

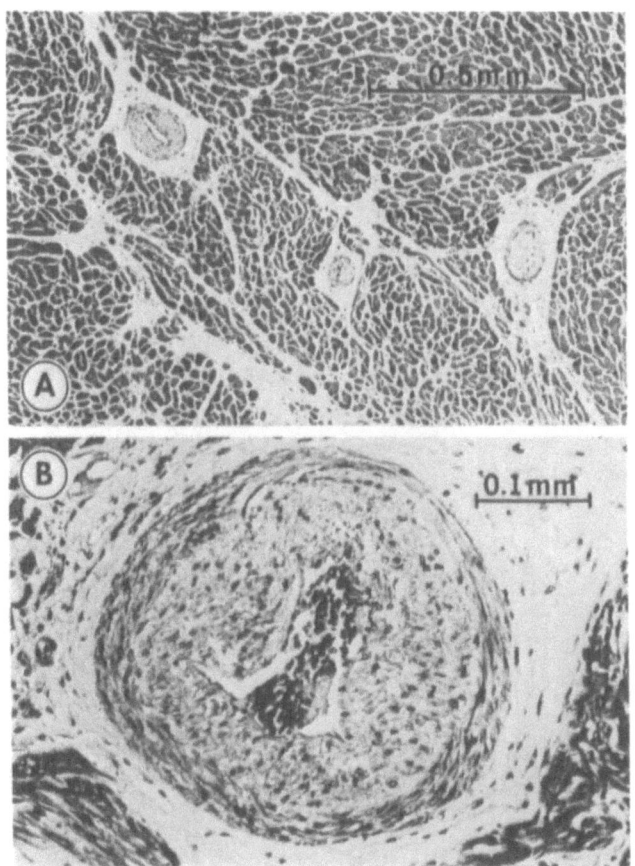

FIGURE 2. Photomicrograph demonstrating focal fibromuscular dysplasia of arteries from the left ventricle (A) and the AV node (B) of a patient dying with scleroderma heart disease. Goldner trichrome stain.

Two familiar abnormalities which narrow the lumen of small arteries are intimal proliferation and focal fibromuscular dysplasia. Intimal proliferation is a prominent component of the arterial response in congenital homocystinuria where it involves both large and small coronary branches (5). It is in part attributable to the known abnormality of platelet function in homocystinuric patients. However, since other diseases characterized by the abnormal aggregation of platelets, such as disseminated intravascular coagulation (6) and thrombotic thrombocytopenic purpura (7), also obstruct small coronary arteries but do not produce much

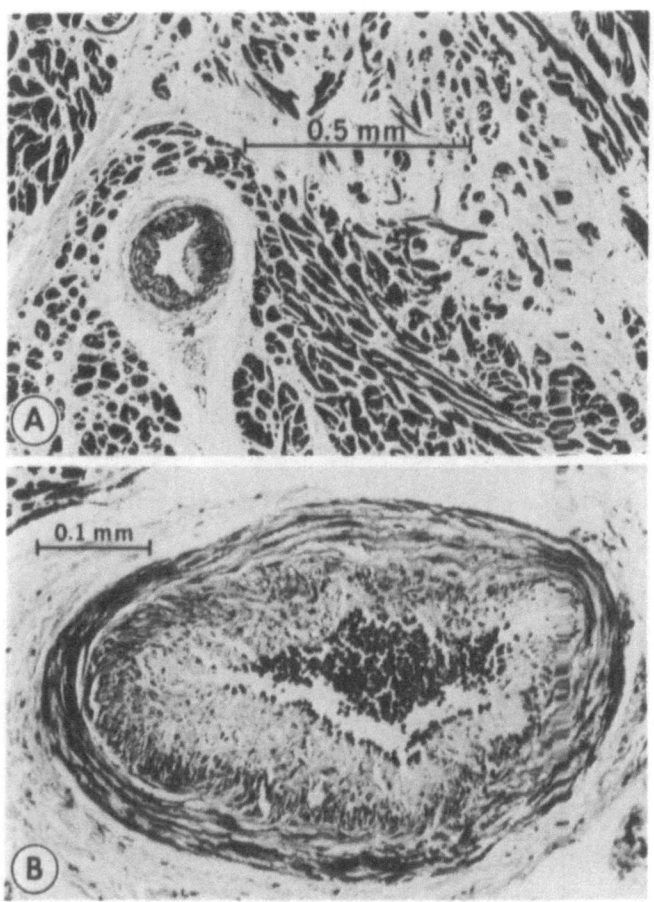

FIGURE 3. Focal fibromuscular dysplasia of small arteries in the left
ventricle (A) and the AV node (B) of a patient dying with asymmetrical
hypertrophy of the heart. Goldner trichrome stain.

intimal proliferative response, one may deduce that an additional
abnormality of the endothelium is present in homocystinuria and this has
been demonstrated (8).   Examples of other diseases in which varying
degrees of intimal proliferation may be observed in small coronary
arteries include polyarteritis nodosa, lupus erythematosus, rheumatoid
arthritis, diabetes mellitus and Whipple's disease (9).

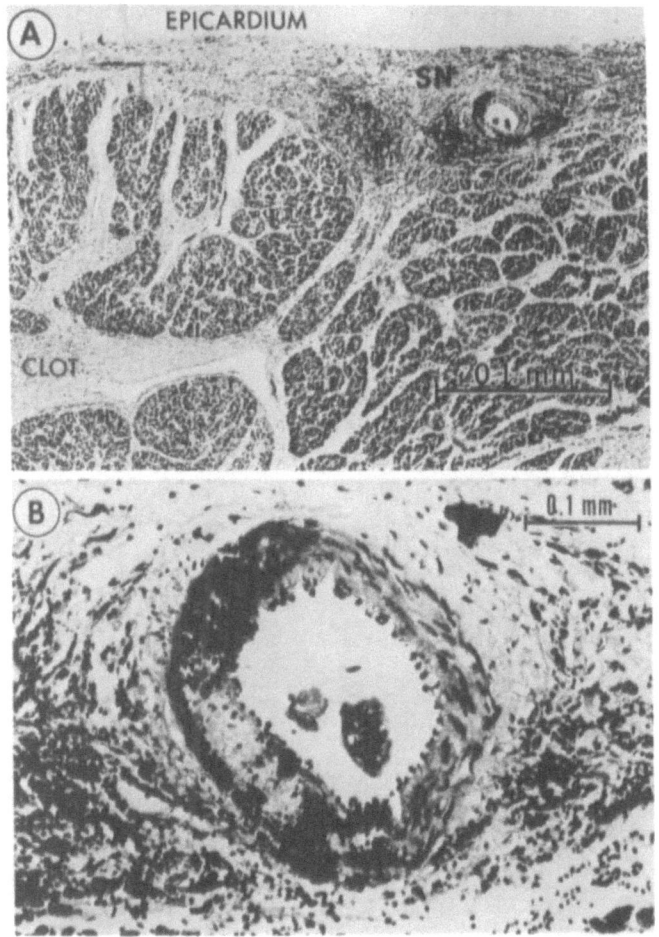

FIGURE 4. Photomicrographs of the sinus node (SN) and adjacent right atrium of a patient dying with primary pulmonary hypertension. The sinus node artery in <u>A</u> is seen at higher power in <u>B</u>, where extensive hemorrhagic degeneration of the tunica media is apparent. Goldner trichrome stain.

Focal fibromuscular dysplasia is found with surprising frequency in a wide variety of diseases narrowing small coronary arteries. These notably include scleroderma (10), hypertrophic cardiomyopathy (11,12), essential hypertension and pheochromocytoma (13). Furthermore, focal fibromuscular dysplasia of small coronary arteries may be seen in the hearts of patients without any recognized systemic illness; for example, it has been found in the sinus node artery and/or the AV (atrioventricular) node artery of otherwise healthy victims of sudden unexpected death (14-16).

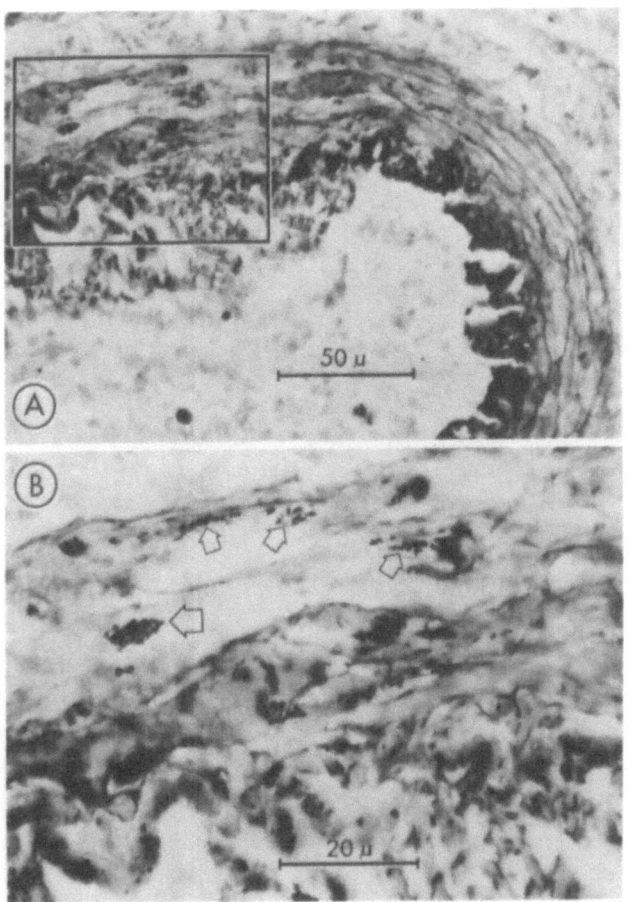

FIGURE 5. Mural destruction by invasion of the tunica media with Whipple bacilli is depicted here in a left ventricular coronary artery of a patient dying with Whipple's disease and cardiomyopathy. Area boxed in A is seen at higher magnification in B where four arrows indicate clumps of bacilli. Periodic acid Schiff stain.

Mural diseases damaging the tunica media of small coronary arteries include degenerative processes such as polyarteritis, lupus or Whipple's disease, but they also include infiltrative conditions such as amyloidosis and the bizarre and almost unique intramural deposits of a PAS-positive material found in the small coronary arteries in Friedreich's cardiomyopathy (17-18). A primary non-inflammatory degeneration of the tunica media of small coronary arteries occurs in patients with primary pulmonary hypertension (19) as well as in the cardiomyopathies associated with certain heritable neuromuscular disorders such as progressive muscular dystrophy (20) and Marfan's syndrome (21). In each of these examples the medial lesions may be minor and focal in only a segment of the circumference of such arteries seen in cross-section, but they may also be extensive and completely encircle the entire vessel.

Finally, there is a miscellany of abnormalities of an embolic nature which may partially or totally obstruct small coronary arteries. If these represent a single or only a few embolic events, their consequences may be negligible unless the artery obstructed supplies the sinus node, AV node or some other crucial structure. However, many embolic processes occur in more extensive showers or recurrent emboli as in DIC (6) or TTP (7) and then the cumulative effect upon the coronary circulation can be profound. At the time of open-heart surgery there is the opportunity for embolization of assorted debris into the small coronary arteries, including not only fibrin and clot fragments, but other products of surgical activity or of the pump perfusion itself. Those cumulative effects have been postulated as one explanation for certain postoperative complications following such surgery (22,23). With the growing use of fibrinolytic efforts within the coronary system and of angioplasic procedures therein, it may be anticipated that embolic showers downstream will be inescapable in many instances. Although the ultimate clinical significance of this is yet to be determined, it would be a grievous mistake to assume that detritemic (23) embolization is easily ignorable.

FUNCTIONAL INTERPRETATIONS

Luminal Caliber. Caliber of the lumen is an important determinant of flow in any artery, but it is only one determinant. Arterial pressure and blood viscosity are other important determinants. Furthermore, in all arteries but particularly smaller ones the caliber varies greatly and repeatedly because of normal vasoreactivity. When the wall of any artery becomes thickened, the effect of vasoconstriction upon the lumen becomes compounded (24,25) almost in a geometric fashion (Figure 6). Among the highly reactive small coronary arteries, therefore, any mural thickening will not only reduce lumen caliber to some extent but will greatly compound the narrowing which occurs with normal degrees of vasoconstriction.

For some diseases with an inflammatory component, such as the coronary arteritis of rheumatoid arthritis or polyarteritis nodosa or Whipple's disease, extension of inflammation to the intima introduces the additional hazard of thrombosis or at the least some local aggregation of platelets. While this can itself cause either luminal narrowing or total occlusion, the stimulative effect of some platelet factors or of leucocyte aggregation upon endothelium can further lead to local cellular proliferative responses which can themselves encroach upon the luminal caliber of the vessel.

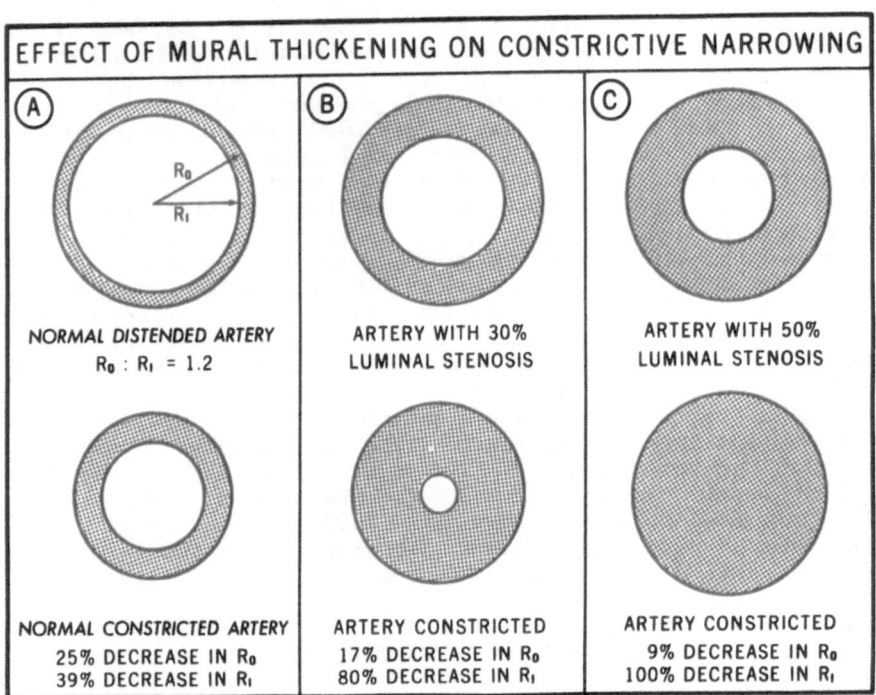

FIGURE 6. Diagrammatic illustration of the compounding effect of mural thickening in worsening the consequences of vasoconstriction of an artery. Modified from reference number 25.

Impaired Vasoreactivity. An opposite consideration must also be included for interpretation of functional significance of small coronary disease and that has to do with the capacity for normal distensibility and/or vasodilatation. Local regulation of arterial blood flow into the myocardium depends significantly upon these properties, the failure of which will at the very least distort normal metabolic and reflex regulatory responses. Small arteries with thickened walls, as in focal fibromuscular dysplasia which itself may narrow the lumen significantly, may thus further derange normal coronary flow not only by their compounded response to vasoconstrictive signals but also by a failure or impairment of their ability to distend and/or dilate when they should.

Still an additional effect can be produced by diseases which damage or destroy the tunica media without thickening it at all. Since both constriction and dilatation depend upon the smooth muscle of the arterial wall, its destruction will prevent effective responses of either constrictive or dilative nature. Such vessels become tubular conduits of fixed caliber, and while they may accommodate normal volumes of arterial blood flow under resting or basal circumstances, it is unlikely that they can respond appropriately to any form of regulation from neural, humoral or metabolic signals. These considerations naturally apply when clinical investigative efforts are made to assess coronary reserve.

Effects of Focal Ischemia. Interpretation of functional significance of small coronary disease may usefully be related to what structures are being supplied. Occlusion of the sinus node artery or the AV node artery may or may not cause sinus arrest or heart block, respectively, but it is highly probable that electrical stability of the heart will be deranged, depending in part upon how much collateral circulation may be available and how soon. Occlusion of one or a few small coronary arteries in the working myocardium may be negligible, since the volume of muscle potentially lost would be so small. However, the cumulative effect of many such lesions would be the development of many foci of degeneration and fibrosis with compensatory hypertrophy ultimately leading to increased ventricular mass in the manner found in most examples of cardiomyopathy.

Importance of Tridimensional Analysis. One of the problems in interpreting the functional significance of small coronary disease in the ventricular myocardium, because of the very large number of such branches, is the matter of quantification. Various strategies for this purpose have been devised, usually based upon the counting of lesions found in histological sections and accepting only those lesions with a certain minimal degree of luminal narrowing. There are two major flaws in such approaches. One is the lack of allowance for the loss of vasoreactivity, which may be totally abolished even in vessels with no significant luminal encroachment as discussed previously. The other flaw is the misconception introduced by thinking in two dimensions about a problem which is in essence three dimensional. Thus, while any lesion completely occluding a small artery would preclude any normal flow beyond that point (except via collateral circulation), the likelihood of detecting such a lesion on random histological sections is surprisingly small.

Small arteries in the human heart are commonly two or three centimeters long and some, such as the sinus node artery or septal branches of the left anterior descending coronary artery, may normally be five centimeters or more in length. If an obstructing lesion in such a vessel were only 100 microns in length, which is not an unusual situation at all, then the chance of encountering a single such lesion in a vessel 50,000 microns in length becomes 1 in 500. Quantitative studies which reject as insignificant the demonstration of narrowing lesions found in 5 or 10% of arteries encountered in histological sections fail to allow for the probabilities of finding such lesions in comparatively long vessels. Furthermore, one may be misled by thinking of "arteries" encountered in histological sections whereas what is actually seen are 8 micron sections of arteries which may be many thousands of microns in length.

Clinical Interpretations. From a clinical standpoint there are certain functional consequences which may assist one in interpreting whether a small coronary lesion was important or not. If there is an atrial arrhythmia of any sort, then the presence of disease in the sinus node artery is probably important. If there is heart block, an obstructed AV node artery may have contributed to that problem. If there are many foci of ventricular myocardial fibrosis, then the presence of multiple narrowings of small ventricular coronary branches is a plausible explanation. With multifocal ventricular myocardial ischemia patients may complain of chest pain which is usually atypical in nature and their electrocardiograms often exhibit widespread inversion of T waves. The latter abnormality is frequently misinterpreted as myocardial infarction or myocarditis.

If there is any basis for predilection for certain specific small coronary arteries by some disease processes, it remains to be established clearly. One may suspect that those arteries in richly innervated areas, such as the sinus node or the coronary chemoreceptor, may be more prone to focal fibromuscular dysplasia, especially if that disease is neurally mediated, but that still remains speculative. It is probably wisest at present to assume that pathologic involvement of small coronary arteries is for practical purposes a random process. On that basis, given enough time, some ventricular arteries, some in the conduction system or the chemoreceptor and some among the coronary anastomoses will sooner or later be involved. With this interpretation one can then understand why certain diseases such as cardiomyopathy (17,18) are clinically characterized by arrhythmias, conduction disturbances and progressive cardiac enlargement and their symptomatic representation as palpitations, syncope, congestive failure and sudden death.

REFERENCES

1. James TN: Anatomy of the Coronary Arteries, Harper and Row, Inc., Hagerstown, Maryland, 1961.
2. James TN: The delivery and distribution of coronary collateral circulation. Chest 58:183-203, 1970.
3. James TN, Isobe JH, Urthaler F: Analysis of components in a hypertensive cardiogenic chemoreflex. Circulation 52:179-192, 1975.
4. Becker AE: The glomera in the region of the heart and great vessels. Pathologia Europaea 1:410-424, 1966.
5. James TN, Carson NAJ and Froggatt P: De Subitaneis Mortibus. IV. Coronary vessels and conduction system in homocystinuria. Circulation 49:367-374, 1974.
6. James TN, Marshall ML and Craig MW: De Subitaneis Mortibus. VII. Disseminated intravascular coagulation and paroxysmal atrial tachycardia. Circulation 50:395-401, 1974.
7. James TN and Monto RW: Pathology of the cardiac conduction system in thrombotic thrombocytopenic purpura. Annals of Internal Medicine 65:37-43, 1966.
8. Harker LA, Harlan JM and Ross R: Effect of sulfinpyrazone on homocysteine-induced endothelial injury and arteriosclerosis in baboons. Circulation Research 53:731-739, 1983.
9. James TN: Small arteries of the heart. The 36th George E. Brown Memorial Lecture. Circulation 56:2-14, 1977.
10. James TN: De Subitaneis Mortibus. VIII. Coronary arteries and conduction system in scleroderma heart disease. Circulation 50:844-856, 1974.
11. James TN and Marshall TK: De Subitaneis Mortibus. XII. Asymmetrical hypertrophy of the heart. Circulation 51:1149-1166, 1975.

12. Maron BJ, Wolfson JK, Epstein SE and Roberts WC: Intramural ("small vessel") coronary artery disease in hypertrophic cardiomyopathy. Journal of the American College of Cardiology 8:545-557, 1986.

13. James TN: De Subitaneis Mortibus. XIX. On the cause of sudden death in pheochromocytoma, with special reference to the pulmonary arteries, the cardiac conduction system and the aggregation of platelets. Circulation 54:348-356, 1976.

14. James TN, Froggatt P, and Marshall TK: Sudden death of young athletes. Annals of Internal Medicine 67:1013-1021, 1967.

15. James TN, Hackel DB and Marshall TK: De Subitaneis Mortibus. V. Occluded AV node artery. Circulation 49:772-777, 1974.

16. James TN and Marshall TK: De Subitaneis Mortibus. XVII. Multifocal stenoses due to fibromuscular dysplasia of the sinus node artery. Circulation 53:736-742, 1976.

17. James TN and Fisch C: Observations on the cardiovascular involvement in Friedreich's ataxia. American Heart Journal 66:164-175, 1963.

18. James TN, Cobbs BW, Coghlan HC, McCoy WC and Fisch C: Coronary disease, cardioneuropathy and conduction system abnormalities in the cardiomyopathy of Friedreich's ataxia. British Heart Journal, in press.

19. James TN: On the cause of syncope and sudden death in primary pulmonary hypertension. Annals of Internal Medicine 56:252-264, 1962.

20. James TN: Observations on the cardiovascular involvement (including the cardiac conduction system) in progressive muscular dystropy. American Heart Journal 63:48-56, 1962.

21. James TN, Frame B and Schatz IJ: Pathology of the cardiac conduction system in Marfan's syndrome. Archives of Internal Medicine 144:339-343, 1964.

22. Morales AR, Fine G and Taber RE: Cardiac surgery and myocardial necrosis. Archives of Pathology 83:71-79, 1967.

23. Ingelfinger FJ: Detritemia. New England Journal of Medicine 292:696-697, 1975.

24. Van Citters RL: Occlusion of lumina in small arterioles during vasoconstriction. Circulation Research 18:199-204, 1966.

25. MacAlpin RN: Relation of coronary arterial spasm to sites of organic stenosis. American Journal of Cardiology 46:143-153, 1980.

This work was supported by the Alabama State Program for Research on Sudden Death and by the Luckie Fund for Cardiovascular Research.

ANATOMY AND PATHOLOGY OF LARGE CORONARY VESSELS

A.V.G. Bruschke and B. Buis

For practical reasons we will define large coronary vessels as coronary arteries that are large enough to be visualized by coronary arteriography in such detail that moderate atherosclerotic changes can be detected. With modern equipment this includes arteries with an internal diameter of about 0.2 mm or more. Assuming that the normal coronary anatomy is generally well known we will focus on nomenclature, standardized interpretation of coronary arteriograms, and the significance of pathologic findings.

Although coronary arteriography has been widely used to evaluate patients with known or suspected ischemic heart disease and coronary arteriographic findings have been the core of numerous clinical investigations for more than 25 years, this has, surprisingly, not led to uniformity of nomenclature and interpretation.

Standardization has many advantages. It improves the quality of interpretations because arteriographers are urged to evaluate every branch of the coronary arterial tree in a similar fashion. It leads to uniformity of reports which is particularly helpful in teaching interpreting coronary arteriograms. Standardization also facilitates clinical comparisons and collaborative studies between institutions.

Recently, a WHO/ISFC Task Force published recommendations for standardization (1,2) which we will follow in this chapter.

Nomenclature
The following terms are recommended for normal coronary anatomy:
Left coronary artery (LCA)
a. Left main coronary artery
b. Left anterior descending artery (LAD)
   diagonal branch(es) (left ventricle)
   septal branch(es)
c. Left circumflex artery (LCX)
   antero-lateral branches   )
   obtuse marginal branch   )   lateral branches
   postero-lateral branch(es))
   posterior descending artery
Right coronary artery (RCA)
   Conus branch (in 50% via separate ostium in aorta)
   Anterior right ventricular branch(es)
   Acute marginal branch
   Posterior right ventricular branch(es)
   Posterior descending artery (or arteries)
   Posterior septal branch(es)
   Posterior left ventricular branches

For practical purposes variations in coronary anatomy can be divided into normal and abnormal variations. We will consider variations normal if they have no pathological meaning and abnormal if they have or may have pathological significance.

Typical examples of *normal variations* are:
1. *Dual left anterior descending artery* (fig. 1) Occasionally the left anterior descending artery divides proximally into two parallel-running branches, one of which may be located intramural. Several terms, such as giant first septal branch, have been used to describe this situation but for practical and theoretical reasons the term "dual left anterior descending artery" is to be preferred.

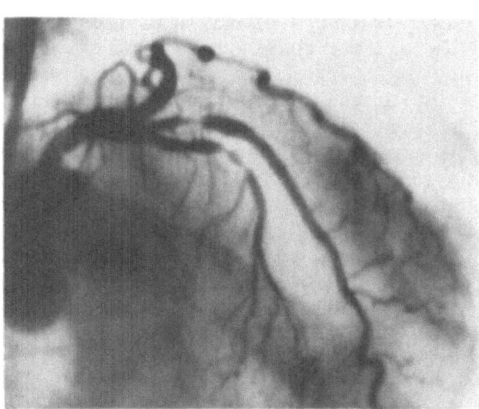

FIGURE 1.
Left coronary artery in right anterior oblique, slightly angulated, view. Dual left anterior descending artery.

2. *Left intermediate artery*. Fairly frequently there is a trifurcation of the left main coronary artery into left anterior descending artery, left circumflex artery, and a third branch between them. The latter branch is neither a true diagonal artery nor a lateral branch of the circumflex artery and should be termed left intermediate artery.
3. *Abnormal origin of the first large septal branch*. The most common abnormal origin of the first large septal branch is the first diagonal branch. Rarely the first septal branch originates from the right coronary artery or the circumflex artery and sporadically it does from the left main coronary artery.
4. *Right anterior diagonal artery*. Occasionally the right coronary artery divides proximally into two almost equally large branches, one branch having a normal course in the atrioventricular groove, and one branch coursing over the right ventricular wall towards the apex. The latter shall be called right anterior diagonal artery.
5. *Right posterior diagonal artery*. The posterior descending artery may have its origin proximal to the posterior interventricular groove, leaving the atrio-ventricular groove near the acute margin of the heart. More commonly this situation exists in combination with a (short) normally originating posterior descending artery, in which case there are two posterior descending arteries in sequence, one supplying the basal portion and the other the apical portion of the inferior part of the interventricular septum.
The term "posterior diagonal artery" is recommended to identify the proximally originating branch.

6. *Separate orifice* of left anterior descending and circumflex arteries from the left coronary sinus. In this situation there is no main left coronary artery.
7. *Left circumflex* from separate orifice in *right* coronary sinus or from right coronary artery coursing posteriorly to the root of the aorta.

Variations are generally considered *abnormal* (or having pathological significance) if they have been associated with cardiac death for which no other cause could be demonstrated. These variations generally include ectopic origin of a coronary artery from the aorta but an intramural course of the left anterior descending artery has also been mentioned as a possible cause of sudden death (3). So far, it remains unsettled which variants of the origin of coronary arteries have pathological significance. In a pathologic-anatomic study of 23 cases Mahowald et al. (4) found that sudden death had occurred in 3 cases; in all of these the right coronary artery and the left main coronary artery arose from the same aortic sinus namely in 1 case from the right and in 2 cases from the left sinus. Reviewing 7,000 coronary arteriograms Kimbiris et al. found 45 cases with ectopic origin of one or more coronary arteries but they reported only one case in which this had led to myocardial infarction (5). There is some controversy as to the mechanism which causes death in these cases. Several investigators have postulated that compression of the anomalous artery between aorta and pulmonary artery is the major cause. Perhaps this is true in some cases but it is unlikely that this is the only mechanism involved and obviously it cannot explain death in patients in whom the abnormally originating artery does not course between aorta and pulmonary artery. A more important factor is probably the acute angle which often exists between an abnormally originating coronary artery and the aorta. This may result in a slit-like orifice and is sometimes associated with a flap of tissue near the arterial ostium (4,5,6,7). Particularly if the proximal portion of the abnormally originating artery is embedded in the aortic wall such a configuration may be marked. In this situation the origin or proximal portion of the coronary artery is liable to become obstructed, for instance by stretch of the aortic wall during episodes of increased blood pressure. Identification of high-risk variations by arteriography alone is difficult, if not impossible. In any case, in the past probably too much emphasis has been placed upon the course of abnormal coronary arteries between the great arteries.
In contrast to the left main coronary artery, a left circumflex artery originating from the right sinus of Valsalva or from the right coronary artery has no pathologic significance.

Rarely gross variations in the distal distribution patterns of the coronary arteries are encountered (fig. 2). It is nearly always impossible to determine solely by the anatomic picture whether these variations have pathological meaning. Assessment of the coronary circulation by other methods, such as Thallium-201 scintigraphy, may be helpful but these tests are of limited value if the anomaly is associated with atherosclerotic obstructions which may determine their outcome.

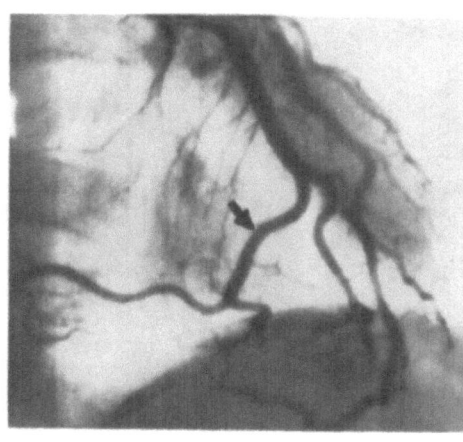

FIGURE 2.
Left coronary artery in right anterior oblique projection. The left circumflex artery, which originates normally, courses towards the apex and divides into two branches, one of which (arrow) courses backward to the atrioventricular groove and terminates as a small posterior descending artery. There appears to be a paucity of vessels supplying the posterior wall. The patient had a severe stenosis of the proximal left anterior descending artery (not visible in this frame) which limited his exercise capacity to such extent that isotope studies were not helpful in determining the significance of the congenital anomaly.

Miscellaneous abnormalities
Apart from atherosclerotic lesions, more or less frequently occurring abnormalities of the coronary arteries are:

1. *Calcifications*
2. *Thrombus*
3. *Dissection*
4. *Ectasia*
5. *Aneurysm*
6. *Myocardial bridging*
7. *Shunts and fistulae*
8. *Origin of either coronary artery from pulmonary artery*

If these abnormalities are present it is usually not necessary to indicate their exact localization. Provisions for a general description of their localization, such as proximal or distal portions of major arteries, can be included in a code form.

The presence of intracoronary thrombus can usually only be proven by its disappearance after thrombolytic therapy but the morphology of certain obstructions may be suggestive.

Dissections can easily be recognized if they occur during transluminal coronary angioplasty but in chronic cases it is often difficult to differentiate between a dissection and a corkscrew-like atherosclerotic lesion.

Evidence of myocardial bridging may be variable (fig. 3) and often disappears after myocardial infarction in the area of bridging.

Myocardial bridging is rare in arteries other than the left anterior descending artery. Its hemodynamic significance is still a matter of debate. Since bridging causes arterial narrowing during systole whereas flow in the left anterior descending artery occurs mainly during diastole it is difficult to understand how bridging could compromise the coronary circulation. It has been postulated that a narrowing due to bridging may still be present during the early part of diastole, particularly at high heart rates. Therefore, it may be relevant to determine arteriographically the duration and severity of the narrowing at various heart rates. Hopefully in these cases more information will be obtained by intracoronary Doppler flow velocity measurements.

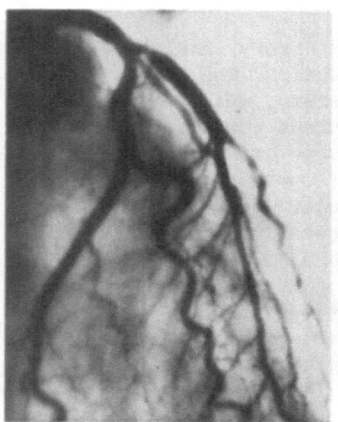 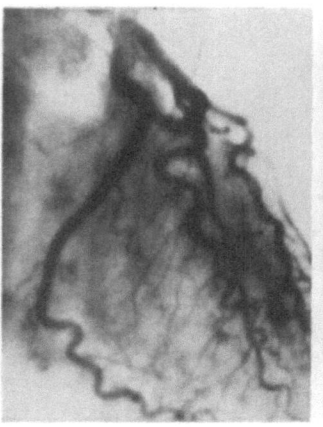 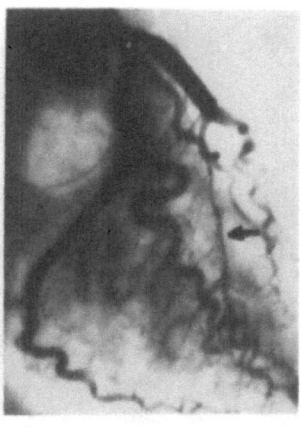

A   B   C

FIGURE 3.
Left coronary artery in right anterior oblique projection.
A. Diastole. Severe stenosis of proximal left anterior descending artery.
B. Systole. No change in caliber of distal left anterior descending artery.
C. Because the possibility of spasm was considered nitroglycerin was administered sublingually. Now the distal left anterior descending artery appears markedly attenuated during systole (arrow) and regains its normal caliber during diastole. A superficial intramyocardial course is suspected.

Coding systems for coronary arteriograms

Coding systems are particularly suitable to achieve standardization and perform clinical investigations in which arteriographic findings are used. To warrant adherence to a coding system it should fulfill the following requirements:

1. It should be easy to use, that is: it should be possible to use the system without having expertise in computer technology and completing the report should not take considerably more time than preparing a verbal report.
2. It must be possible to generate automated reports to obviate the need to make additional verbal reports.
3. The computer generated reports should suffice to describe the coronary anatomy accurately in the vast majority (at least 90%) of the cases.
4. Access to the system should be immediate and coding must be possible at all places where this is needed.
5. Only one system should be used, which should therefore be suitable for reporting and practically all clinical investigations.

To avoid the extra costs and possible errors of copying coded information, it is advisable to use either optical readable forms or to enter the data via computer terminals. The use of optical readable forms has the advantage that the arteriograms can be coded at any time wherever a film viewer is available whereas the use of computer terminals has the advantages of more flexibility, easier correctability, and the possibility to incorporate error messages for incompatible or incomplete codings.

Coding anatomical variatons.

In our opinion the most appropriate method to achieve such a degree of
flexibility that all major anatomical variations can be coded accurately,
consists of including all potential segments from which those are deleted
that are not present in an individual case. If, in addition, the
possibility is provided to indicate if a branch is unusually large, it is
relatively easy to program the computer in such a manner that an accurate
report of the coronary anatomy is generated. An example is given in
figure 4.

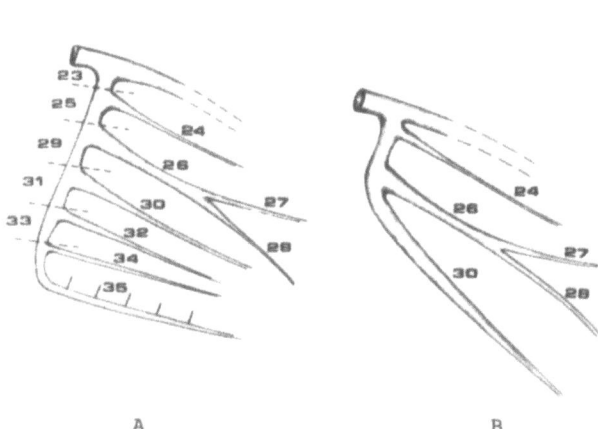

A   B

FIGURE 4.
A. The left circumflex
artery is divided into 12
potential segments.
B. In this patient
segments 23, 29 and 31 to
35 are coded "absent" and
segment 30 is coded
"large". The computer-
generated report states
that there is an inter-
mediate artery and that
the circumflex terminates
as a large lateral branch
originating immediately
distal to the obtuse
marginal branch.

Grading of stenoses

Interpretation of narrowing lesions optimally should be based upon multiple
views. If a lesion appears more severe in one view than in others, as is
the case in excentric lesions, some investigators grade the narrowing
according to the projection in which the greatest reduction of lumen
diameter is observed. In our opinion it is more accurate to use the average
degree of narrowing in all views that provide a good longitudinal view of
the arterial segment involved.

Quantitation of arterial narrowing generally refers to percentage reduction
of lumen diameter. In clinical practice this yields acceptable results although interpretations are subject to errors, for instance when the
portions of the artery adjacent to the narrowing show significant atherosclerosis and are therefore unsuitable for comparison or when these
portions appear arteriographically normal but in reality are narrowed.
These pitfalls may be present irrespective of the method of measurement
used. Ideally actual lumen size should be determined additonally but at
present this is not commonly done and to be sufficiently accurate requires
intricate measuring techniques. Likewise, it is difficult to include
quantitative descriptions of the morphology, such as length of stenoses and
excentricity of narrowings.

Particularly if optical readable code forms are used it is much easier to
divide narrowings into categories than it is to enter the exact estimated
or measured percentage of lumen diameter reduction. To this end several
coding systems use large incremental steps, for instance, normal, 0-25
percent, 20-50 percent, 50-75 percent, 75-99 percent and 100 percent.
Arguments to do so are that broad categories are adequate for clinical

purposes and that visual estimates (currently still the commonly used method of interpretation) have a certain inaccuracy anyway. This is probably true but using such a division implies that for specific purposes (for instance studying progression of disease and evaluating results of percutaneous transluminal coronary angioplasty) a different coding system is required which is in disagreement with the advisability to have only one system.

We also doubt whether the inaccuracy of assessments of narrowings is a valid reason to use broad categories as this certainly does not improve accuracy and, in fact, may enhance inaccurate categorization of lesions that cause percentages reduction of lumen diameter lying around the separation points. We therefore recommend incremental steps of small percentages or the actual estimate of narrowing (if the data are stored via a computer terminal) be used. If for clinical purposes one chooses to use broader categories the computer can easily be programmed to provide the categorization desired.

It is not always possible to determine with reasonable accuracy the degree of narrowing caused by atherosclerotic lesions. Apart from the reasons mentioned above this may be due to inadequate visualization of the arterial branch involved or the artery being too small to allow precise evaluation of narrowing lesions. It is also hazardous to grade narrowings in occluded arterial segments that are solely opacified by collaterals. Comparison of pre- and postoperative arteriograms in patients who underwent bypass surgery has shown that narrowings in arteries distal to occlusions can easily be grossly over- or underrated. In these cases general descriptive terms, such as: "probably normal", "markedly narrowed", etc. rather than unreliable estimates of percentages should be used, and the coding system should provide the possibility to do so.

Although the interpretation of postoperative arteriograms is beyond the scope of this chapter we will discuss briefly grading of narrowings in vein and internal mammary artery bypass grafts. The diameter of venous grafts is highly variable and usually considerably larger than the diameter of the recipient vessel(s). Consequently, narrowings expressed as precentage reduction of the lumen diameter have variable physiological significance and even marked reductions may not significantly compromise flow. From physiological standpoint it is more logical to grade narrowings in relation to the size of the recipient vessel(s) but this may provide insufficient information about changes in the bypass graft itself. Therefore, narrowings in grafts can best be described by taking both aspects into consideration, which would yield statements like: "The saphenous vein graft is x% narrowed; the residual lumen corresponds with y% of the lumen of the recipient vessel". The same principle may be applied in cases in which internal mammary artery grafts have been used. However, in contrast to saphenous vein grafts the diameter of the internal mammary artery is usually not much larger and occasionally even smaller than that of the recipient vessel. Although the hemodynamic consequences of this are not yet fully known it may be advisable to describe not only narrowings but to indicate the diameter of internal mammary arteries in relation to the diameter of the recipient vessel(s) also.

Collateral flow

Frequently it is impossible to identify accurately all sources of collateral flow and occasionally collateral pathways cannot be clearly defined although collateral filling obviously is present. As, moreover, a detailed description of collaterals is of limited, if any, clinical consequence it suffices to indicate the presence or absence of collateral flow and, if possible, its major source. Its magnitude may be recorded in general terms (e.g. good - moderate - poor) but one should realize that the arteriogram is a poor indicator of the physiological significance of collaterals, partly because opacification of occluded arteries is as much dependent on the outwash as it is on the inflow of contrast medium.

Some investigators consider the presence of "jeopardized collaterals" a particular risk. Although this term has not always been used in the same sense it generally indicates that collaterals originate from from an artery which is significantly narrowed proximal to their take-off. Supposedly, in such cases progression of the narrowing to occlusion will lead not only to loss of perfusion of the area supplied by the parent vessel but also of the area supplied by the collaterals. This may be a logical presumption, however, in a study dealing with patients who underwent repeated coronary arteriographies we related progression of obstructions to changes of left ventricular contractions and found no difference between patients with jeopardized and those with unjeopardized collaterals. This subject deserves further study and we suggest to indicate the presence of jeopardized collaterals in cases in which these are the sole source of collateral filling of arterial segments distal to occlusions.

Spasm

If coronary arterial spasm is observed symptoms and ECG changes and whether spasm occurs spontaneously or after provocation should be coded in addition to arteriographic findings. Coding of arteriographic evidence of spasm should include the severity of narrowing (e.g. in steps of 25% reduction of lumen diameter), a general description of localization, and whether or not spasm is superimposed upon a fixed lesion.

REFERENCES

1. James TN, Bruschke AVG, Böthig S, Dodu SRA, Gil JF, Kawamura K, Paulin SJ, Piessens J: Report of WHO/ISFC Task Force on nomenclature of coronary arteriograms. Circulation 74:451A-455A, 1986.
2. James TN, Bruschke AVG, Gyárfás I, Neufeld HN, Paulin SJ, Rafflenbeul W, Schmuziger M: Report of WHO/ISFC Task Force on coronary arteriograms and coronary interventions. Circulation 75:895A-897A, 1987.
3. Morales AR, Romanelli R, Boucek RJ: The mural left anterior descending coronary artery, strenuous exercise and sudden death. Circulation 62:230-237, 1980.
4. Mahowald JM, Blieden LC, Coe JI, Edwards JE: Ectopic origin of a coronary artery from the aorta. Sudden death in 3 of 23 patients. Chest 89:668-672, 1986.
5. Kimbiris D, Iskandrian AS, Segal BL, Benies CE: Anomalous aortic origin of coronary arteries. Circulation 58:606-615, 1978.
6. Gittenberger-de Groot AC, Bogers AJJC, Bartelings MM: Aspects of normal and abnormal development of the main coronary arteries. This book, chapter 4.
7. Roberts WC, Siegel RJ, Ziper DJ: Origin of the right coronary artery from the left sinus of Valsalva and it functional consequences: analysis of 10 necropsy patients. Am. J. Cardiol. 49:863-868, 1982.
8. Visser RF, van der Werf T, Ascoop CAPL, Bruschke AVG: The influence of anatomic evolution of coronary artery disease on left ventricular contraction: An aniographic follow-up study of 300 nonoperated patients. Am. Heart J. 112:963-971, 1986.

ASPECTS OF NORMAL AND ABNORMAL DEVELOPMENT OF THE MAIN CORONARY ARTERIES

A.C. GITTENBERGER-DE GROOT, A.J.J.C. BOGERS, M.M. BARTELINGS

INTRODUCTION
 Knowledge of the normal development of the main coronary arteries in man is still incomplete. This implies that abnormal development can only be discussed at a mainly theoretical level. In the present chapter data on normal development of the coronary arteries will be presented from our own studies and literature data concerning investigations of both human and animal material. Thereafter nomenclature and classification followed by data on abnormal coronary arterial development will be discussed. This latter information will mainly be based on casuistic data from teratology.

NORMAL DEVELOPMENT
 During development of the coronary arterial system in general three connecting vascular beds can be distinguished. First there is an intramural (intramyocardial) system of endocardium lined trabeculae that comes into contact with a second network of subepicardial vessels. The origin of the endothelial cells of the subepicardial network most probably relates to the origin of the extracardiac mesenchyme that spreads over the myocardial heart tube with the formation of the epicardium (1). The subepicardial network of vasculature forms a peritruncal ring of vessels that surrounds the arterial orifice region (2). The third phase of development shows the sprouts from the arterial orifice contacting this peritruncal ring and thus completing the coronary vascular system.
 With development of the coronary arterial sprouts from the orifice region the site of origin of the coronary arteries is given. In hearts with normally related great vessels the coronary arteries usually arise from two semilunar sinuses of the aorta. These semilunar sinuses and cusps develop from the two opposed endocardial outlet ridges in the outlet of the heart. On both sides these outlet ridges are flanked by intercalated valve swellings. Septation of the arterial orifice level results thus in the formation of three future semilunar cusps in each arterial orifice, two of which face the other arterial orifice (Figure 1). The coronary arteries arise from the two facing sinuses of the aorta.
 There are two major theories that explain a normal and abnormal origin of a coronary artery (e.g. from a pulmonary orifice) (Figure 1). The first one is by Abrikossoff (3) who explains septation abnormalities to account for abnormal sites of coronary orifices. A second theory by Hackensellner (4) indicates that there is a potential for coronary arterial sprout formation along the complete arterial orifice level, in general only two sprouts from the facing sinuses of the aorta really contact the epicardial vasculature. This latter theory allows a better explanation for the variations that can be encountered. However, neither theory gives a sufficient explanation for the consistency of the normal

origin and branching pattern of the coronary arteries nor for their abnormal variations.

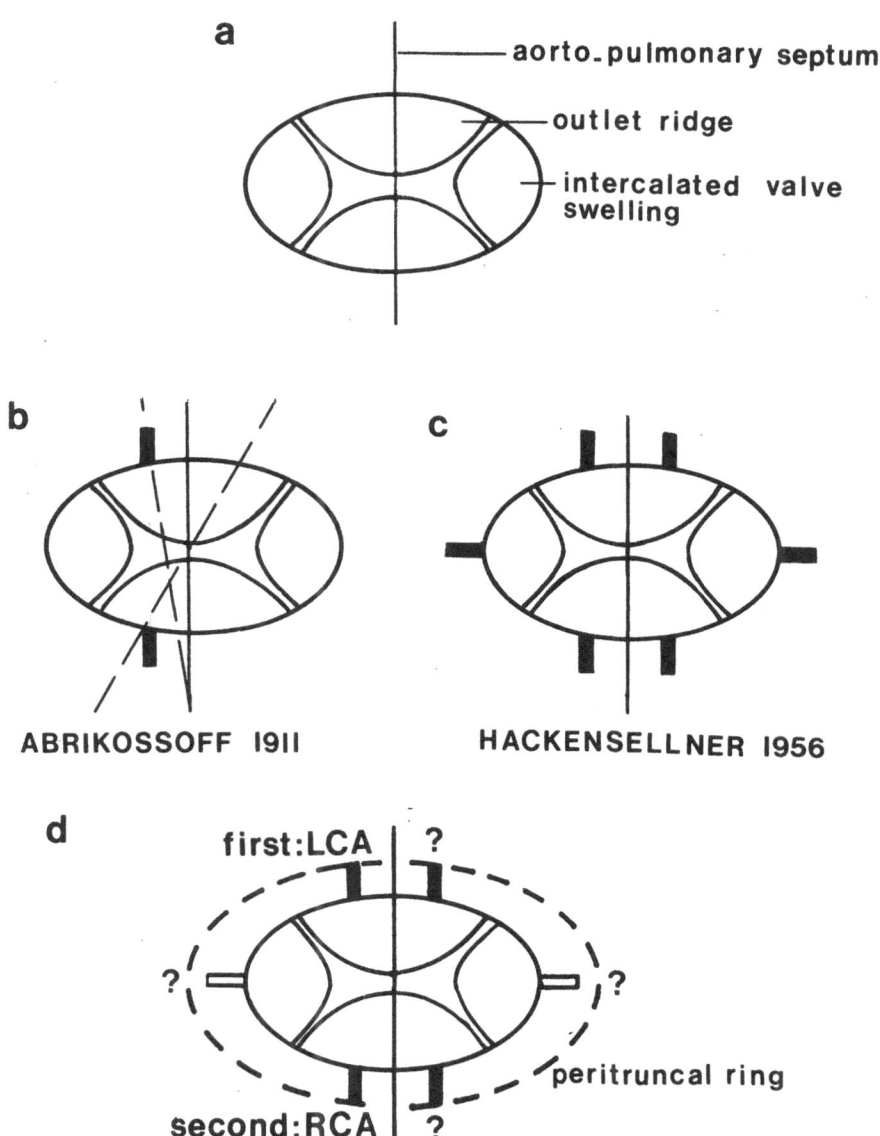

FIGURE 1. a-d) Schematic drawing of septation of the arterial orifice level during development a). Drawings b) and c) show the main theories for potential normal and abnormal origin. Scheme d) brings data from our own observations combined with recent literature (2,5,6).

Own research of septation of the outlet of the arterial orifice level in man (25 specimens, 6-25 mm C-R length), mouse (5 specimens, 13-17 days gestation) and rat (11 specimens, 14-20 days gestation) embryos learned that septation of this level takes place well before the first indication of coronary arterial sprouts (Table 1).

TABLE 1. Relation between time of septation of the aortic and pulmonary orifice and the first detection of coronary arterial sprouts.

	septation aortic/pulm. orifice	first indication coron. art. sprouts
MAN	8 mm C-R length	15-16 mm C-R length
MOUSE	10-12 days	14 days
RAT	12-13 days	16 days

This invalidates the theory of Abrikossoff (3). Furthermore, in our material, studied by light microscope in 5-10 μm sectioned embryos we could not detect more sprouts than eventually necessary. Actually the first indication was that of a left coronary artery (LCA) already possessing a small lumen (Figure 2a,b), shortly after followed by the development of a right coronary artery (RCA). This is in accordance with recent human (2) and animal studies (5,6). There is information from the literature that mentions the development of more sprouts than necessary for the LCA and the RCA (6). However, these data are not sufficiently detailed to be convincing. For instance nobody mentions whether there are actually also sprouts arising from the area above the intercalated valve swellings, being the future site of a non-facing sinus. From a developmental point of view this is of importance as in general both in normal and abnormal hearts a coronary artery does not arise from a non-facing sinus (thus usually referred to in the aorta as the non-coronary sinus).

Recent observations from our own institute on development of outlet septation of the heart also learned that the arterial orifice level of the heart is not as is generally depicted in the literature (7) in one plane but already before septation (6 mm C-R length human embryo) there is an angled configuration of the future aortic and pulmonary orifice (8). After septation, which actually starts at orifice level, the pulmonary orifice lies in a more horizontal plane whereas the aortic orifice has a lower, more upright position (Figure 3). As a consequence the intercalated valve swelling (future non-facing coronary cusp) is in close proximity to the superior endocardial cushion, that is to the future atrioventricular orifice.

A direct initiating effect of the extracardiac mesenchyme of the aorto-pulmonary septum, which is thus closest to the facing semilunar sinuses, on the development of the coronary arterial cannot be excluded and needs further investigation.

NOMENCLATURE FOR SEMILUNAR SINUSES

In hearts with normally related great arteries it is customary to name the semilunar valves of the aorta in a positional way, referring to a left, right and posterior sinus. From the first two the LCA and the RCA arise respectively, the posterior sinus being the non-coronary sinus. The left and right sinus are in fact the facing semilunar sinuses, the poste-

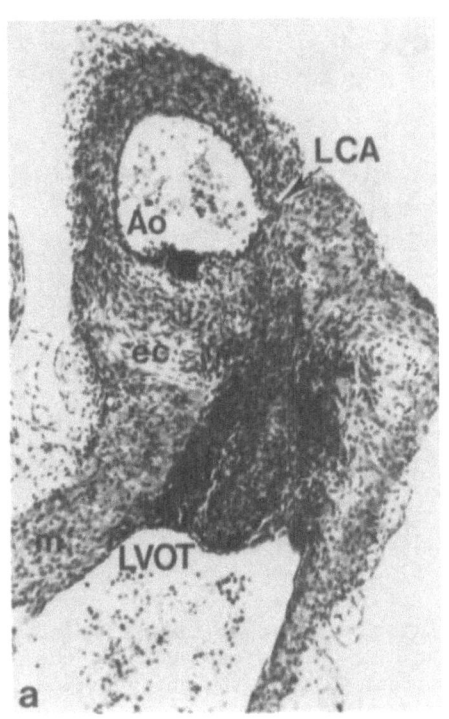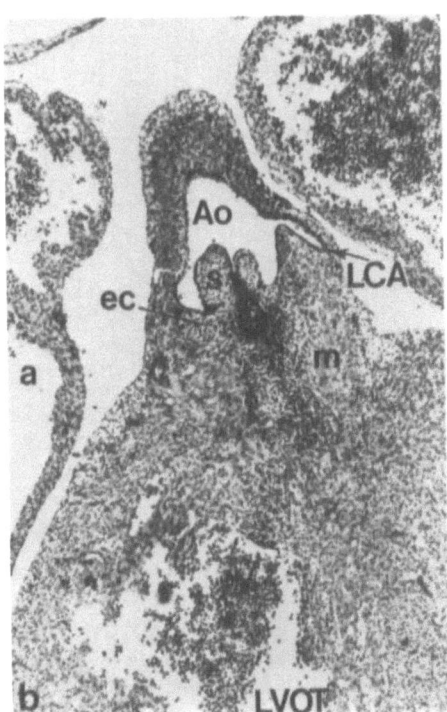

FIGURE 2. a) First indication of the left coronary artery (LCA) in a 16
mm human embryo. b) LCA in a 17 mm human embryo, which already possesses
in contrast of the embryo a) a right coronary artery.
Ao: aorta; ec: endocardial cushion tissue of valve region; m: myocardium;
LVOT: left ventricular outflow tract; s: semilunar cusp; a: atrium.

rior or non-coronary sinus is the non-facing one. A relative change in
position of the arterial orifices as often encountered in congenital
heart disease will also change the position of the semilunar sinuses, and
therefore their nomenclature. For instance in transposition of the great
arteries (TGA) this results in a completely different description of the
origin of the coronary arteries if these are designated after the semilunar sinus they originate from. To overcome this problem we have chosen
a nomenclature for the semilunar cusps which is not positional in nature
(9,10). The basic rule is that the coronary arteries in general originate
from the facing sinuses (10,11). These are given a numerical indication
of 1 and 2 which is independent of the relative position of the arterial
orifices (Figure 4).
If one than takes position in the non-facing semilunar cusp (in general
the non-coronary cusp) of the aorta and looks towards the pulmonary
orifice, the facing sinus 1 is on the right-hand side and the facing
sinus 2 on the left-hand side (Figure 5a). The notation is that the
coronary arterial origin is indicated by the number of the sinus followed

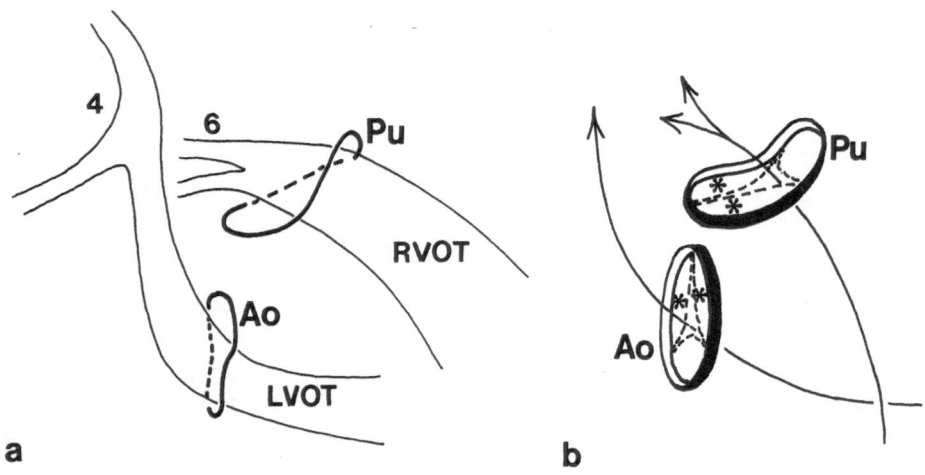

FIGURE 3. Schematic drawings of the position of the aortic (Ao) and pulmonary orifice (Pu) in a 9 mm human embryo. a) Figure a) indicates the left (LVOT) and right ventricular outflow tract (RVOT) with the position of the orifices in relation to the long ascending aorta (connecting to the 4th arches) and the short pulmonary trunk which separates into pulmonary arteries and the 6th arches. b) Shows the position of the future semilunar valves. The LVOT and the RVOT are here indicated by drawn lines and arrows. The facing semilunar valves are indicated by an asterisk.

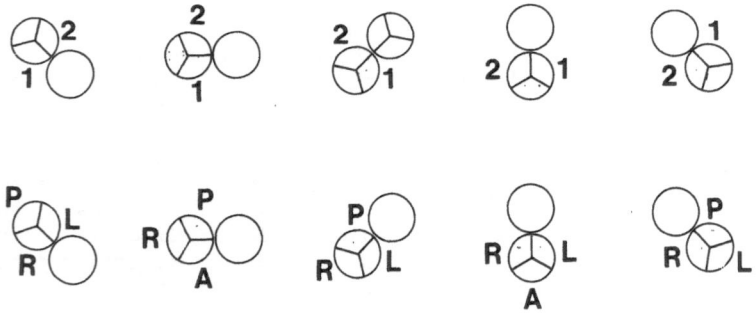

FIGURE 4. Schematic drawing showing that the indication of the facing semilunar sinuses by 1 and 2 makes them independent of the relative positions of the arterial orifices.

by the main coronary arterial branch (es) that originate from it. In a normal heart this would be: 1 RCA, 2 LAD, LCx (Figure 5b).

The main coronary arteries in fact consist of three main branches, i.e. the RCA, the LAD and the LCx, which can originate in any given combination from the two facing semilunar sinuses. This allows for six basic types of origin (Figure 6). The number and position of the orifices in their respective sinus is not taken into account.

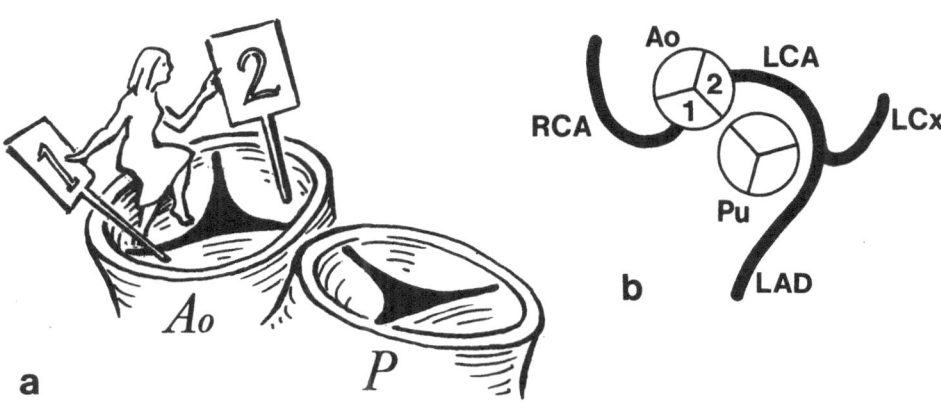

FIGURE 5. a) Drawing showing how to define facing sinus 1 and 2. b) Indication of the main coronary arterial branches. The LCA in fact only exists if the LAD and the LCx have a common stem. Ao: aortic orifice; Pu: pulmonary orifice; RCA: right coronary artery; LCA: left coronary artery; LAD: left anterior descending artery; LCx: left circumflex artery.

ABNORMAL DEVELOPMENT

With regard to abnormal development there can be variations in origin and proximal course of the main coronary arterial branches. The origin abnormalities relate to the aortic and or the pulmonary orifice(s) which give rise to coronary arteries. More than one coronary orifice can be found in one sinus. Furthermore there is the possibility of an ectopic position which can be abnormally high and or eccentric. Whether a double orifice in one sinus is the result of either a separate development of the coronary orifices or an incorporation and remodeling of a main stem, is not clear. Literature data are not conclusive (12,13). It has been shown, however, that during prenatal and postnatal development changes in the number of orifices may develop (13,14).

Abnormalities in proximal course are relatively rare in hearts with normally related great arteries (15) because here also a general rule exists that the coronary arteries take the shortest course from the sinus they originate from to the nearest subepicardial artery. This is well illustrated by congenital heart anomalies in which the relative position of the orifices of the great arteries is such that no obvious shortest

38

VARIATIONS IN ORIGIN FROM AORTIC ORIFICE

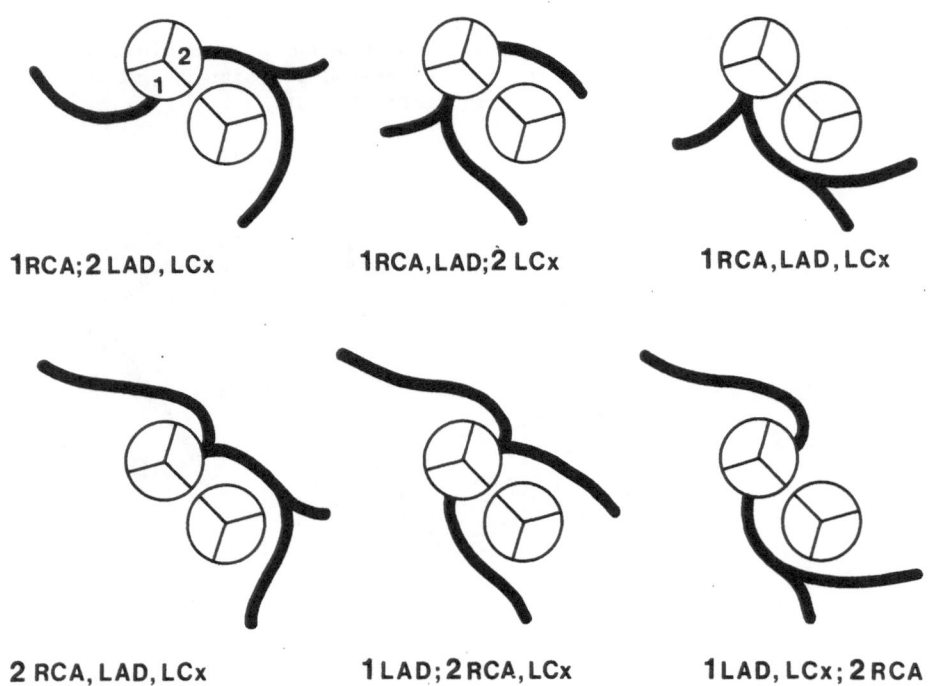

1RCA;2 LAD, LCx   1RCA,LAD;2 LCx   1RCA,LAD, LCx

2 RCA, LAD, LCx   1 LAD;2 RCA, LCx   1 LAD, LCx;2 RCA

FIGURE 6. Six basic types of origin of the three main coronary arterial
branches from the aortic orifice.

course exists. TGA with a side-to-side position of the great arteries is
a good example (9,10).

Literature data on abnormal coronary arterial development mainly
concern casuistic data from teratology. In this respect the work of
Rychter and colleagues forms an exception in that coronary arterial
development has been studied in experimentally induced right- and left
hypoplastic chick-hearts (5). In the experimentally induced hypoplastic
left heart the LCA develops in contrast to normal after RCA formation.
However, the main part of the septum and the posterior ventricular wall
are in general perfused by the LCA. A satisfactory explanation for this
finding is not provided. A similar lack of explanation exists for the
finding of absence of proximal coronary arteries in e.g. pulmonary
atresia (16) or severe hypoplasia and atresia of the coronary artery as
we observed it in specimens with this anomaly.

From a developmental point of view there can be variations in the
origin and proximal course of the coronary arteries. If there are no
clinical implications, we refer to those cases as having a normal variation. Abnormal variations are those that have clinical consequences. The
developmental error need, however, not be essentially different.

VARIATIONS IN ORIGIN FROM PULMONARY ORIFICE

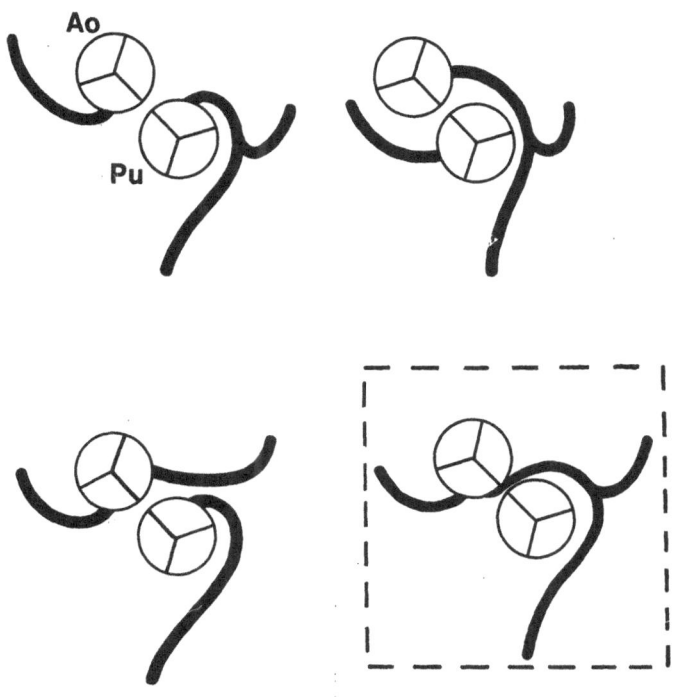

FIGURE 7. Schematic drawing of the variations in origin of the main branches from the pulmonary orifice. The hatched line encloses a case with an in-between course of a coronary artery, in which the coronary artery runs partially intramural in the aortic wall.

Two examples of such conditions will be shortly referred to in this chapter. First the origin of one or more main branches from the pulmonary orifice has serious side-effects (17). From a developmental point of view it is not acceptable that an asymmetric septation of the arterial orifice level is responsible (3). As explained in the paragraph on normal development the possibility that sprouts can develop on both sides of the aorto-pulmonary septum seems a better explanation. In general the abnormally originating artery is the LCA (Figure 7), but solely a LAD or RCA have also been reported. The clinical description of this anomaly may be found under the term "Bland-White-Garland syndrome" (17).

The second example concerns the course of a coronary artery in between the aortic and pulmonary orifice. This can be a life-threatening situation. This anomaly is not exclusively found in normally related great arteries (18); recently we have described it in TGA (19). The abnormal coronary orifice was always found very close to the interostial commissure (the commissure between the two facing sinuses) or just above this level. Furthermore the coronary artery was in part intramural in the aortic wall. In TGA this provides a problem for the arterial switch procedure (10). It cannot be excluded that this configuration is also typical for the in between course in normally related great arteries.

CONCLUSION

Research of normal development of the coronary arterial system is still necessary. Thin sectioning and immunohistochemical staining techniques in animal models are the first steps in further analysis. Some attempts have been made to do experimental work on abnormal development. Our knowledge in that field, however, is mainly based on case reports and clinical and post-mortem series. Nonetheless, a descriptive nomenclature is presented that is simple and allows an unambiguous description of variations in origin and branching pattern of the main coronary arteries in hearts with normally and abnormally related great arteries.

REFERENCES

1. Shimada Y, Ho E, Toyota N: Epicardial covering over myocardial wall in the chicken embryo as seen with the sacnning electron microscope. Scanning Electron Microscopy 11: 275-280, 1981.
2. Hirakow R: Development of the cardiac bloodvessels in staged human embryos. Acta Anat 115: 220-230, 1983.
3. Abrikossoff A: Aneurysma des linken Herzventrikels mit abnormer Abgangsstelle der linken Koronararterie von der Pulmonalis bei einem fünfmonatlichen Kinde. Virch Arch Path Anat 203: 413-420, 1911.
4. Hackensellner HA: Akzessorische Kranzgefässanlangen der Arteria pulmonalis unter 63 menschlichen Embryonen - Serien mit einer grössten Länge von 12 bis 36 mm. Z Mikrosk Anat Forsch 62: 153-164, 1956.
5. Dbalý J, Rychter Z: The vascular system of the chick embryo. XVII. The development of the branching of the coronary arteries in the chick embryos with experimentally induced left-half heart hypoplasy. Folia Morphologica 4: 358-368, 1967.
6. Zuber M: Die Entwicklung der Koronararterien bei der Maus. Inaugural Diss. Freien Universität Berlin. 1-45, 1984.
7. Kramer TC: The partitioning of the truncus and conus and the formation of the membranous portion of the univentricular septum in the human heart. Am J Anat 71: 343-370, 1942.
8. Gittenberger-de Groot AC, Bartelings MM, Wenink ACG: Developmental considerations with regard to normal and abnormal arterial valve formation. 4th Einthoven Meeting on Past and Present Cardiology: Valvular Disease, held in Leiden, December 1985. Arntzenius AC, Dunning AJ, Snellen HA (eds). Assen/Maastricht, The Netherlands, Wolfeboro, New Hampshire 03894-2069 USA, pp 27-34, 1986.
9. Gittenberger-de Groot AC, Sauer U, Oppenheimer-Dekker A, Quaegebeur J: Coronary arterial anatomy in transposition of the great arteries: A morphologic study. Ped Cardiol 4: 15-24, 1983.
10. Quaegebeur J: The arterial switch operation. Rationale, results, perspectives. Thesis, Leiden, 1986.
11. Anderson RH, Becker AE: Coronary arterial patterns a guide to identification of congenital heart disease. Paediatric Cardiology 3, Becker AE, Losekoot G, Marceletti C, Anderson RH (eds), Edinburgh, Churchill Livingstone: 251-262, 1981.
12. Aikawa E, Kawano J: Formation of coronary arteries sprouting from the primitive aortic sinus wall of the chick embryo. Experientia 38:

816–818, 1982.
13. Edwards BS, Edwards WD, Edwards JE: Aortic origin of conus coronary artery. Br Heart J 45: 555–558, 1981.
14. Miyazaki M, Kato M: The developmental study on the third coronary artery of human being. Gegenbaurs Morph Jahrb. Leipzig 132: 195–204, 1986.
15. Ogden JA: Anomalous aortic origin. Circumflex, anterior descending or main left coronary arteries. Arch Path 88: 323–328, 1969.
16. Sauer U, Bindl L, Pilossoff V, Hultisch W, Bühlmeyer K, Gittenberger-de Groot AC, de Leval MR, Sink SD: Pulmonary atresia with intact ventricular septum and right ventricle-coronary artery "fistulae" selection of patients for surgery. In: Doyle EF, Engle ME, Gersony WM, Rashlund WJ, Talmer NS (eds). Pediatric Cardiology. New York, Springer, 566–578, 1986.
17. Bogers AJJC, Quaegebeur JM, Huysmans HA: The need for follow-up after surgical correction of abnormal left coronary artery from the pulmonary artery. J Cardiovasc Surg, in press.
18. Cheitlin MD, de Castro CM, McAllister HA: Sudden death as a complication of anomalous left coronary origin from the anterior sinus of valsalva 50: 780–787, 1974.
19. Gittenberger-de Groot AC, Sauer U, Quaegebeur J: Aortic intramural coronary artery in three hearts with transposition of the great arteries. J Thorac Card Surg 91: 566–571, 1986.

II
Myocardial perfusion

LOCAL CONTROL OF CORONARY FLOW

Jos AE Spaan, Isabelle Vergroesen, Jenny Dankelman, Henk Stassen.

INTRODUCTION

The heart needs coronary flow for its oxygen supply. Myocardial oxygen usage can vary over a wide range. In the potassium arrested heart O_2 consumption is as low as 21 ul O_2/s/100 g (14) whereas in dogs during severe exercise it may increase to 1 ml O_2/s/100 g (27, 13). Coronary flow adapts to the level of oxygen usage required. This adaptation is not strictly proportional because oxygen extraction from the coronary blood is not constant. It is generally suggested that oxygen extraction by the myocardium is maximal and therefore the only way for the heart to receive more O_2 would be to increase flow. This is (in general) not true as we will see below. It seems more likely that over a significant range of O_2 consumption the coronary venous oxygen pressure is related to the control signal responsible for coronary flow regulation (11, 10).

The mechanism responsible for local coronary control is as yet unrevealed. There is even doubt whether the mechanism is based on a single mediator or on complex interaction between many. The list of possible factors involved is long and contains: oxygen, adenosine, carbondioxide, potassium, prostaglandins, endothelial relaxant factor, myogenic response, etc. For extensive reviews on the estimated effect for the different factors the reader is referred to Feigl (13) and Belloni (3). The hypotheses which we will consider more closely are the first two in the list. This is not a random choice but it concerns the mechanisms that are considered as the major candidates for control.

The flow to the myocardial micro-circulation is not steady but pulsatile because of the effect of systole. The effect of contraction depends on the level of vasoconstriction (34).

If a stenosis is present in a major coronary artery the perfusion pressure on the coronary bed is decreased. For moderate stenoses, the local control mechanism will be able to compensate for this pressure drop by the induction of vasodilation.

EXPERIMENTAL CHARACTERIZATION OF LOCAL CORONARY FLOW CONTROL

In a recent study of our group (37) the local control of coronary flow could be characterized by a simple formula:

$$CBF = a \cdot Pp + b \cdot MVO_2 + c \qquad (1)$$

where Pp equals coronary arterial pressure, MVO_2 = oxygen consumption and a, b and c are constants representing the sensitivity of coronary flow for coronary arterial pressure and oxygen consumption respectively. Obviously it is impossible to test a relation as eq. 1 without being able to manipulate arterial pressure and oxygen consumption independently.

In the literature often only one of both independent variables has been altered without control of the other one (e.g. 12, 26). In our study we have manipulated coronary arterial pressure in two ways, which is cannulation and partial occlusion of the main coronary artery. Both techniques were employed in anesthetized open chest dogs and goats. Arterial-venous oxygen content difference was monitored continuously by the method of Shepherd and Burger (32). Low levels of oxygen consumption were obtained by the administration of examethonium bromide and high levels by the administration of epinephrine. Within each animal eq. 1 was fitted to the experimentally found data of CBF, Pp and MVO_2. Both CBF and MVO_2 were normalized to 100 g of tissue.

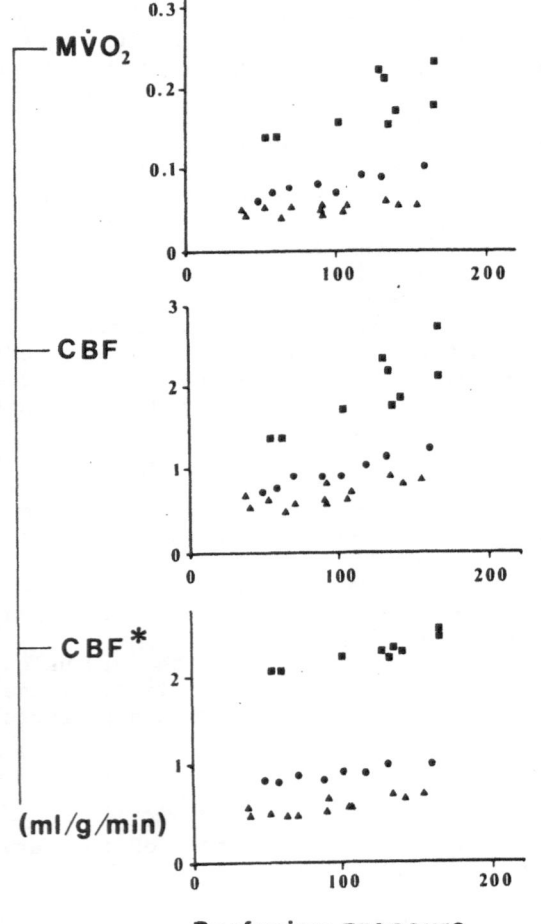

Fig. 1

Autoregulation curves corrected for the Gregg effect. MVO_2 = oxygen consumption, CBF = coronary blood flow, CBF* = corrected coronary blood flow. MVO_2 and CBF were measured. CBF* was calculated from eq. 1 after fitting the equation to the MVO_2 and CBF data. For overall results on these experiments, we refer to Vergroesen (37).

In a cannulated left main preparation it is not difficult to vary oxygen consumption at constant perfusion pressure. However, varying perfusion pressure without affecting oxygen consumption is based on experimental luck. The Gregg effect (17) makes this virtually impossible. The Gregg effect refers to the effect of perfusion pressure on oxygen consumption. This effect is indirect and acts via mechanical alterations of the ventricular wall, probably via the gardenhoose effect (1). The arterial pressure has an erectile effect on the vascular bed, which the myocardium has to overcome during systolic change of shape and therefore represents an extra workload. In a non-cannulated preparation it is even hard to keep coronary arterial pressure constant and to vary oxygen consumption independently at the same time. However, for the fitting procedure, using eq. 1, it is not relevant whether the data were obtained by varying only one or two variables at the same time.

Pressure flow relations obtained at different levels of oxygen consumption are shown in fig. 1. In the top panel the oxygen consumption is given as a function of perfusion pressure. Since the mechanical parameters like heart rate, systolic and diastolic pressures were almost not altered, this relationship shows the Gregg-effect. In the middle panel the flow data as actually measured have been depicted. In the bottom panel the flow data, corrected for perfusion pressure dependent MVO_2 changes, are presented. In fact, these corrected flow data were calculated using the regression formula obtained by fitting the experimental model equation to all the data of the specific animal. The corrected pressure flow lines are indeed parallel.
Since the pressure flow lines at constant O_2 consumption have a slope different from zero, oxygen extraction decreases with increasing perfusion pressures. Hence, especially at the higher perfusion pressures an increase in oxygen consumption could be met with an increase in oxygen extraction from the coronary blood. Moreover, it is known that at severe exercise coronary venous oxygen saturation can become as low as ten percent, which is much lower than the values found in experimental studies, like ours and those of others, in anesthetized animals.

MECHANISMS

Oxygen and coronary flow control
As stated above, the key factor responsible for flow control is not yet known. In this section we will analyse the oxygen and adenosine hypothesis for coronary flow control. The oxygen model is based on the assumption that interstitial oxygen tension is the controlling factor. In words: the model assumes that when interstitial or tissue pO_2 falls, coronary resistance will decrease. This may be due to either a direct effect of oxygen on arteriolar smooth muscle or by an intermediate substance. Hence, those factors that influence tissue pO_2 will effect coronary resistance in a similar manner.
Via the tissue pO_2 coronary resistance can be influenced by perfusion pressure and oxygen consumption. When perfusion pressure is increased from a stationary value, coronary flow and therefore oxygen supply will increase. This will result in an increase in tissue pO_2 and consequently in vasoconstriction reducing the increase in flow. In this way autoregulation can be explained. If oxygen consumption of the myocardium rises, tissue pO_2 decreases.

48

According to the oxygen model this decrease in tissue pO_2 will give
rise to vasodilation and consequently to an increase in coronary flow
and oxygen supply, which can explain metabolic adjustment of coronary
flow.

Above the oxygen hypothesis is formulated in words. However, a
quantitative evaluation of this hypothesis can only be performed when
the hypothesis is translated into equations. In this case this is not
too difficult. The mathematics of the model are discussed in more
detail in the chapter of Wieringa et al. in this book.

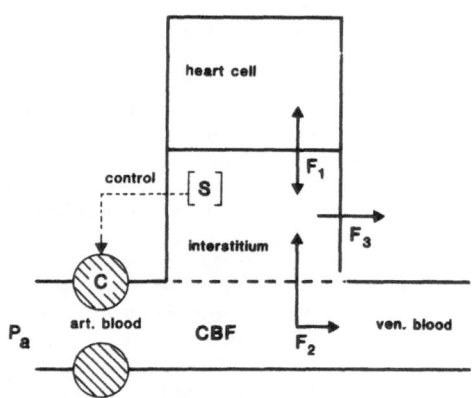

Fig.2   Schematic representation of a steady state mass balance
         model; $[S]_i$ = concentration of flow regulating substance
         in the interstitium. F_1, F_2, F_3 fluxes of the regulating
         substance in and out the interstitium. In steady state
         these fluxes are in balance with each other:
         --   Mass balance of Oxygen model:
                   $$MVO_2 = CBF \cdot [O_2]_{(a-v)} \qquad 1)$$
              Control function:
                   $$(P_a - P_v)/CBF = K_1 + K_2 \cdot [O_2]_i \qquad 2)$$
              Result: $CBF = b_0 + b_1 \cdot MVO_2 + b_2 \cdot P_a$ 3)
              where MVO_2 = oxygen consumption, CBF = coronary
              blood flow, $[O_2]_{(a-v)}$ = arterio-venous oxygen
              content difference, P_a = arterial pressure, P_v =
              venous pressure, $[O_2]_i$ = interstitial oxygen
              concentration, K_1, K_2, b_0, b_1, b_2 = parameters.
         --   Mass balance of adenosine model:
                   $$C_1 \cdot MVO_2 = CBF \cdot [A]_i + C_2 \cdot [A]_i \qquad 4)$$
              Control function:
                   $$CBF/(P_a - P_v) = C_3 \cdot [A]_i \qquad 5)$$
              Result:
                   $$CBF^2 + C_2 \cdot CBF = C_1 \cdot C_3 \cdot MVO_2 \cdot (P_a - P_v) \qquad 6)$$
              where $[A]_i$ = interstitial adenosine concentration.
              C_1, C_2, C_3 are parameters.

The oxygen model predicts the parallel shift of the autoregulation
curves with a variation in oxygen consumption as was found
experimentally. This, of course, is not proof that coronary

flow is regulated by tissue pO_2. However, comparison between model prediction and experimental results indicates that coronary resistance is more tightly coupled to tissue pO_2 than to oxygen consumption per se.

Adenosine and coronary control

The adenosine hypothesis has been very popular for a long time as an explanation for coronary flow control (4). In words the hypothesis is as follows.

Adenosine is a break down product of ATP. Hence, if oxygen consumption increases, ATP usage and consequently the adenosine production will increase. Adenosine will then diffuse to the arteriolar smooth muscle and will relax it. The vasodilation will result in a decrease of coronary resistance and increase in coronary flow. This could be the basis for the explanation of metabolic flow adjustment. An increase in perfusion pressure would result in increase in coronary flow and therefore, in an increased washout of adenosine. The washout of adenosine would then result in vasoconstriction and therefore, in a reduction of the original increase in coronary flow. In this way, autoregulation would be explained.

We also formulated the adenosine hypothesis mathematically. The notions used for this are illustrated in fig. 2. The equations are non-linear and do not predict a parallel shift of autoregulation curves with an increase in oxygen consumption. The result of a fit of these model equations to the experimental data is shown in fig. 3. The conclusion is that the adenosine model, as formulated above, does not provide such a nice fit as well as the oxygen model did.

A variation of the original adenosine hypothesis of Rubio and Berne was described by Granger et al. (15). They assumed that the adenosine production was proportional to the oxygen demand-to-supply ratio. However, the mathematical equivalent of this assumption does not provide a linear equation between flow on the one hand and perfusion pressure and oxygen consumption on the other hand.

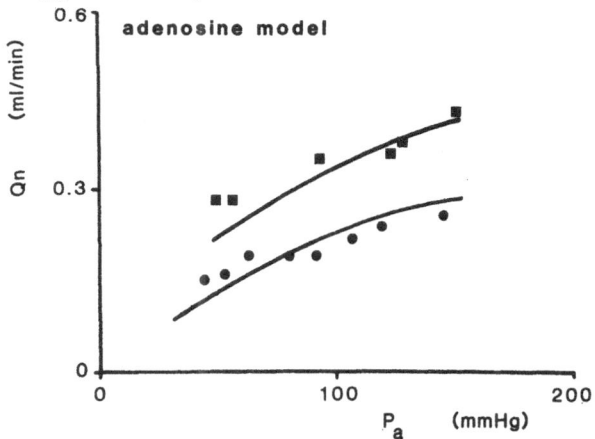

Fig. 3   Fit of adenosine model to experimental data Qn = normalized flow. Pa = coronary arterial pressure.
Qn = 1 at Pa = 100 mm Hg and at peak reactive hyperemic flow.

We then searched for an adenosine hypothesis that provided a mathematical equation compatible with the experimental characterization of the local coronary flow. The linear equation could be obtained by assuming that tissue adenosine can not be washed out by flow and that adenosine production is determined by the oxygen supply to demand ratio. However, these assumptions are incompatible with experimental findings which show that tissue adenosine is washed out by flow (28).

Experimental evaluation of the adenosine hypothesis

Experimental evidence of the adenosine hypothesis was found in the concomitant increase in adenosine production and oxygen consumption. This has been measured by determining the concentrations of adenosine and its purine derivatives in coronary venous outflow (e.g. 33). Tissue adenosine increased proportionally with the duration of coronary occlusion as was the peak reactive hyperemic flow (28).

However, the adenosine hypothesis has been under severe attack, not only by theoretical analyses as presented above (e.g. 24) but also by experiments. Several experiments have been designed to effect interstitial adenosine by adenosine deaminase infusion into the coronary blood. The underlying idea is that if adenosine plays a major role in local coronary flow control, then coronary flow should decrease if tissue adenosine would be decreased by the enzyme. Saito et al. (30) were the first to attempt to study the role of adenosine by the infusion of adenosine deaminase. Control flow and peak reactive hyperemic flow were not affected by the deaminase infusion. However, reactive hyperemic flow volume was reduced by about 30%, showing that adenosine plays a role in this response. Studies have shown (23, 9, 18) that deaminase infusion indeed does not affect coronary flow control. From assaying either cardiac lymph or pericardial fluid, it was clear that adenosine deaminase came into the interstitial space in a sufficient amount to effect interstitial adenosine. Hence, the conclusion from these experimental studies must be that adenosine does not play a major role in the normal control of coronary blood flow. However, it may play a role as a reserve mechanism if normal control fails to increase supply sufficiently to meet demand.

DYNAMICS OF CORONARY FLOW CONTROL

Reactive hyperemia

A very well known phenomenon of dynamic response of the coronary circulation is reactive hyperemia, the response of coronary flow to an arterial occlusion. A typical example is shown in fig. 4. When the artery is occluded for about ten seconds, coronary flow increases by a factor of about 4. In the middle panel coronary venous oxygen saturation is shown as measured by a fiber optics. Obviously, this signal provides no information about capillary oxygen exchange during the occlusion. After release of the occlusion, the venous oxygen saturation signal shows a delay and a dip. The dip is due to the blood that was within the capillaries during the occlusion and hence had lost more than usual of its oxygen. Then, oxygen extraction decreases, reaches a minimum and returns to control.

From flow and oxygen extraction the oxygen disappearance from the blood between the arterial and venous measuring sites can be calculated.

The formula to be used in this calculation is:

$$MVO_2 = Qa(t) * Sa - Qv(t) * Sv(t)$$

where MVO_2 = Oxygen consumption, Qa, Sa are arterial flow and arterial oxygen saturation respectively. Sa is assumed to be constant. $Qv(t)$, $Sv(t)$ are venous flow and venous oxygen saturation respectively.

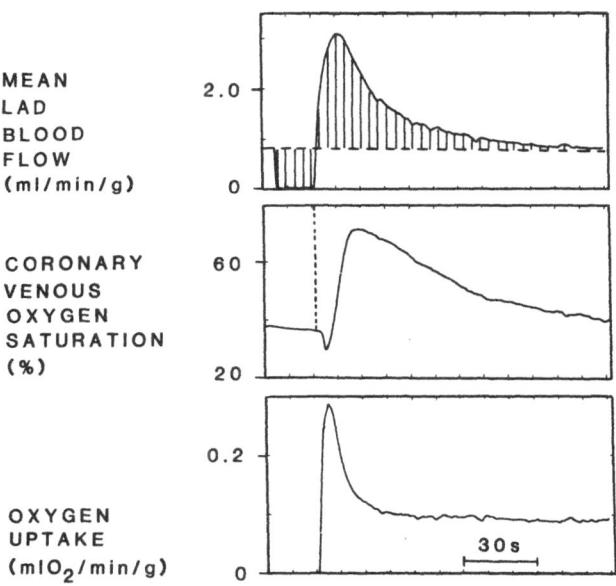

Fig. 4   Reactive hyperemia, resulting from 15 s occlusion of a coronary artery. Note the low overpayment of oxygen. For explanation see text (according to 29).

This formula has to be applied with care. $Sv(t)$ is delayed with respect to the coronary flow signal because of two reasons. In the first place it takes some time, about 1.5 s, after the release of a coronary occlusion before venous flow starts again. When venous flow has been restored it takes some time for the blood to travel from the capillaries to the venous measuring site. In order to compensate for these delay times, we shifted the venous oxygen saturation signal in time such, that the onset of the decrease of this signal coincided with the onset of coronary arterial flow.

Oxygen Repayment Ratio, ORR, is used to characterize the oxygen consumption response to the coronary occlusion. It is defined as the ratio between the total oxygen consumption above control in the reactive hyperemic response and the lack of oxygen uptake during the occlusion.

52

In formula this yields;

$$ORR = (\int_{t=0}^{t=T} MVO_2 dt - TMVO_{2c})/(MVO_{2c} \cdot T_{occ}) \tag{3}$$

where $t = 0$ at the moment of release, MVO_{2c} = control oxygen consumption, T = integration time, T_{occ} = duration of the occlusion. We are so explicit with this formula since a serious error previously has been made in calculating this oxygen repayment ratio (6, 17). The subtle cause of this error has been discussed by Ruiter (29). It is related to the fact that the mean of a product of two terms is not equal to the product of the mean of these two terms.

1) The old studies reported a repayment ratio of about 300%. 2) In some recent text-books this value is still taught to be the accurate data. In the study of Ruiter et al. where the correct equation was used, the repayment ratio was about one. It was calculated that this repayment could be explained for a large part by the restoration of blood and tissue oxygen buffers in between arterial and venous measuring sites.

Coronary flow response to heart rate change.
     The rate of metabolic flow adjustment is slow. Following Belloni and Sparks (2) we measured the coronary response to a sudden change in heart rate. Our experiments are different from their in that Belloni and Sparks applied a constant flow perfusion whereas we applied a constant pressure perfusion.

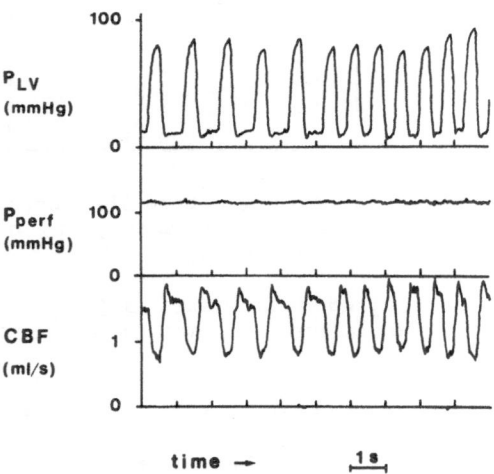

Fig. 5   Response of coronary flow to a sudden change in heart rate from 60 to 90 beats/minute. P_{LV} = left ventricular pressure, P_{perf} = perfusion pressure, CBF = coronary blood flow. The initial phase of diastole at the low heart rate is not different from diastolic flow at the high heart rate.

The initial response of coronary flow to the heart rate change is shown in fig. 5. As is shown, not much happens during the first few beats following the change in heart rate. This casts some doubt on those studies reporting a very fast response time for coronary control. We will come back to those discrepancies below. We have quantified the change in the coronary vascular tone in two ways: a Diastolic Coronary Index, DCI and a Beat Coronary Index, BCI. The diastolic index is defined as mean diastolic pressure divided by mean diastolic flow. The BCI is defined as the ratio between mean pressure and mean flow both averaged over the heart beat. The normalized responses of these indices are presented in fig. 6. The responses shown, are the averaged data of 14 experiments obtained by changing the heart rate from 60 into 90 beats per minute. Both indices show a slow response. The $t_{1/2}$ of the response is in the order of 15 seconds. The conclusion to be drawn from this finding is that all responses, much slower than the regulation constant, must be due to mechanical phenomena.

Beat and Diastolic Indices

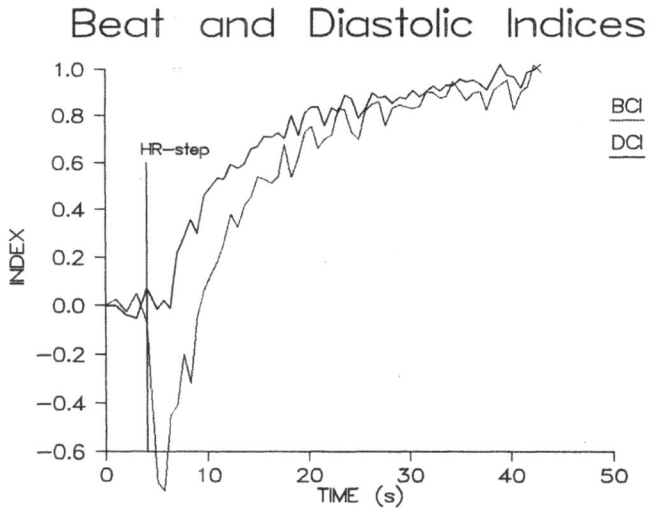

Fig. 6   The regulatory response of coronary indices to a sudden change in heart rate (60-90 beats/min.). DCI = Diastolic Coronary Index, BCI = Beat Coronary Index.

For the interpretation of the difference in the initial transient of the DCI and BCI, one can not ignore the discussion of how cardiac contraction affects the coronary micro-circulation. The hypotheses, directed to this interaction, are distinguishable by the time constants assumed to be necessary to establish pressure equilibrium within the coronary micro-circulation (see also Downey's chapter in this book). The scientific discussion in this field is vivid and far from conclusive yet. Analysis of arterial inflow responses alone to e.g. a perfusion pressure step or sudden cardiac arrest have led to conclusions that these time constants are in the order of 0.1 sec. (25, 8, 21, 22). However, those studies that are directed to the coronary venous outflow provide evidence that these time constants are much longer (36, 5, 20).

According to the theory based on short time constants, systole and diastole can be considered as independent parts of the cycle as far as coronary perfusion is concerned. Diastole would then be a phase where coronary flow is determined by the properties of the vascular bed alone, unaffected by cardiac contraction. In that case the Diastolic Coronary Index is the index of choice. The drop in BCI then is easily explained by the reduction in diastolic and hence inflow time. In this conception BCI is a meaningless index. In the other concept, diastolic coronary flow is affected by the preceding beats of the heart. The dip in index then can be explained on the basis of a combination of two effects:
1) a capacitance effect due to a change in average compression of the micro-circulation by the change in heart rate, and
2) by an increase in resistance in the micro-circulation because some blood volume will be squeezed out on account of the increased compression.

It is beyond the scope of this chapter to go into this discussion in detail. In the opinion of the authors the second concept will appear to be correct in the end, be it that the different effects still need to be quantified. This would mean that in the cyclic scientific views we will be back to the original interpretation of Scaramucci in 1695 (31), who claimed that the diastolic inflow of the coronary bed is influenced by the preceding systole.

CORONARY RESERVE WITH A CORONARY STENOSES

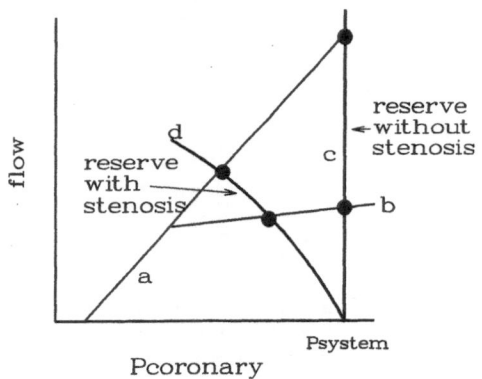

Fig. 7   Effect of stenosis on coronary reserve. The vertical axis reflects both the actual flow and flow demand (curves c and d) of the myocardium. Curve a = pressure-flow relation at maximal vasodilation. Curve b = autoregulation curve, depending on oxygen consumption as shown in fig. 1. Curve c = the relation between flow demand and the systemic pressure if systemic pressure remains constant. Curve d = the relation between flow demand and coronary arterial pressure in the presence of a stenosis. The horizontal distance between curves a and c at a certain level of flow is the pressure drop over the stenosis.

An important notion that is used in several chapters of this book is coronary reserve. This is defined as the amount of blood flow above control which the coronary circulation is capable of recruiting. However, this definition is vague and is hardly suitable for quantitative analysis, since both the maximal flow and control flow are dependent on a variety of conditions. These points are best illustrated graphically as done in fig. 7 (e.g. 19, 35).

The vertical line (c) shows that flow can increase above control at constant pressure. However, in the presence of a stenosis, the pressure distal to the stenosis is the effective perfusion pressure of the micro-circulation. Because of the hydrodynamic resistance of the stenosis, the pressure drop across it will increase with flow. With severe stenoses this drop is not linear with flow as shown in fig. 7.

The impeding effect of the stenoses on coronary reserve is apparent from fig. 7. However, in reality the situation is more complex. As said, the maximal dilated line, a, is not unique. Pharmacologically the bed can be dilated further than with an ischemic stimulus (16). Moreover, the position of the curve depends on the mechanical compression of the heart as discussed by Downey in this book. It is even more important that this compression effect is extreme in the sub-endocardium but absent in the sub-epicardium. Therefore (flow) measurements in large coronary branches may indicate a considerable coronary reserve, even in the absence of reserve in the most vulnerable part of the heart, the sub-endocardium.

The uncertainty of the definition "control flow" is evident as well. In order to assess the physiological significance of a stenosis, one ought to know the oxygen consumption at the moment of measurement but also the oxygen requirement of the heart of the specific patient out of bed at rest and during exercise.

DISCUSSION
In this chapter some dynamic and static characteristics of coronary flow control were discussed. These characteristics are relevant to several practical problems. We have discussed the relevance for coronary reserve studies above. However, the analysis is also of importance to pharmacological studies. For example, in order to draw a justified conclusion whether a drug causes vasodilation or not, its effect on oxygen-consumption of the myocardium should be known. Moreover, the response of the coronary control system is slow and sufficient time between control and intervention measurement should be allowed. On the other hand, the effect of mechanical interventions can be studied, not affected by vascular smooth muscle tone variations, if the measurements are done within a few seconds.

56

REFERENCES

1. Arnold G, Morgenstern O, Lochner W: The autoregulation of the heart work by the coronary perfusion pressure. Pfluegers Arch., 321: 34-55, 1970.
2. Belloni FL, Sparks HV: Dynamics of myocardial oxygen consumption and coronary vascular resistance. Am. J. Physiol. 233 (Heart and Circ. Physiol. 2.): H34-H43, 1977.
3. Belloni FL: The local control of coronary blood flow. Cardiovasc. Res. 13: 63-85, 1979.
4. Berne RM: Cardiac nucleotides in hypoxia: possible role in regulation of coronary blood flow. Am. J. Physiol. 204: 317-322, 1963.
5. Chilian WM, Marcus ML: Coronary venous outflow persists after cessation of coronary arterial inflow. Am.J.Physiol. 247 (Heart and Circ. Physiol. 16.): H984-H990, 1984.
6. Coffman JD, Gregg DE: Reactive hyperemia characteristics of the myocardium. Am. J. Physiol. 199: 1143-1149, 1960.
7. Dole WP, Monteville WJ, Bishop VS: Dependency of myocardial reactive hyperemia on coronary artery pressure in the dog. Am. J. Physiol., 240: H709-H715, 1981.
8. Dole WP, Alexander GM, Campbell AB, Hixson EL, Bishop VS: Interpretation and physiological significance of diastolic coronary artery pressure-flow relationships in the canine coronary bed. Circ.Res. 55: 215-226, 1984.
9. Dole WP, Yamada N, Bishop VS, Olsson RA: Role of adenosine in coronary flow regulation after reductions in perfusion pressure. Circ. Res. 56: 517-524, 1985.
10. Dole WP, Nuno DW: Myocardial oxygen tension determines the degree and pressure range of coronary autoregulation. Circ. Res. 59: 202-215, 1986.
11. Drake-Holland AJ, Laird JD, Noble MIM, Spaan JAE, Vergroesen I: Oxygen and coronary vascular resistance during autoregulation and metabolic vasodilation in the dog. J. Physiol. Lond. 348: 285-299, 1984.
12. Eckenhoff JE, Hafkenschiel JH, Landmesser CM, Harmel M: Cardiac oxygen metabolism and control of the coronary circulation. Am. J. Physiol. 149: 634-649, 1947.
13. Feigl EO: Coronary Physiology. Physiol. Rev., 63: 1-205, 1983.
14. Gibbs GL, Papadoyannis DE, Drake AJ, Noble MIM: Oxygen consumption of the non-working and potassium chloride-arrested dog heart. Circ. Res. 47: 408-417, 1980.
15. Granger HJ, Shepherd AP jr.: Intrinsic microvascular control of tissue oxygen delivery. Microvasc. Res. 5: 49-72, 1973.
16. Grattan MT, Hanley FT, Stevens MB, Hoffman JIE: Transmural coronary flow reserve patterns in dogs. Am. J. Physiol. 250 (heart 19), H276-H283, 1986.
17. Gregg DE: Effect of coronary perfusion pressure or coronary flow on oxygen usage of the myocardium. Circ. Res., 13: 497-500, 1963.
18. Hanley FL, Grattan MT, Stevens MB, Hoffman JIE: Role of adenosine in coronary autoregulation. Am. J. Physiol. 250 (Heart and Circ. Physiol. 19): H558-H566, 1986.

19. Hoffman JIE, Grattan MT, Hanley FL, Messina LM: Total and transmural perfusion of the hypertrophied heart. In: Cardiac Left Ventricular Hypertrophy. H.E.D.J. ter Keurs, J.J. Schipperheyn (Eds). Martinus Nijhoff, Boston 130-151, 1983.

20. Kajiya F, Tsujioka K, Goto M: Evaluation of phasic blood flow velocity of the great cardiac vein by a laser doppler method. Heart and Vessels 1: 16-23, 1985.

21. Klocke FJ, Weinstein IR, Klocke JF, Ellis AK, Kraus DR, Mates RE, Canty JM, Anbar RD, Romanowski RR, Wall KW meyer, Echt MP: Zero-flow pressure and pressure-flow relationship during single long diastoles in the canine coronary bed before and during maximum vasodilation. J. Clin. Invest. 68: 970-980, 1981.

22. Klocke FJ, Mates RE, Canty JM jr., Ellis AK: Coronary pressure-flow relationships, controversial issues and probable implications, Circ. Res. 56: 310-323, 1985.

23. Kroll K, Feigl EO: Adenosine is unimportant in controlling coronary blood flow in unstressed dog heart. Am. J. Physiol. 249 (Heart & Circ. Physiol. 8): H1176-H1178, 1985.

24. Laird JD, Breuls PNWM, Meer P van der, Spaan JAE: Can a single vasodilator be responsible for both autoregulation and metabolic vasodilation. Basic. Res. Cardiol. 76: 354-358, 1981.

25. Lee J, Chambers DE, Akizuki S, Downey JM: The role of vascular capacitance in the coronary arteries. Circ. Res. 55: 751-762, 1984.

26. Mosher P, Ross J, McFate PA, Shaw RF: Control of coronary blood flow by an autoregulatory mechanism. Circ. Res. 14: 250-259, 1964.

27. Restorff W von, Holtz J, Bassenge E: Exercise induced augmentation of myocardial oxygen extraction in spite of normal coronary dilatory capacity in dogs. Pfluegers Arch. 372: 181-185, 1977.

28. Rubio R, Berne RM: Release of adenosine by the normal myocardium in dogs and its relationship to the regulation of coronary resistance. Circ. Res. 25: 407-415, 1969.

29. Ruiter JH, Spaan JAE, Laird JD: Transient oxygen uptake during myocardial reactive hyperemia in the dog. Am. J. Physiol. 235 (Heart Circ. Physiol. 4) H87-H94, 1978.

30. Saito D, Nixon DG, Vomacka RB, Olsson RA: Relationship of cardiac oxygen usage, adenosine content, and coronary resistance in dogs. Circ. Res. 47: 875-882, 1980.

31. Scaramucci J: De Motu Cordis, Theorema Sextum. In: Theoremata Familiaria de physico-medicis lucubrationibus. Iuxta leges mecanicas. 70-81, 1695.

32. Shepherd AP, Burgar CG: A solid state arterio-venous oxygen difference analyzer for following whole blood. Am. J. Physiol. 232: H437-H440, 1977.

33. Schrader J, Haddy FJ, Gerlach E: Release of adenosine, Inosine and Hypoxantine from the isolated guinea pig heart during hypoxia, flow- autoregulation and reactive hyperemia. Pfluegers Arch. 369: 1-6, 1977.

34. Spaan JAE, Breuls NPW, Laird JD: Forward coronary flow normally seen in systole is the result of both forward and concealed back flow. Basic Res. Cardiol. 76: 582-586, 1981.

58

35. Spaan JAE, Bruinsma P, Laird JD: Coronary flow mechanics of the hypertrophied heart. In: Cardiac Left Ventricular Hypertrophy. H.E.D.J. ter Keurs, J.J. Schippenheyn (Eds). Martinus Nijhoff, Boston 170-193, 1983.

36. Spaan JAE: Coronary diastolic pressure-flow relation and zero flow pressure explained on the basis of intramyocardial compliance. Circ. Res. 56: 293-309, 1985.

37. Vergroesen I, Noble MIM, Wieringa PA, Spaan JAE: Quantification of oxygen consumption and arterial pressure as independent determinants of coronary flow. Am. J. Physiol. 252 (Heart and Circ. Physiol. 21). H545-H553, 1987.

THE EXTRAVASCULAR RESISTANCE

JAMES M. DOWNEY

1. INTRODUCTION

Two phenomena determine the heart's resistance to coronary blood flow - the caliber of the resistance vessels as determined by smooth muscle in the walls of the coronary vessels and external compression of those vessels by the mechanical motion of the beating heart. The smooth muscle is controlled by cardiac nerves and local metabolic processes in the heart and is the effector for a rapid and efficient control system which matches blood flow to metabolic requirements under a wide variety of hemodynamic and contractile states.

The second process is not part of any purposeful control system, but rather represents a necessary evil with which the heart must contend. As the heart contracts, stresses are created within the myocardium which deform the coronary vessels in a way that increases their resistance to flow. This mechanical impediment to flow has been termed the "extravascular resistance," since its origins are outside the vessels. In the normal heart the control systems easily compensate for these periodic blood flow deficits by modifying the vascular smooth muscle's tone so that the time-averaged perfusion to any region of the heart remains in the proper range to insure adequate nutrition.

The magnitude of the extravascular resistance is quite large. Under normal hemodynamic conditions a third of the coronary resistance is extravascular in origin (47). In many forms of heart disease coronary dilatory reserve will be lost such that the vascular smooth muscle may no longer be able to compensate the extravascular component. Animal experiments indicate that this can occur with stenotic coronary arteries (41), valvular dysfunction (8) or hypotension (17). When coronary reserve has been exhausted, the extravascular resistance indeed becomes the major determinant of regional perfusion. If the physician manages such patients so as to minimize the extravascular resistance, ischemic injury to the heart in turn can be reduced. To accomplish such management requires an understanding the origins and the determinants of the extravascular resistance. This chapter will attempt to summarize those factors.

2. AN HISTORICAL PERSPECTIVE

The influence of the heart beat on coronary flow has only recently begun to be understood. At first physiologists believed that the beating heart, like other muscle pump systems in the body, actually helped to propel blood through the coronary system by a massaging action (45). This "massaging" theory was supported by the observation that coronary sinus outflow came forth in spurts coincident with contraction. These spurts persisted even when the coronary circulation was perfused from a nonpulsatile source. In 1940, Gregg and Green developed an orifice-plate flow meter which had sufficient fidelity to measure phasic coronary flow

(22). They found that coronary flow was greatly reduced during systole. The massaging theory began to fall out of favor with most scientists in light of the phasic coronary flow data.

The massaging theory was laid to rest in 1957 by the classic experiment of Sabiston and Gregg (47). The heart was fibrillated while the coronary blood vessels were perfused from a pressurized reservoir. Asystole was always accompanied by an abrupt and dramatic increase in blood flow as shown in Figure 1. The conclusion was clear: removal of the coordinated heart beat also lowered the coronary artery´s resistance to flow.

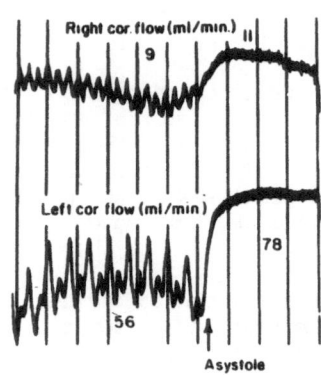

FIGURE 1. The effect of asystole on coronary flow when perfusion pressure is maintained. Note that flow increases abruptly indicating that coronary resistance had fallen. Reprinted from (47) with permission from the American Heart Association.

3. EXTRAVASCULAR RESISTANCE HAS ITS PEAK VALUE IN THE SUBENDOCARDIUM

It has long been recognized that the subendocardium is a favored site for myocardial infarction in patients with diseased coronary arteries. The vulnerability of the subendocardium is now believed to directly result from a high degree of extravascular resistance in that region which reduces its nutritionl flow. Although the transmural distribution of blood flow across the wall of the normal heart has been found to be nearly uniform (21), Griggs and Nakamura (23) demonstrate that partial occlusion of a coronary artery consistently results in a preferential reduction in the subendocardial blood flow. The coronary stenosis caused a greater percentage of the coronary inflow to occur during systole, a time when flow is distributed away from the subendocardium by the extravascular factors. Buckberg et al. changed the partitioning of flow between systole and diastole with valvular lesions (8). Again, they demonstrated that any maneuver which selectively reduced inflow during the diastolic period distributed flow away from the subendocardium.

The distribution of the systolic blood flow can be visualized by perfusing the coronary arteries with ventricular pressure (14). Diastoic flow is eliminated because this pressure falls to near zero during diastole. Tracers injected during those conditions reveal a steep blood flow gradient across the heart wall with flow to the subendocardial layers approaching zero.

The relative magnitude of the extravascular resistance at each depth can be revealed by repeating the Sabiston and Gregg experiment and making regional blood flow measurements using microspheres. Figure 2 reveals that arresting the heart has virtually no effect on flow to the subepicardium while it nearly doubles flow to the subendocardium. The effect on flow in the mid-wall is intermediate between those two extremes. While extravascular factors double the subendocardial resistance they are negligable at the subepicardium.

4. VASCULAR WATERFALL HYPOTHESIS

Although it is not difficult to appreciate that the contracting heart muscle can compress the coronary blood vessels and inhibit flow, it would be helpful if this process could be quantified. To do that requires a knowledge of the fundamental processes involved. Three possible mechanisms can be proposed. The first involves shear strains in the heart wall. Note that strains refer to the actual deformation of the tissue and are to be differentiated from stresses - the forces giving rise to those deformations. Adjacent muscle fibers may contract in such a way that they slide past one another, creating a region of shear between them. Any blood vessel passing through this region would then be pinched at the interface, thereby increasing its resistance to flow, or perhaps even totally occluding it. The muscle-fiber orientation changes as one passes from the epicardium toward the endocardium by about 120 degrees (54). Some shear likely exists between these nonparallel fibers.

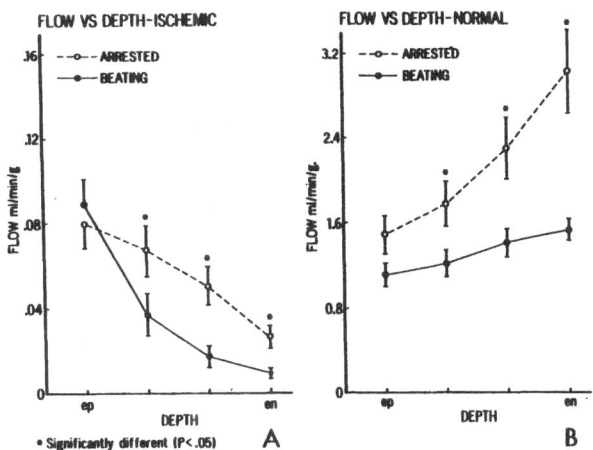

FIGURE 2. The effect of asystole on regional coronary flow for both a collateral dependent region (A) and a normaly perfused region (B) of the heart. Note that in both regions asystole doubles flow to the subendocardium but has no significant effect on flow to the subepicardium. Reprinted from (46) with permission from the American Physiological Society.

Extravascular resistance might also be related to traction forces on the blood vessels. Increasing the length of a vessel increases its resistance through both length and diameter effects. Since the ventricular wall thickens during systole, any vessels oriented at right angles to the epicardial surface will experience an increased length at this time and, thus, an increased resistance.

A third possibility is that compressive stresses within the myocardium are responsible for deforming the coronary blood vessels. Compressive stesses in the subendocardium must at least equal the pressure in the ventricular lumen and could theoretically even exceed it. Attempts to measure the intramyocardial forces (see below) indicate that these stresses are substantial.

It is now believed that stress development accounts for the major portion of the extravascular resistance. Both shear and traction are a consequence of strains in the heart wall resulting from myocardial fiber shortening. The contribution of strains can be examined by comparing the distribution of the systolic blood flow across the wall of the isovolumetrically beating heart to that of hearts ejecting against zero afterload (16). In the isovolumetric state, pressure development is near normal but strains are minimal. Yet flow is diverted away from the subendocardium as effectively by isovolumetric contractions as by normal ejections. Conversely, the systolic coronary flow distribution of the empty beating heart, which should experience maximal strains, experiences no redistribution away from the subendocardium (16).

If a compressive stress in the tissue is clearly above the perfusion pressure then the blood vessels are obliged to collapse obliterating flow to that region. But what happens to vessels in regions where the tissue pressure is elevated above venous pressure but is still less than perfusion pressure? This condition has been extensively studied in the lung (44) and elsewhere (25) and it has been found that the blood vessels respond to an elevated tissue pressure by forming waterfalls.

The waterfall theory, as presented by Holt (27,28), says that, when the pressure surrounding a collapsible tube is between the inflow and the outflow pressures, there must be a point along the tube´s length where the pressure inside the vessel falls below that outside the vessel. The vessel, being a non rigid structure, is obliged to collapse at that point. If the region completely collapsed, however, the system would be unstable. Flow would cease, causing the pressure drop along the proximal segment of the tube to be lost. The full inflow pressure would then be transmitted to the region of collapse and reopen the tube.

The equilibrium which is finally achieved causes a region of partial collapse to form near the outflow end of the tube. The orifice formed at the region of collapse will adjust its resistance so that it will drop the pressure inside the vessel from tissue pressure to venous pressure. Because only a very small portion of the vessel´s distal segment is involved in the partial collapse, the resistance of the patent upstream portion closely approximates the overall resistance of the vessel before the tissue pressure was elevated. Since the pressure gradient across the upstream resistance is known - arterial pressure minus tissue pressure - flow can easily be calculated by the following equation:

$$Q = \frac{(\text{Perfusion pressure} - \text{Back pressure})}{\text{Resistance}}$$

Resistance in the equation refers to the resistance to flow as measured when tissue pressure is zero. Back pressure is either the tissue pressure, if Arterial pressure> tissue pressure > venous pressure or; venous pressure, if tissue pressure < venous pressure. In essence, whenever local tissue pressure exceeds venous pressure, tissue pressure is simply substituted for back pressure in the above equation. Resistance in the equation is independent of tissue or venous pressure. Note that this equation is discontinuous in that flow becomes zero when arterial pressure is less than back pressure.

5. EVIDENCE FOR THE WATERFALL HYPOTHESIS IN THE CORONARY BED

The waterfall hypothesis was the first attempt at quantitating the extravascular resistance. Although the validity of this hypothesis has yet to be proven, its attractivness is its ability to explain many aspects of the extravascular resistance in the coronary bed. The strongest evidence that waterfalls may actually be forming in the heart is the coronary pressure-flow relationship. The pressure-flow characteristics between a vascular waterfall system and a simple resistance are very different. Figure 3 shows the pressure-flow curve for a vascular waterfall. Since the resistance of the blood vessel upstream of the collapsed region is not affected by changes in the surrounding pressure, the slope of the pressure-flow curve is independent of the surround pressure. Changes in the surround pressure only shift the pressure-axis intercept. Changes in resistance, in turn, should have no effect on the pressure-axis intercept – only the slope of the line. Figure 4 shows that, when the pressure flow curve of the coronary artery of a beating heart was compared with that for the same heart in an arrested state, the curves are only shifted in parallel fashion (15). This indicates that the contribution from contraction had no affect on the resistance, only the pressure-axis intercept. The conclusion again was that only waterfall phenomena were contributing to the extravascular resistance. It should be noted that the two curves in figure 4 are only parallel in the region of perfusion pressures above peak ventricular pressure. The convergence at low perfusion pressures can be explained by the complete collapse of vessels in those regions where perfusion pressure has fallen below the extravascular compression.

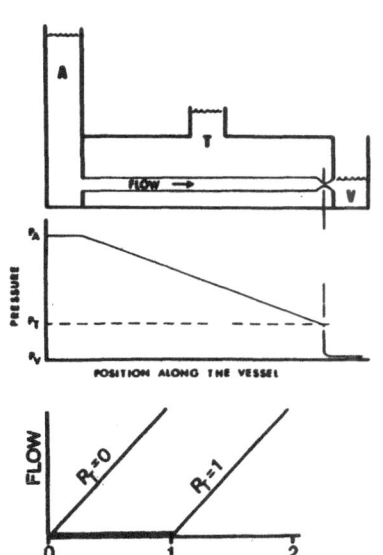

FIGURE 3. The upper panel shows the waterfall model. If the pressure sur-rounding the vessel, T, is between arterial pressure, A, and venous pressure, V, then a region of collapse will form at the outflow end. The middle panel shows the pressure gradient along the length of the vessel. Note that pressure drops abruptly from T to V in the region of partial collapse. The bottom panel shows the pressure flow curves for the vessel when T=0 and when T=1. Note that increasing T shifts the curve to the right but does not change the slope.

The waterfall hypothesis has been challenged by Spaan et al. (52). The criticism revolves around the magnitude of the capacitance of the

64

coronary arteries. These investigators propose a large capacitance (the change in intravascular volume which results from a given change in intravascular pressure) in the coronary microcirculation. Their data suggest that this capacitance exists deep in the coronary bed with an appreciable resistance between either the coronary ostium or the coronary sinus and this capacitance.

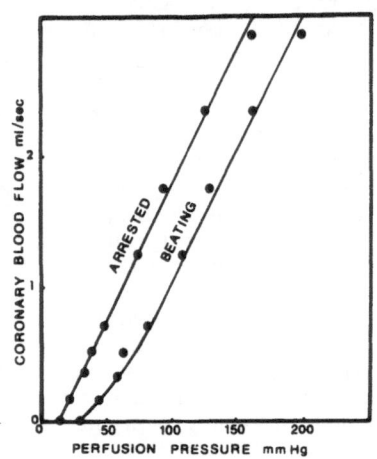

FIGURE 4. The pressure-flow relationship for a canine coronary artery. Peak ventricular pressure remained constant at 100 mmhg and the vessels were dilated with adenosine. Note that beating shifts the curve to the right in a parallel fashion in the range of perfusion pressures above peak ventricular pressure. Reprinted from (15) with permission from the American Heart Association.

Since the capacitance vessels in the deep layers have intramyocardial pressure as their surround pressure, that compression will initially be transmitted through the vessel wall to the contained blood with the onset of each beat. The pressure within the vessel would not fall to a value below the tissue pressure and allow waterfall formation until that capacitance site had emptied. The capacitance would have to empty through the proximal and distal resistances, and the time constant for that emptying was thought to be about 3 seconds. The effect would be to force blood both retrograde into the arterial side, causing a reduction in inflow throughout systole even though the resistance to flow had not actually changed. Blood would also be forced antegrade toward the venous side, causing an increased coronary sinus flow during systole. Furthermore, if the time constant is as large as they reported (3 seconds) then only a small percentage of that blood would empty with a single beat, and the pressures within the vessels would never fall to a value low enough to allow waterfall formation. Most importantly, although phasic flow at the coronary ostium would be reduced by contraction of the ventricle, nutritional flow at the capillary level would continue unaffected throughout the cardiac cycle.

The critical point then hinges on the magnitude of this time constant. If it is much shorter than the duration of systole, then the pressure within the vessels would be quickly dissipated and waterfalls would be allowed to form. Several studies have since addressed the coronary capacitance using more sophisticated approaches. When the coronary artery was presented with either a sine wave (10) or a step function (11,18,35,37) a time constant of less than 100 ms was determined. Such a time constant would indeed allow waterfalls to form early in the systolic period. The time constant appears much longer when coronary sinus outflow is examined, however (51) and the controversy is yet to be resolved.

It should be noted that if waterfall formation was being prevented by a long capacitive time constant then the effect of the heart beat on coronary blood flow would not be to inhibit flow, only make it appear pulsatile. If that were the case it would be hard to reconcile the fact that asystole is associated with a sustained decrease in coronary resistance (47) or that systole diverts blood flow away from the subendocardium (8,14).

6. THE INTRAMYOCARDIAL PRESSURE

Since current evidence strongly supports the hypothesis that the extravascular resistance is the result of the coronary vessels responding to intramyocardial pressure through either capacitance or waterfalls, we must ask what is the magnitude of this pressure? Many investigators have attempted to measure it over the years by inserting some pressure-sensitive element directly into the beating myocardium. Johnson and Dipalma (29) were the first to try this approach. They implanted segments of carotid artery into the ventricular wall and estimated the pressure tending to collapse them. They concluded that intramyocardial pressure during systole reached a peak of about twice ventricular pressure in the subendocardium but had very low values near the subepicardium. This basic protocol has been repeated using needles (32,36,57), open catheters (7,21), and catheter-tipped manometers (3,4,5,53). Most of these investigators arrived at a similar result: subendocardial pressure appreciably exceeded the pressure in the ventricular lumen. This point continues to be a matter of considerable controversy.

Brandi and McGregor (7) demonstrated that the pressure experienced by a foreign body in the heart wall is a function of its size. Furthermore, when they extrapolated their data to zero volume, the extrapolated subendocardial pressure was equal to ventricular pressure. They concluded that there is an inescapable artifact associated with any direct measurement of intramyocardial pressure.

Three reports support the concept that subendocardial pressure does not exceed ventricular pressure. Heineman et al. (24) attempted to measure intramyocardial pressure using a micropipette and a Servo-nulling device. The size of the pipette tip was several orders of magnitude smaller than any previous device tried. All of the pressures measured with the micropipette were equal to or less than ventricular pressure.

When Downey and Kirk (15) derived a model based on multiple parallel vessels at various depths in the heart, each exhibiting waterfall behavior. That model predicted that inflow should be a linear function of pressure when perfusion pressure is above the highest tissue pressure present in the heart wall. The model predicted that the curves would have a break point below which flow would become a nonlinear function of perfusion pressure. This would represent the range of perfusion pressures below the peak tissue pressure. Analysis of the actual curves from anesthetized dogs in figure 4 showed that the predicted break point was clearly present and that it occurred at or very near peak ventricular pressure.

A waterfall-based model can accurately predict regional blood flow to the subendocardium of a dog but only when a value for intramyocardial pressure equal to ventricular pressure is used in the calculation (42). When a value of twice ventricular pressure is employed for the tissue pressure, the correlation between predicted and actual blood flow is poor. While the controversy over the magnitude of the intramyocardial pressure is far from resolved, it is this author´s opinion that current evidence favors the concept that intramyocardial pressure approaches but does not exceed the pressure in the ventricular lumen.

The term intramyocardial pressure is a misnomer. The coronary deformation is undoubtly the result of compressive stresses rather than hydrostatic pressure in the heart wall. Pressure is a scalar quantity which denotes a force which is equal in all directions, while a stress is a vector quantity representing a force within the material in a single direction. Widely differing stresses coexist in the ventricle. A tensile stress results from the Laplace relationship in the circumferential direction (40). A tensile stress is negative, tending to pull the material apart. If a vertical cut were made in the epicardial surface, the cut would gape during each systole, illustrating that the stress in that orientation is tensile and not compressive. Although the circumferential stress may exceed ventricular pressure in magnitude, this stress - being tensile - would not be expected to collapse coronary vessels but, rather, to pull them open.

A radially oriented stress is also obligatory in the heart wall (40). This is a compressive stress and represents the accumulative inward force of each muscle layer pressing on the layer below it. This stress should increase monotonicaly from a value of zero at the epicardial surface, where no layers overlay it, to a maximal value at the subendocardium. At the subendocardium it represents the sum total from all of the layers and must equal the pressure opposing it, ventricular pressure. The radial stress, unlike the circumferential stress, is compressive. If a cut could be made in the ventricle at mid-wall and parallel to the epicardial surface, the radial stress would force this cut closed with each beat. Similarly, any blood vessels oriented normal to this stress would tend to be collapsed by it. This author suggests that the radial stress is responsible for coronary vessel compression.

Although the two stresses described are obligitory, it is not impossible to envision still other stresses in the heart which could have a greater magnitude. These stresses could result from the complex geometry of the muscle fibers. Such stresses have been formally proposed (32) but never proven.

7. CRITICAL CLOSING BEHAVIOR IN THE CORONARY SYSTEM

In the above discussion it was proposed that compression in the ventricular wall might be causing the formation of vascular waterfalls. Up to this point it has been assumed that the coronary vessels, in the absence of any compression, behave as simple linear resistors. That may not be the case, however. In 1978, Bellamy measured the pressure-flow relationship in the coronary artery during diastole, a time when extravascular compression is thought to be negligible (6). Although he found a linear relationship between the instantaneous flow and the instantaneous pressure, these plots had a projected zero flow intercept of 40-50 mmHg. One dog which had an unusually slow heart rate even showed complete cessation of coronary flow in late diastole. Furthermore, it was found that the zero-flow intercept was a function of coronary tone. When the coronary arteries were dilated, either pharamacologically or by reactive hyperemia, the intercept fell to 15-20 mmHg.

This apparent waterfall behavior is obviously not due to extravascular compression, since all evidence indicates that intramyocardial pressure is quite low during diastole. Rather, it seems to be associated with forces in the blood vessel wall itself. The fact that the pressure-flow curves are linear indicates that a waterfall type of behavior associated with vascular tone is occurring, similar to that described by Permutt and Riley (43). This will be refered to as critical closing pressure in this chapter to distinguish it from waterfall behavior associated with systole. This is a fundamentally different process than the critical closing hypothesis forwarded by Burton (9) several decades ago in which the vessel was assumed to be either patent or completely collapsed. The fact that the collapsing forces originate within the vessel walls further complicates our understanding. Because of the Laplace relationship, the pressure required to open the vessel should be much higher than that required to keep it open. This expected hysteresis makes it difficult to understand how such seemingly perfect regulation of the back pressure to flow could occur in such a system.

Physiologists, embarrassed that such a fundamental aspect of hemodynamics had gone unnoticed for so many years, immediately speculated that the observation may have been an artifact. One possible artefact was that the pressure-flow curve had been altered by vascular capacitance. Since flow was measured at a time when pressure was falling, some back flow must occur as the capacitance in the coronary arteries empties. Since this back flow was mixed with a forward flow to the microcirculation, it would have been in essence "concealed". The net effect would be an apparent shift in the pressure-flow curve towards higher pressures (18)

Several recent studies indicate that the concealed back flow from arterial capacitance does cause the zero flow pressure measurement to be artifactually high but arterial capacitance alone cannot fully account for the phenomenon. Kirkeeide et al. (33) caused the aortic pressure to oscillate by rapidly pumping blood into and out of the aorta. Under these conditions, some diastoles found the aortic pressure rising instead of falling. If the perfusion pressure were rising, then the concealed back flow would be negative and in the same direction as the microcirculatory flow and the curves would be shifted to abnormally lower pressures. The difference between curves plotted with a rising perfusion pressure and those with a falling perfusion pressure should reveal the magnitude of the artifact. Capacitance was found to be less than 10 mmHg. Attempts to measure the magnitude of the small vessel capacitance by perturbations in the arterial pressure indicate that its time constant is in the range of milliseconds (10,19,37) which argues against the capacitance artifact (see Figure 5).

Capacitance deep in the microcirculation, having a long time constant, could also serve as an apparent back pressure to arterial inflow by maintaining an elevated pressure in the region of the capillaries for several seconds after perfusion pressure was changed (51). Measurements made from the venous side do give much longer time constants (51). The problem arises in that coronary autoregulation also has a time constant of several seconds so that a constant state of tone cannot be maintained while the venous capacitance is allowed to decay. As a result the controversy is far from resolved.

Finally, collateral anastomoses have been offered as a source of error in these studies. If the pressure in only one coronary branch is manipulated, collateral anastomoses would create an apparent back pressure to flow. Direct measurements reveal that collateral connections could only raise the zero flow intercept pressure by 10 mmHg or less (39). Furthermore, the collateral artifact would not apply to those studies where the entire coronary bed was manipulated (37).

An important ramification of the non-zero intercept hypothesis of the diastolic pressure-flow relationship is that classical resistance measurements would have little utility in the coronary bed. Resistance, as traditionally calculated by perfusion pressure divided by flow, was conceived to reflect the state of smooth muscle tone in a vascular bed. Even if coronary tone does not change, the calculated resistance is clearly pressure dependent in both the beating and the arrested heart. Thus, it would not be possible to equate a change in the calculated resistance - even if that calculation were made in late diastole - with changes in vascular tone unless the measurement were made at the same perfusion pressure.

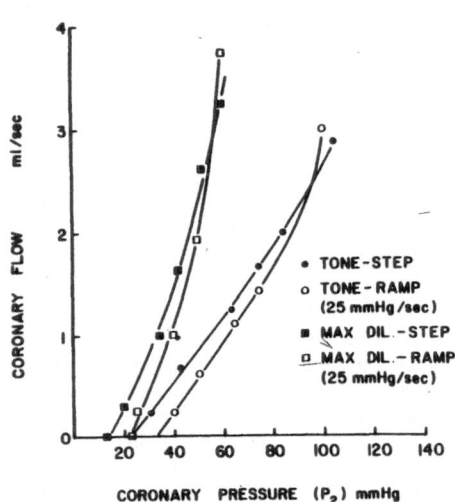

FIGURE 5. Pressure-flow curves from the heart during a long diastole with tone (squares) or maximally dilated (circles). Open symbols were collected by the falling pressure method and have a capacitance artifact. The solid symbols were collected with a step method thought to eliminate the arterial capacitance artifact. Even when that capacitance was eliminated, the zero-flow pressure was still above left atrial pressure. Reprinted from (37) with permission from the American Heart Association).

It is this author's opinion that current evidence supports the concept of an apparent waterfall associated with the coronary vessels which provides an effective back pressure of between 20-30 mmHg when tone is present and 10-20 mmHg when tone is absent. Unfortunately the exact site for this collapse is still not understood. It has been presumed (but not yet proven) that compression outside the blood vessel will be additive to the forces originating within the vessel wall. Because the extravascular forces are much greater than the intravascular closing forces, the frormer clearly predominate in the beating heart with the latter only exerting a minor effect.

8. CORONARY FLOW IN THE BEATING HEART

Coronary tone is low to absent in the presence of severe coronary stenosis. Under these conditions mechanical factors become the primary determinants of regional perfusion. Because numerous studies indicate that the severity of ischemic injury is reciprocally related to the residual flow, effective patient management requires that steps be taken to minimize the extravascular resistance in the beating heart.

By far the largest single determinant of the extravascular resistance is ventricular pressure. All reports agree that intramyocardial pressure is proportional to ventricular pressure. Furthermore, because the perfusion pressure to the coronary vessels during systole is not likely to exceed left ventricular pressure, cessation of flow is predicted for the subendocardium, regardless of whether subendocardial compression just equals or actually exceeds ventricular pressure. Stoppage of flow during systole limits subendocardial flow to the diastolic period. That is not the case for mid-wall or subepicardial regions, but because the subendocardium is clearly the most vulnerable region of the heart to ischemia, it is worthwhile to consider it separately.

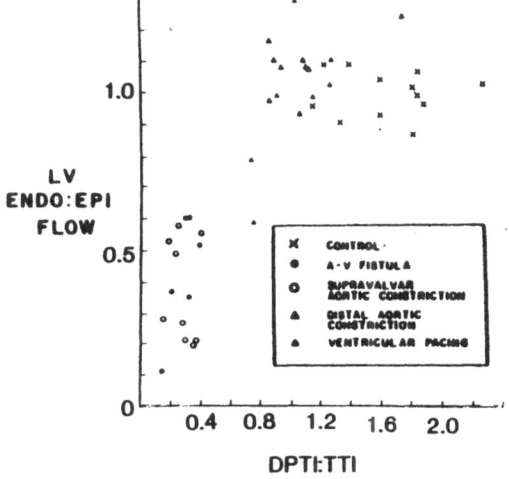

FIGURE 6. Subendocardial ischemia is indicated whenever the inner to outer blood flow ratio in the heart wall falls below 1. That condition predictably occurs whenever the DPTI:TTI ratio falls below 0.8 regardless of the cause. Reprinted from (8) with permission from the American Heart Association.

Cessation of flow to the subendocardium during systole predicts that subendocardial flow per beat is in proportion to the area between the ventricular pressure and the coronary perfusion pressure curves. Buckberg et al. (8) termed this the diastolic pressure time index (DPTI). Furthermore, the metabolic requirements per beat can be roughly determined by the area under the ventricular pressure curve, Sarnoff's tension time index (TTI) (48). The ratio of DPTI to TTI should describe the supply-demand status of the subendocardium (8). Indeed, subendocardial ischemia results whenever this ratio falls below 0.8 in dog experiments (see Figure 6). The results of this and subsequent studies suggest that the DPTI TTI ratio is an effective indicator of the adequacy of myocardial perfusion in the ischemic patient. Conditions which reduce this ratio include: tachycardia, which reduces the percent of the cardiac cycle spent in diastole; aortic stenosis, which causes ventricular systolic pressure and, thus, demand to increase but diastolic perfusion pressure to fall; or aortic regurgitation, which causes a rapid run-off of aortic diastolic pressure. Conversely, maneuvers which augment the DPTI:TTI should be beneficial; these include counterpulsation (55), which reduces afterload and augments diastolic aortic pressure. Unfortunately, this index has never gained wide application for patients with coronary artery disease since the coronary perfusion pressure, the pressure distal to a stenosis, can not be easily measured in patients. Nevertheless, a simple calculation substituting arterial pressure for the coronary perfusion pressure makes a useful guide for patient management. Maneuvers which increase the value of the ratio should improve perfusion, while those which decrease it will exacerbate the ischemia.

9. CORONARY FLOW DURING DIASTOLE

The average coronary perfusion is uniformly distributed across the wall of the heart (20). Because the subendocardium is underperfused during systole, it must be compensated by a reverse gradient of flow during diastole. Intramyocardial pressure is quite low during diastole, and the reverse gradient results from a gradient of vascular resistance. When perfusion pressure is adequate, this compensatory gradient is the result of local autoregulation adjusting resistance in each region to achieve an appropriate overall perfusion (41). This flow gradient favoring the subendocardium in diastole persists even when autoregulation is abolished (12). That finding indicates that there is also a greater vascular density in the subendocardium.

One would expect an elevated diastolic pressure as seen in the the failing heart to be transmitted through the myocardium and impede diastolic perfusion. Kjekshus (34) actualy was able to produce subendocardial ischemia by elevating diastolic pressure to 18 mmHg by volume loading. More recently, Archie (2) has attempted to quantify the diastolic intramyocardial pressure by direct examination of regional pressure-flow curves in arrested hearts. Since waterfall theory predicts that the pressure-flow curve will intercept the pressure axis at a pressure equal to the surrounding pressure, he interpreted the projected intercept from each region to reflect intramyocardial pressure. He found that the full lumenal pressure was experienced in the subendocardial region and that this fell to about half the lumenal value in the mid-wall and epicardium. It is noteworthy that appreciable impediment to flow persisted in the outer layers, rather than falling to zero, as appears to be the case with a normal systole. One explanation offered was that a large portion of the circumferential stress in the passive diastolic state is carried by the visceral pericardium rather than being dissipated in the ventricular wall. Another explanation is that they simply were observing the normal critical closing pressure in the outer layers.

It should be noted that the DPTI:TTI as presented by Buckberg et al. (8) assumes pressure in the ventricular lumen to be the compressional component to the subendocardium through out diastole (26). This concept was supported by the study of Munch and Downey (42) in which subendocardial blood flow with maximally dilated coronaries was correlated with predictions from DPTI calculations under conditions of elevated diastolic pressure, and the correlation was found to be excellent. Thus, we must conclude that elevated diastolic ventricular pressure does inhibit subendocardial perfusion, and that the degree of inhibition will be approximately of the same proportion as diastolic pressure is to coronary perfusion pressure.

10. THE EFFECT OF CONTRACTILITY ON CORONARY FLOW

The contribution of contractile state to the extravascular resistance is not yet clear. If, indeed, the radial equilibrium stress is the primary source of compression in the heart wall, then contractility would not be expected to greatly influence it. The radial stress is only determined by pressure in the ventricular lumen. On the other hand, if the predominant component of compression is due to stress resulting from interactions between contracting muscle fibers, it might be very sensitive to the contractile state.

Snyder et al. (50) approached this problem by examining the effect of changes in contractility on the magnitude of the extravascular resistance. A small coronary branch was cannulated and perfused at constant flow, the branch was maximally dilated with an infusion of adenosine, and contractility was either increased or decreased by injections of isoproterenol or pentobarbital directly into the perfusate. Because only a small portion of the ventricle received the inotropically active agent, overall ventricular dynamics and, thus, ventricular pressure was not altered. Since perfusion rate was held constant, changes in the extravascular resistance were reflected by changes in perfusion pressure. Only very small changes in perfusion pressure accompanied the contractility changes. Yet, vagal asystole revealed that almost half of the resistance in this preparation was extravascular in origin (see Figure 7).

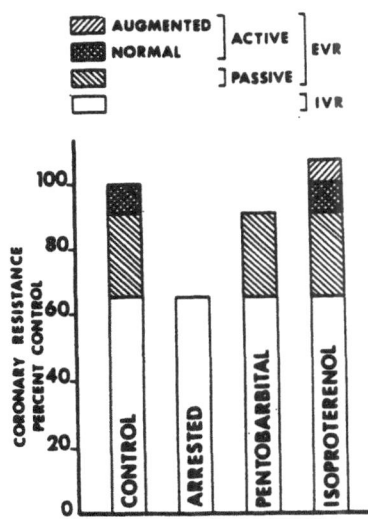

FIGURE 7. The conrtibution of contractility to the extravascular resistance. When active shortening was prevented in the segment with pentobarbital the coronary resistance decreased by only the amount indicated by the cross hatching (active – normal). Similarly, when contractility was augmented with isoproterenol, resistance increased only by the amount shown (active – augmented). Asystole caused resistance to change by the largest amount. Pressure development in the ventricle clearly has the more pronounced effect on coronary resistance. Reprinted from (50) with permission from the British Medical Association.

The Snyder et al. study was repeated by Trimble and Downey (56), this time using a constant pressure perfusion and measuring regional flow changes with microspheres. Regional flow data revealed that about a 20 percent decrease in the mid-wall flow had occurred following isoproterenol, but with little change in subendocardial flow, even when perfusion pressure was much higher than peak ventricular pressure. The interpretation again was that the massive increase in contractility had caused little change in compression at the subendocardium and that compressional increases were limited to the mid-wall. Rendering the region akinetic with pentobarbital, however caused subendocardial flow to increase, indicating that compression had been reduced in that region.

A similar study was simultaneously reported by Marzilli et al. (38). Although Trimble and Downey found very little dependence of subendocardial flow on regional contractile state, Marzilli et al. reported large changes. In that study, abolition of contractility reduced subendocardial flow by 43 percent. The only real difference in the two models is that Marzilli et al. waited five minutes for the animals to equilibrate to the inotropic intervention before injecting the microspheres for flow measurement. Trimble and Downey injected the microspheres within 60 seconds of the intervention. Other than the possible involvement of some time related stress-relaxation phenomenon, no explanation for the divergent data is apparent.

Whatever contractility's exact effect on flow turns out to be, contractility does have a profound effect on the oxygen demand of the heart and positive inotropic drugs can clearly drive the heart into ischemia by increasing demand. Judicious reduction of the inotropic state can in appropriate cases be an important means of managing ischemic heart disease.

11. THE COLLATERAL CIRCULATION

The coronary arteries are interconnected by numerous anastomoses which comprise a collateral circulation. If a major branch becomes occluded, flow does not completely stop in the region supplied by that artery, but continues at a reduced rate. This residual flow is delivered by the collateral vessels and, in the dog, averages about 20 percent of normal flow. Collateral flow in the human with normal coronary arteries is thought to be much lower than that in the dog (49), but collaterals are known to develop in patients with myocardial ischemia and can be substantial. Anrep and Hausler (1) inserted a catheter into the distal segment of a dog's occluded coronary artery. It was noted that oxygenated arterial blood flowed from this catheter when it was vented to the atmosphere. This represented arterial blood which had entered the main coronary trunk via collateral channels. Normally, it would have been forced through the microcirculation subtended by that artery, but instead it took the low-resistance pathway retrograde through the catheter. These collateral connections exist high in the coronary tree since microsphere measurements confirm that flow will not enter the microcirculation during the collection of retrograde flow (31,59).

Wyatt et al. (58) examined the linearity of coronary collateral resistance and found that it closely approximates a fixed resistance running between the major arterial branches. Collateral flow ceased, however, when pressure in the ischemic artery was 20 mmHg below aortic pressure. It was concluded that this simply represented the pressure at the origin of the collateral vessels in the donor bed but an alternative explanation may exist. Eng and Kirk (19) propose that waterfall dynamics exist in the collateral bed and that flow does not occur in them until a sufficient gradient exists to open them. In a recent study Messina (39) examined collateral flow with microspheres as a function of the pressure gradient between the circumflex and the left anterior descending coronary arteries. Collateral flow seemed to cease abruptly whenever the gradient fell below 60 mmHg. Thus, a waterfall may exist in the collateral vessels as well. The factors which contribute to this behavior have yet to be clearly identified.

Are the collateral vessels affected by mechanical compression? That must be answered with both a yes and a no. When aortic pressure is mantained, the prolonged diastole of cardiac arrest does not increase retrograde flow as is the case in the antegrade bed, but rather, usually depresses it (13). This occurs because the collaterals escape comression compression during systole so eliminating the systolic period does not decrease their resistance. Increasing left ventricular diastolic volume, however, does increases the collateral resistance probably by increasing their length (13,30). The collateral vessels in the dog probably escape compression as a result of their epicardial location (49). In the human, intramural collaterals have been described (49), and this location may cause them to be more sensitive to compression. No data are available on this latter point.

To say that the collateral vasculature is unaffected by contraction of the heart is not to say that collateral flow is unaffected by systole, however. The vessels which the collateral channels supply are very much affected by cardiac contraction. Even though the collateral-dependent segment may be akinetic due to ischemic depression, ventricular pressure will continue to be transmitted through that portion of the wall so that waterfalls would still be expected to form. It has been shown that systolic compression impedes collateral flow to the inner layers of an ischemic segment to a simmilar degree as occurs in a normally perfused region (46). For that reason, the percentage of the cardiac cycle spent in systole is an important determinant of collateral flow as well as for antegrade flow.

It should be noted that the inhibition to perfusion experienced during systole in collateral dependent tissue is not compensated by a reverse gradient of flow in diastole. The collateral flow to myocardium distal to an arterial occlusion will always be distributed so that the subendocardium will receive only about one third of that received by the subepicardium (46). This gradient of flow is thought to be primarily responsible for the subendocardium's proclivity for infarction.

REFERENCES

1. Anrep GV and Hausler H: The coronary circulation. I. The effect of changes of the blood pressure and the output of the heart", J. Physiol. 65:357-373, 1928
2. Archie JP, Jr: Transmural distribution of intrinsic and transmitted left ventricular diastolic intramyocardial pressure in dogs. Cardiovasc. Res. 12:255-262, 1978
3. Armour JA and Randall WC: Canine left ventricular intramyocardial pressures. Am. J. Physiol. 220:1833-1839, 1971
4. Baird RJ, Adeseshiah M, Okumori M: The gradiennt in regional myocardial tissue pressure in the left ventricle during diastole: its relationship to regional flow distribution. J. Surg. Res. 20:11-16, 1976
5. Baird RJ, Dudka F, Okumori M, de la Roche A, Goldbrock MM, Hill TJ and MacGregor DC: Surgical aspects of regional myocardial blood flow and myocardial pressure. J. Thorac. Cardiovasc. Surg. 69:17-29, 1975
6. Bellamy RF: Diastolic coronary artery pressure-flow relations in the dog. Circ. Res. 43:93-101, 1978
7. Brandi G and McGregor M: Intramural pressure in the left ventricle of the dog", Cardiovasc. Res. 3:472-475, 1969
8. Buckberg GD, Fixler DE, Archie JP and Hoffman JIE: Experimental subendocardial ischemia in dogs with normal coronary arteries. Circ. Res. 30:67-81, 1972
9. Burton AC: On the physical equilibrium of small blood vessels. Am. J. Physiol. 164:319-329, 1950
10. Canty JM, Klocke FJ, Mates RE: Pressure and tone dependence of coronary diastolic input impedance. Am J. Physiol 248:H700-H711, 1985
11. Dole WP, Bishop VS: Infleunce of autoregulation and capacitance on diastolic coronary artery pressure-flow relationships in the dog. Circ Res 51:261-270, 1982
12. Downey HF, Bashour FA, Boatwright RB, Parker PE and Kechejian SK: Uniformity of transmural perfusion in anesthetized dogs with maximally dilated coronary circulation. Cir. Res. 37:111-117, 1975
13. Downey JM and Chagrasulis RW: The effect of cardiac contraction on collateral resistance. Circ. Res. 34:286-292, 1976

14. Downey JM and Kirk ES: Distribution of the coronary blood flow across the canine heart wall during systole. Circ. Res. 34:251-257, 1974

15. Downey JM and Kirk ES: Inhibition of coronary blood flow by a vascular waterfall mechanism. Cir. Res. 36:753-760, 1975

16. Downey JM, Downey HF and Kirk ES: Effects of myocardial strains on coronary blood flow. Circ. Res. 34:286-292, 1974

17. Downey JM, Kirk ES, Cowan DF, Sonnenblick EH and Urschel CW: The adequacy of coronary blood flow during acute hypotension. Circ. Shock. 3:83-91, 1975

18. Eng C, Jentzen JH and Kirk ES: Coronary capacitive effects on the high estimates of coronary critical closing pressure. Circulation 62:974, 1980

19. Eng C, Kirk ES: Flow into ischemic myocardium and across coronary collateral vessels is modulated by a waterfall mechanism. Circ Res 55:10-17, 1984

20. Feigl EO: Coronary Physiology. Physiological Reviews 63:1-205, 1983

21. Gregg DE and Eckstein RW: Measurements of intramyocardial pressure. Am. J. Physiol. 132:781-790, 1941

22. Gregg DE and Green HD: Registration and intrepretation of normal phasic inflow into a left cornary artery by an improved differntial manometric method. Am. J. Physiol. 130:114-125, 1940

23. Griggs DM and Nakamura Y: Effect of coronary constriction on myocardial distribution of iodoantipyrine-I131. Am. J. Physiol. 215:1082-1088, 1968

24. Heineman F, Grayson J, and Bayliss ce: Intramyocardial pressure distribution in the left ventricular wall. Fed. Proc. 38:1038, 1979

25. Hinshaw LB, Brake CM, Iampietro PF and Emerson TE: Effect of increased venous pressure on renal hemodynamics. Am. J. Physiol. 204:119-123,1963

26. Hoffman JIE: Determinants and prediction of transmural myocardial perfusion. Circulation 58:381-391, 1978

27. Holt JP: Collapse factor in the measurement of venous pressure: Flow of fluids through collapsible tubes. Am. J. Physiol. 134:292-299, 1941

28. Holt JP: Flow through collapsible tubes and through in situ veins", IEEE Trans. Biomed. En. 16:274-283, 1969

29. Johnson JR and DiPalma JR: Intramyocardial pressure and its relation to aortic pressure. Am. J. Physiol. 125:234-243, 1939

30. Kattus AA and Gregg DE: Some determinants of coronary collateral flow in the open-chest dog. Cir. Res. 7:628-642, 1959

31. KIrk ES: Equivalence of retrograde blood flow and collateral flow following acute coronary occlusion in the dog. Circulation 52 (Supp III):66, 1980

32. Kirk ES and Honig CR: Experimental and theoretical analysis of myocardial tissue pressure. Am. J. Physiol. 207:261-267, 1964

33. Kirkeeide R, Puschmann S and Schaper W: Diastolic coronary pressure flow relationships investigated by induced long-wave pressure oscillations. Basic Res. Cardiol. 76:564-569, 1981

34. Kjekshus JK: Mechanism for flow distribution in normal and ischemic myocardium during increased ventricular preload in the dog. Cir. Res. 33:489-499, 1973

35. Klocke FJ, Weinstein IR, Ellis AK, Kraus DR, Mates RE, Canty JM, Anbar RD, Romanowski RR, Walllmeyer KW, Echt MP: Zero flow pressure and pressure flow relationships during long diastoles in the canine coronary bed before and during maximal vasodilation: Limited infleunce of capacitive effects. J. Clin Invest 68:970-980, 1981

36. Laszt VL and Muller A: Der myokardial druick. Helv. Physiol. Pharmacol. Acta. 16:88-106, 1958

37. Lee J, Chambers DE, Akizuki S, Downey JM: The role of vascular capacitance in the coronary arteries. Circ Res 55: 751-762, 1984.

38. Marzilli M, Goldstein S, Sabbah HN, Lee T and Stein P: Modulating effect of regional myocardial performance on local myocardial perfusion in the dog. Cir. Res. 45:634-640, 1979
39. Messina LM, Hanley FL, Uhlig PN, Baer RW, Gratten MT, and JIE Hoffman: Effects of pressure gradients between branches of the left coronary artery on the pressure axis intercept and the shape of the steady state circumflex pressure-flow relations in dogs. Circ Res 56:11-19, 1985
40. Mirsky I: Left ventricular stresses in the intact human heart. Biophysics J. 9:189-208, 1969
41. Moir TW: Subendocardial distribution of coronary blood flow and the effect of antianginal drugs. Circ. Res. 30:621-627, 1972
42. Munch DF and Downey JM: Prediction of regional myocardial blood flow in dogs. Am. J. Physiol. 239:H308-H315, 1980
43. Permutt S and Riley RL: Hemodynamics of collapsible vessels with tone: Vascular waterfall. J. Appl. Physiol 18:924-932, 1963
44. Permutt S, Bromberger-Barnea B and Bane HN: Alveolar Pressure, pulmonary venous pressure and vascular waterfall. Med. Thorac. 19:239-260, 1962
45. Porter WT: The influence of the heart beat on the flow of blood through the walls of the heart. Am. J. Physiol. 1:145-163, 1898
46. Russell RE, Chagrasulis RW and Downey JM: Inhibitory effect of caardiac contraction on coronary collateral blood flow. Am. J. Physiol. 233:H541-546, 1977
47. Sabiston DC, Jr. and Gregg DE: Effect of cardiac contraction on coronary blood flow. Circulation 15:14-20, 1957
48. Sarnoff SJ, Braunwald E, Welch GH, Case RB, Stainsby WB and Marcruz R: Hemodynamic determinants of oxygen consumption of the heart with special reference to the tension-time index. Am. J. Physiol. 192:148-156, 1958
49. Schaper W: Collateral circulation of the heart (Elsevier, New York, 1971)
50. Snyder R, Downey JM and Kirk ES: The active and passive components of extravascular coronary resistance. Cardiovasc. Res. 9:161-166, 1975
51. Spaan JAE: Coronary diastolic pressure-flow relation and zero flow pressure explained on the basis of intramyocardial compliance. Circ Res 56:293-309, 1985
52. Spaan JAE, Breuls NPW and laird JD: Diastolic-systolic coronary flow differences are caused by intramyocardial pump action in the anesthetized dog. Circ. Res. 49:584-593, 1981
53. Stein PD, Marzilli M, Sabbah HN and Lee T: Systolic and diastolic pressure gradients within the left ventricular wall. Am. J. Physiol. 238:H625-630, 1980
54. Streeter DD, Jr, Spotnitz HM, Patel DP, Ross J, Jr and Sonnenblick EH: Fiber orientation in the canine left ventricle during diastole and systole. Circ. Res. 21:65-74, 1969
55. Swank M, Singh HM, Flemma FJ, Mullen DC and Lepley D: Effect of intraaortic balloon pumping on nutrient coronary flow in normal and ischemic myocardium. J. Thorac. Cardiovasc. Surg. 76:538-544, 1978
56. Trimble J and Downey JM: Contribution of myocardiall contractility to myocardial perfusion. Am. J. Physiol. 236:H121-H126, 1979
57. Van Der Meer JJ, Reneman RS, Schneider H and Weibendink J: Technique for estimation of intramyocardial pressure in acute and chronic experiments. Cardiovasc. Res. 4:132-140, 1970
58. Wyatt D, Lee J, and Downey JM: Determination of collateral flow by a load line analysis. Circ Res 50:663-670, 1982
59. Yoshida S, Akizuki S, Gowski D, and Downey JM: Discrepancy between microsphere and diffusable tracer estimates of perfusion to ischemic myocardium. Am J Physiol 249: H255-H264, 1985

CORONARY BLOOD FLOW CONTROL AND HETEROGENEOUS OXYGENATION
OF TISSUE

Peter A. WIERINGA, Henk G. Stassen, Jos A.E. Spaan.

1. INTRODUCTION

Measurements on extraction of substances from coronary blood are often performed to obtain information about the condition of the myocytes. Mostly, these measurements are interpreted by means of models that must predict the microscopical conditions from the macroscopical measurements. For very good reasons modelers tend to keep the models simple. In particular the vascular anatomy of the heart is simplified to either well mixed compartments in which the biochemical reactions take place (5, 8, 15), or to a parallel aligned number of vessels (9, 10, 11).

After a quick look at the coronary capillary network anatomy one may put questions upon the usefulness of these models when they are used to study tissue oxygenation or metabolite distribution. It is known that the three-dimensional capillary network contains many bifurcations and short capillary anastomoses (1, 13). The blood flow distribution through these numerous channels is not trivial and so is the spatial oxygen distribution in the tissue space between the capillaries. It is plausible that capillary flow is not the same in all capillaries (2). A spatial heterogeneity in flow limits the usefulness of compartment models since the compartments are not well mixed. Meanwhile, the interconnections at the capillary level limit the application of a parallel capillary model as well.

This chapter aims to convey the following three points :
1) the interconnectedness of the coronary capillary network causes microcirculatory flow and cellular pO2 to be heterogeneous,
2) this spatial heterogeneity is concealed from observations on coronary arterial and venous blood flow and other blood properties,
3) that because of the heterogeneity an important fraction of tissue has a pO2 at a level capable of controlling arteriolar smooth muscle tone.
This analysis will be based on the incorporation of a control model of the coronary circulation describing globally measured coronary control and the classical Krogh cylinder model into a new model based on the capillary topology.

2. MODEL FOR CONTROL OF BLOOD FLOW

The intrinsic property of the heart to regulate coronary blood flow is called local control (6). Local control is distinguished from the extrinsic neural and humoral effects on the coronary flow. The characteristics of local control are defined globally from observations of coronary blood flow in the large coronary arteries. The local control of coronary blood flow is demonstrated by the behavior of the vasculature after a quasi steady state change in 1) perfusion pressure (autoregulation), and 2) oxygen uptake (metabolic regulation). The measurements on the global system may consist of arterial and venous pressure, coronary blood flow, and arterial-venous oxygen pressure difference. The autoregulation curves, that can be constructed from these global measurements of the coronary perfusion, demonstrate a change in the mean of the coronary blood flow after quasi steady state changes in perfusion pressure, at constant oxygen consumption rate. Vergroesen (15) used the model of Laird and Spaan (8) to interpret such measurements. Laird and Spaan came to the conclusion that a three-compartment model consisting of a linear relationship between tissue oxygen pressure and coronary resistance may be used to predict the parallel shift in autoregulation curves and metabolic regulation curves that is commonly observed. This is discussed in a different chapter in this book.

Local blood flow may be regulated by the condition of the tissue cells that affects the smooth muscle tone in the vascular wall. This is called the metabolic hypothesis for local control of blood flow. The condition of the cells in this respect may be defined as the magnitude of concentration of certain substances, among which oxygen is one of the favored (6). The hypothesis for the control mechanism for local control by means of oxygen as a controlling agent is called the oxygen hypothesis.

The three-compartment model of Laird and Spaan assumes that the controlling pO_2 equals the venous pO_2. This restriction is not necessary to show that if tissue pO_2 is a major determinant for the control of blood flow than the parallel shift in autoregulation and metabolic regulation curves can be explained using the model. The three compartment model becomes more generally applicable when it is extended so that it can deal with a controlling pO_2 different from venous pO_2. This will be shown in section 2.1. In section 2.2 we will see how the model may still be useful despite a spatial heterogeneity in controlling pO_2.

2.1. CONTROLLING pO_2 DIFFERENT FROM VENOUS pO_2

Drake-Holland et al. (3) found a strong correlation between venous pO_2 and coronary resistance. Laird and Spaan (8) used a linear relationship between these two variables in their model (see appendix 1 Eq. 9). If we assume that a controlling pO_2, p_{con}, in the tissue exists that is linearly related to the venous pO_2, p_{ven}, we can write :

$$p_{con} = c \cdot p_{ven} + d \quad , \qquad (1)$$

where c and d are parameters. The controlling pO_2 is controlling the resistance according to :

$$R = a' \cdot p_{con} + b' \quad , \qquad (2)$$

where a' and b' are parameters. If Eq. 1 is substituted into Eq. 2 we can write :

$$R = a' \cdot c \cdot p_{ven} + (a' \cdot d + b') = a \cdot p_{ven} + b \quad . \qquad (3)$$

Hence, the global measurements may indicate that the venous pO_2 is an important intermediate for local flow control, but Eq. 3 shows that in fact any tissue pO_2 that is linearly correlated to the venous pO_2 may as well predict the same results. One can not distinguish between these two variables from global measurements only. Assuming that a controlling pO_2 in the tissue exist that may be different from the venous pO_2 makes the model more generally applicable.

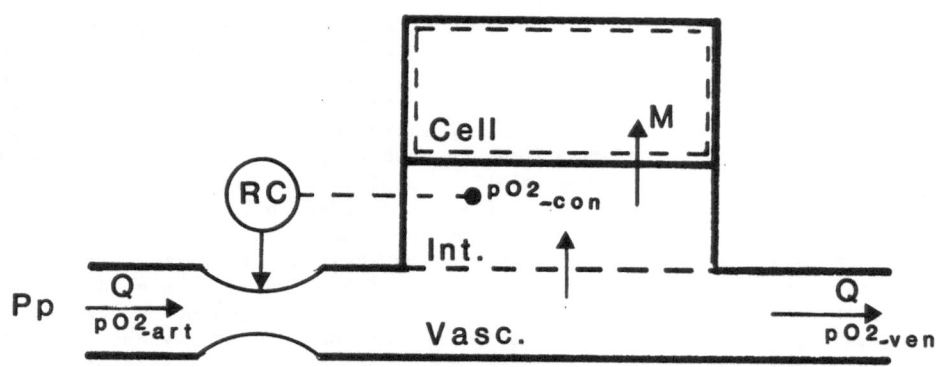

FIGURE 1 : *Three compartment model as proposed by Laird and Spaan (8). The compartments are a vascular compartment (Vasc.), an interstitial compartment (Int.), and a cell compartment. For the steady state the oxygen flows over the boundary of the compartments are equal. See appendix 1 for the symbols and the mathematical formulation of the model.*

2.2. HETEROGENEOUS pO_2 ALONG AN ARTERIOLE

Arterioles are several hundred micrometers long. The total resistance of the arteriole is not established at one location but is distributed along the arteriole. One may assume that the arteriole consists of many small controlling units in series. The total resistance is established by addition of the resistances of all the units :

$$R = R_1 + R_2 + \ldots + R_i + \ldots + R_n \quad , \tag{4}$$

where n is the number of units that make one arteriole. Each controlling unit receives information from a restricted tissue volume around the arteriole. We may say that a controlling units "sees" one controlling pO_2 that is representative for the small tissue volume around the unit :

$$R_i = a'' \cdot p_{con\ i} + b''/n \quad . \tag{5}$$

Putting all the units together results in :

$$R = a'' \cdot [\sum_{i=1}^{n} p_{con\ i}] + b'' \quad . \tag{6}$$

If each $p_{con\ i}$ is linearly related to the venous pO_2 Eq. 6 will result in :

$$R = a'' \cdot [\sum_{i=1}^{n} c_i \cdot p_{ven} + d_i] + b'' \tag{7}$$

$$= [a" \cdot \sum_{i=1}^{n} c_i] \cdot p_{ven} + [a" \cdot \sum_{i=1}^{n} d_i] + b" = a \cdot p_{ven} + b .$$

Hence, for this case one can not distinguish from global measurements whether one or more controlling pO_2s exist that are proportional to the venous pO_2.

3. CAPILLARY NETWORK

Capillary networks in skeletal and heart muscle tissue are characterized by a capillary orientation that is predominantly in parallel (1, 13). This main capillary orientation is willingly used by physiologists in models to study the oxygen supply to the tissue (9, 10, 11, 16, 17). The stacking of parallel capillaries has been applied to introduce symmetry in these models. Many models have been defined on the basis of the solution to the two-dimensional diffusion equation with the specific boundary conditions that were firstly proposed for use in the field of physiology by Krogh and Erlang (9, 10).

The so-called Krogh tissue cylinder model is summarized in appendix 2. It is an useful model to study oxygen supply to the tissue of various organs. The model describes the oxygen diffusion in the microcirculation. A capillary is surrounded by a tissue layer. Oxygen is consumed in the tissue at a constant rate. The transport of oxygen occurs by axial convection by the blood in the capillary and by radial diffusion in the tissue space perpendicular to the axes of the capillary. The parameters are the capillary and tissue cylinder radius, capillary length, diffusion and solubility coefficient.

The classical model assumes that the saturation of the blood at the entrance of the capillary is 100 %, and that the capillary length equals the mean distance between an arteriole and venule in the microcirculation. Both assumptions neglect the importance of a capillary network. In a network the blood is distributed among or collected from the branches of capillary bifurcations. Hence, the oxygen saturation of the blood at the entrance of a capillary is only 100 % when the capillary branches off from an arteriole. Furthermore, the network consists of capillary segments that have different lengths.

In the next two sections we will discuss the properties of a network consisting of Krogh tissue cylinders. The Krogh model will be extended so that oxygen exchange between adjacent tissue cylinders can be studied. This will be discussed in section 3.2. Total network blood flow and oxygen consumption will be important variables in these approaches.

3.1. NETWORK OF KROGH TISSUE CYLINDERS

A three dimensional capillary network was defined (16, 17) in which a main capillary orientation could be distinguished. These so-called *main-capillaries* where hexagonally stacked and interconnected by short, so-called *cross-capillaries*, to their nearest neighbors. The locations at which the cross-capillaries where defined was chosen at random, but such that the lengths of the unbranched segments of the main-capillaries satisfied the findings of Bassingthwaighte et al. (1). The length of a cross-capillary was 19 μm. A typical blood flow pattern through such a network can be seen in Fig. 2.

80

Around each capillary segment in the network a tissue cylinder was
defined according to the Krogh model. The minimum length of the capillary
segments was 31 μm. All cylinders were a multiple of these so-called *tissue
units*. The tissue pO_2 was defined as the average pO_2 in a unit.

A histogram of the tissue pO_2s is plotted in Fig. 3. Due to the different
capillary paths, that can be followed by the blood to perfuse the network,
the tissue units have different pO_2s. The degree of heterogeneity is large
and is predominantly determined by the heterogeneity in capillary flow.
Note that the mean tissue pO_2 is lower than the venous effluent pO_2 of the
network.

The model has a serious shortcoming in that it predicts negative pO_2s.
This is due to the assumed oxygen consumption rate in the tissue, that is
constant despite low and even "negative" pO_2s. In the next section this
shortcoming is overcome.

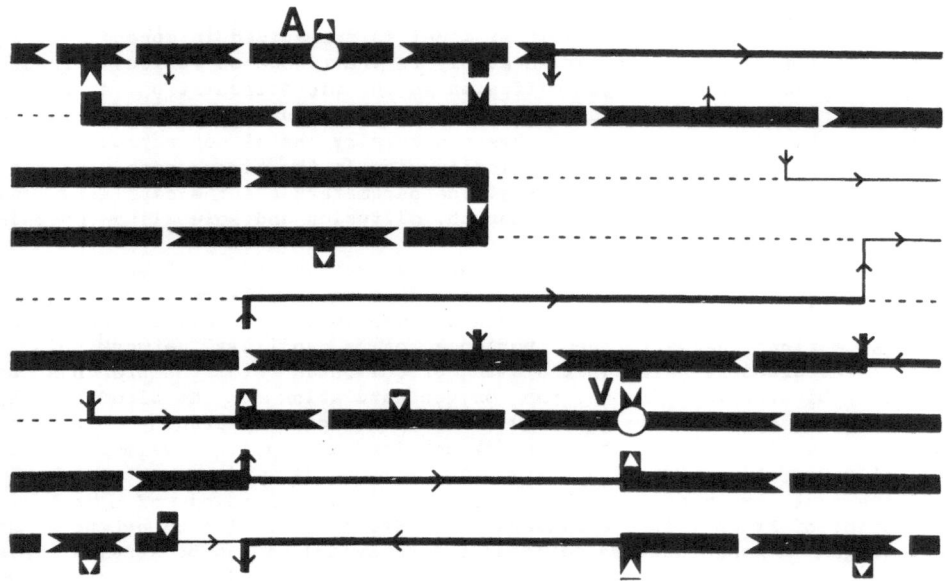

*FIGURE 2 : A typical flow pattern in longitudinal section of a
capillary network is shown an the basis of a theoretical model
(16, 17). The flow directions are marked with arrow heads. The
flow velocity magnitudes are divided in four classes. Above 142
μm/s: heavy lines; between 47.5 and 142 μm/s: dark lines; between
23.7 and 47.5 μm/s: thin lines; and under 23.7 μm/s: broken
lines. The figure shows only one layer of the network. The short
vertical branches, that seem to terminate suddenly, are in fact
connected to layers above or beneath the plane of observation.*

3.2 DIFFUSIONAL SHUNTING BETWEEN ADJACENT CAPILLARIES

The heterogeneity in tissue pO_2 will also exist between neighbor units.
Hence, an oxygen pressure difference will exist at the borders of a tissue
unit. Due to this pressure difference the oxygen flux at the borders of the

tissue cylinder will not be zero, as is assumed in the Krogh model.

We introduced the possibility for radial oxygen exchange between neighbor tissue units in the network model (17). This can be done on the basis of the solution to the two dimensional diffusion equation that consists of a homogeneous part and a non-homogeneous part. The non-homogeneous part of the solution describes the tissue oxygen pressure due to the consumption in the tissue. The homogeneous part describes the oxygen pressure in the

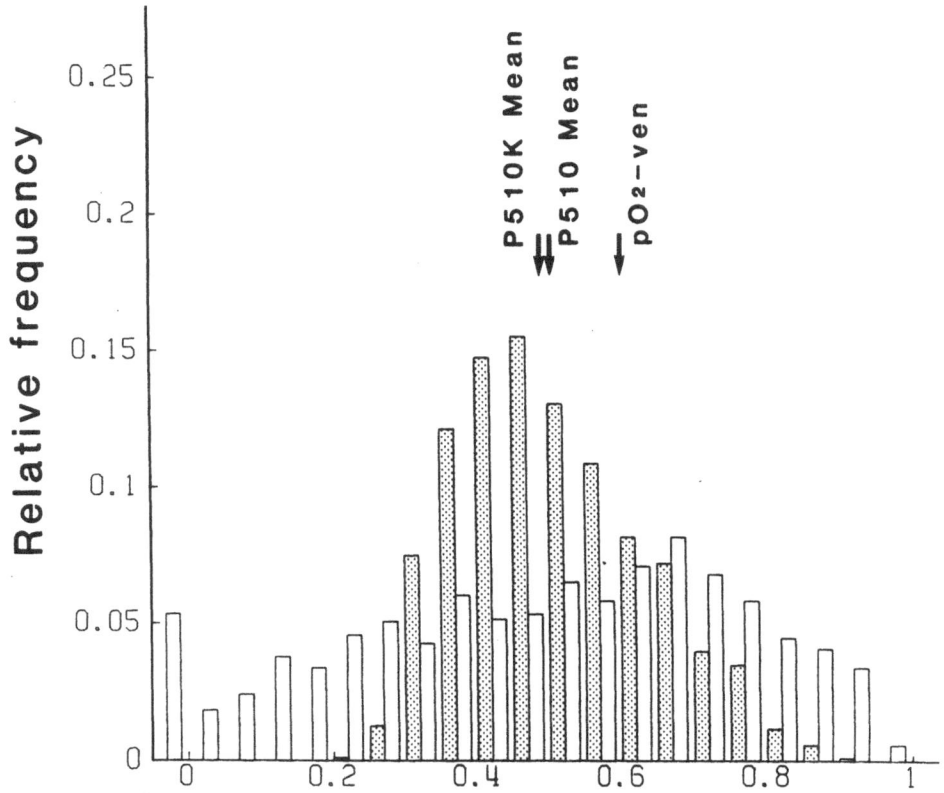

Normalized tissue unit pO2

FIGURE 3 : The histograms for the tissue pO_2s in a network are shown. The open bar histogram shows the results of a network that consists of Krogh tissue cylinders. Diffusional shunting of oxygen between adjacent tissue cylinders was not possible according to the definition of the Krogh model. The histograms with shaded bars was computed from a network in which diffusional shunting was included. This histogram shows a less heterogeneous spatial oxygen distribution. Both histograms show tissue pO_2s that are lower than venous pO_2. The pO_2s were normalized to the arterial pO_2 of 50 mmHg.

tissue space due to an oxygen flux that is the results of an oxygen pressure difference between adjacent capillaries. Both parts are superimposable.

A second histogram has been added to Fig. 3. This histogram represents the tissue unit pO_2s in the network after the possibility for diffusional shunting between adjacent capillaries was implemented in the network model. One can see that the heterogeneity of tissue pO_2s is reduced compared to the network without diffusional shunting. The negative pO_2s no longer appear in the network. However, the mean tissue pO_2 is still lower than the venous pO_2.

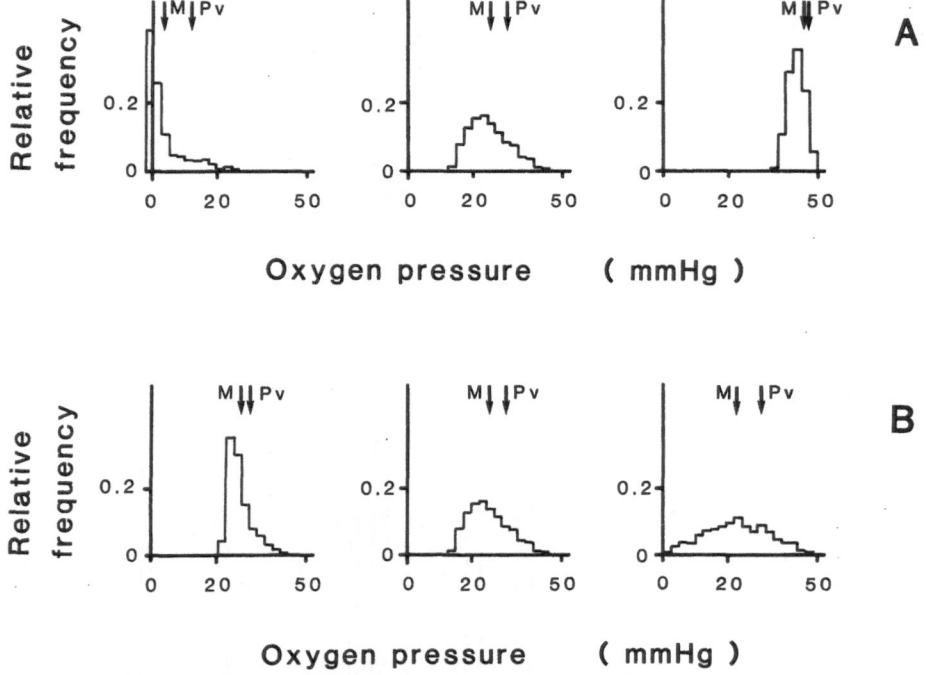

Oxygen pressure   (mmHg)

FIGURE 4 : Oxygen pressure histograms at different values of the oxygen consumption rate and blood supply to the network are drawn. The upper three histograms (A) are computed after a four fold increase (upper right) or decrease in blood supply (upper left). The histograms in the middle of both rows are the same and represent the control condition. The lower three histograms show the effect when the oxygen consumption rate and blood flow are increased (lower right) or decreased (lower left) simultaneously by a factor of four.

4. DISCUSSION

The analysis of the three compartment model that was presented in section 2, shows that one can not distinguish from global measurements whether the coronary resistance is 1) controlled by a controlling pO_2 that is different from the venous pO_2, or 2) is in fact controlled by more than one controlling pO_2 in the tissue. The properties of the model are still valid if more realistic relationships between arteriolar diameter and pO_2 (7) are included (17). The capillary network analysis has shown us that 1) tissue

pO₂s, that are lower than the venous pO₂, may exist under seemingly normal
physiological condition, and 2) that diffusional shunting between neighbor
capillaries may play an important role in the distribution of oxygen in the
tissue. These conclusions are important if one wants to deduce information
about the condition of the myocytes from measurements of coronary flow,
perfusion pressure, and arterial-venous oxygen difference.

The network model has also been used to predict spatial oxygen distribution at different values of the oxygen consumption rate and total blood
flow. These results are plotted in Fig. 4. The upper three histograms are
the result of a change in coronary blood flow at constant oxygen consumption rate in the network. The change in spatial pO₂ distribution after a
four fold increase (upper right histogram) or decrease (upper left histogram) in blood supply to the network is plotted. The histogram in the
middle is the same as the histogram with shaded bars in Fig. 3 and represents the control condition. As expected all tissue pO₂s follow the change
in blood flow. The dispersion, that may be used as a degree of heterogeneity for the spatial oxygen distribution, changed proportionally to the
flow.

The lower three histograms in Fig. 4 were computed after a simultaneous
change in oxygen consumption rate and blood flow. Hence, from the mass-
balance of the network it may be understood that the venous pO₂ stays constant. The dispersion however, changed proportional to the change in blood
flow. One may use these histograms as an example of the change in spatial
oxygen distribution during metabolic regulation.

The venous pO₂ remains constant during these interventions. One is not
able to measure the change in dispersion from global measurements. So very
low tissue pO₂s may exist despite a seemingly normal overall condition of
the heart. Steenbergen et al. (12) showed that ischemic areas in the heart
may exist under certain conditions that are physiologically normal. The
network model simulations show that the total size of the ischemic areas
should increase when the workload of the heart is increased. The area that
suffers from minor ischemia is increased and is at risk to become an area
with severe ischemia, despite a normal local control of coronary blood
flow.

APPENDIX 1 : MODEL FOR THE LOCAL CONTROL OF BLOOD FLOW

Models, designed on the basis of oxygen as a controlling intermediator,
are capable of describing the qualitative features of auto and metabolic
regulation in the heart and in other tissue. The model that will be used is
given in Fig. 1. It is based on the steady state mass-balance for oxygen
over the boundaries of three compartments. The three compartments are 1) a
vascular or blood compartment, 2) an interstitial compartment, and 3) a
cell compartment. The oxygen is transported into the vascular compartment
by the blood via a resistance, R, that equals :

$$R = Pp/Q \ ,$$
(8)

where Pp is the hydraustatic pressure drop over the vascular compartment,
and Q is the coronary blood flow. The pressure drop will be called the
perfusion pressure.

In the model the resistance, R, is assumed to be controlled by the
interstitial pO₂. In general we may assume that a controlling pO₂, $pO_{2_{con}}$,
exists that effects a change in resistance. This relationship is called the
control law for the coronary resistance. The following linear function is
proposed as the control law :

$$R = a' \cdot pO_{2_{con}} + b' \quad . \tag{9}$$

The parameters a' and b' may be found experimentally by perturbations around the working point of the system. Eq. 9 does not satisfy the definition of a linear system. Hence the control system is a nonlinear system.

In general we may propose that the interstitial space of the model is in equilibrium with the plasma of the blood that has a pO_2 that is related to the venous pO_2. For the sake of simplicity we assume a linear relationship between the controlling pO_2 and the venous pO_2 :

$$pO_{2_{con}} = c \cdot pO_{2_{ven}} + d \quad . \tag{10}$$

Substitution of Eq. 10 in Eq. 9 results in a linear relation between the resistance and the venous pO_2 :

$$R = a \cdot pO_{2_{ven}} + b \quad , \tag{11}$$

with $a = a' \cdot c$ and $b = a' \cdot d + b$.

The venous pO_2 is determined by the overall mass-balance for oxygen of the system. In the steady state, the oxygen uptake by the cell, M (consumption rate) is balanced by the oxygen flow over the wall of the compartments. Hence, M equals the arterial-venous oxygen content difference, $S_{art} - S_{ven}$, of the blood multiplied by the coronary blood flow :

$$M = (S_{art} - S_{ven}) \cdot Q \quad . \tag{12}$$

Blood saturated with oxygen enters the large arteries of the heart. When it arrives at the terminal arterioles the saturation may be dropped by about 15% (4). For values of the saturation between 10 and 85 % the saturation curve of blood for oxygen may be linearized by the following equation :

$$S = \alpha \cdot pO_2 + \beta \quad . \tag{13}$$

Eqs 8, 11, 12, and 13 result in :

$$Q = Pp/R_{max} + a \cdot M/R_{max} \quad , \tag{14}$$

where : $R_{max} = a \cdot pO_{2_{art}} + b$.
Eq. 14 Represents a plane in the three-dimensional space defined by Q, Pp, and M. Autoregulation curves are the lines of intersection between this plane and a plane defined by different values for M, independently of Pp and Q. Hence, the autoregulation curves will shift parallel at different consumption rates. By analogy, the metabolic regulation curves are obtained from the line of intersection with a plane defined by M, and Q at different Pp. The shift of auto- and metabolic regulation curves which is in parallel is consistent with experimental observations.

APPENDIX 2 : PRINCIPLES OF THE KROGH TISSUE CYLINDER MODEL

Global mass-balance

We consider a capillary network to which oxygenated blood is transported. The magnitude of the blood flow, F, is proportional to the tissue volume, so that :

$$F = \pi \cdot R_t^2 \cdot L \cdot Q \quad , \tag{15}$$

where R_t is the radius of an imaginary tissue cylinder around the capillaries, L is the sum of lengths of all capillaries in the network, and Q is the flow per unit volume, the so-called bulk flow.

The tissue around the capillaries extracts oxygen at a constant consumption rate. The amount of oxygen that is extracted from the blood, C, equals:

$$C = \pi \cdot (R_t^2 - R_c^2) \cdot L \cdot M \quad , \tag{16}$$

where M is the oxygen consumption per unit tissue volume, and R_c is the capillary radius.

From the oxygen dissociation curve the relation between oxygen content of the blood and the capillary pO_2, p_c, can be found. For the sake of simplicity we will consider a working range for capillary pO_2s for which the oxygen saturation of the blood is near linear. This is the case for partial oxygen pressures between 5 and 50 mmHg. The oxygen supply by the blood, J, equals :

$$J = F \cdot \{\alpha \cdot p_c + \beta\} \quad , \tag{17}$$

where α equals the slope of the linearized oxygen saturation curve, β equals the intercept, and F equals the capillary blood flow.

THE KROGH TISSUE CYLINDER MODEL

The Krogh tissue cylinder model consists of a capillary that lies in the center of a tissue cylinder. Axial diffusion in both capillary and tissue space are neglected. The Krogh-Erlang equation describes the tissue pO_2, p_t, in a thin layer of the tissue as a function of the capillary pO_2, p_c, the oxygen consumption in the tissue, M, the tissue cylinder radius, R_t, and the capillary radius, R_c. The capillary pO_2 is the rotation symmetric driving force for the oxygen diffusion into the tissue and is a function of the axial position along the capillary, z. The oxygen consumption in the tissue space is constant. The tissue pO_2 in a tissue layer with thickness δz, equals the solution to the two-dimensional diffusion equation :

$$p_t(r,z) = p_c(z) - \{\tfrac{1}{2} \cdot M/(D_t \cdot \alpha_t)\} \cdot \{R_t^2 \cdot \ln(r/R_c) - \tfrac{1}{2}(r^2 - R_c^2)\} \quad , \tag{18}$$

$$\text{for } R_c \leq r \leq R_t ,$$

where D_t is the tissue diffusion coefficient, α_t is the solubility for oxygen in muscle tissues.

The oxygen consumption in the tissue space is constant for pO_2s higher than about 3 mmHg. Hence, the oxygen flow across the capillary wall equals the product of the variable M times the volume of the observed tissue. This product is the oxygen delivery of the blood, $\delta J(z)$, as a function of the axial position in the capillary :

$$\delta J(z) = -M \cdot \pi \cdot (R_t^2 - R_c^2) \cdot \delta z \quad . \tag{19}$$

Eq. 19 can be solved if the oxygen content of the blood that supplies the capillary, J(0), is known. Hence :

$$J(z) = J(0) - M \cdot \pi \cdot (R_t^2 - R_c^2) \cdot z \quad . \tag{20}$$

Substitution of Eq. 20 into Eq. 17 results in the capillary pO_2 as a linear function of z :

$$p_c(z) = \{J(0)/F - \beta \quad -M \cdot \pi \cdot (R_t^2 - R_c^2) \cdot z\}/(F \cdot \alpha)$$

$$= p_c(0) \quad -M \cdot \pi \cdot (R_t^2 - R_c^2) \cdot z/(F \cdot \alpha) \quad . \tag{21}$$

Note that Eq. 21 is independent on the intercept, β, of the saturation curve.

Substitution of Eq. 21 into Eq. 18 gives the tissue pO_2 as a function of the distances into the tissue and the the position along the capillary :

$$p_t(r,z) = p_c(0) - M \cdot \pi \cdot (R_t^2 - R_c^2) \cdot z/(F \cdot \alpha) +$$

$$-\{\tfrac{1}{2} \cdot M/(D_t \cdot \alpha_t)\} \cdot \{R_t^2 \cdot \ln(r/R_c) - \tfrac{1}{2} \cdot (r^2 - R_c^2)\} \quad . \tag{22}$$

Note that Eq. 22 is a linear function of the pO_2 of the supplying blood and the oxygen consumption rate. We will substitute F by the formula given by Eq. 15 for the bulk flow.

The mean capillary pO_2, $\bar{p}_c$ along the capillary equals :

$$\bar{p}_c = \int_0^L p_c(z) \cdot \delta z \,/L = p_c(0) - K' \cdot M/Q \quad , \tag{23}$$

with : $K' = \tfrac{1}{2}(1 - R_c^2/R_t^2)/\alpha_c$.

The mean tissue pO_2, $\bar{p}_t$, can be found by integrating Eq. 22 over the tissue space :

$$\bar{p}_t = \{\int_0^L \int_{R_c}^{R_t} p_t(r,z) \cdot 2 \cdot \pi \cdot r \cdot \delta r \cdot \delta z \}/\{L \cdot \pi \cdot (R_t^2 - R_c^2)\}$$

$$= p_c(0) - K' \cdot M/Q - K'' \cdot M \quad , \tag{24}$$

with : $K'' = \tfrac{1}{2} \cdot R_t^2/(D_t \cdot \alpha_t)\} \cdot \{(R_t^2/(R_t^2 - R_c^2)) \cdot \ln(R_t/R_c) + \tfrac{1}{4} \cdot R_c^2/R_t^2 - \tfrac{3}{4}\}$.

The pO_2 of the collected effluent blood flow can be calculated by substituting z=L in Eq. 21 and equals :

$$p_c(L) = p_c(0) - (1/\alpha) \cdot (M/Q) \quad . \tag{25}$$

Note that $p_c(L)$, which may represent the venous pO_2, does not depend on geometrical parameters of the network that are encountered in the parameters K' and K".

ACKNOWLEDGEMENT
   I like to acknowledge J.D. Laird, D.Phil, and Dr. I. Vergroesen for their
stimulating discussions that were of great importance to this study.

REFERENCES

1. Bassingthwaighte, JB, Yipintsoi, T, Harvey, RB: Microvasculature of the
   dog left ventricular myocardium. Microvasc. Res. 229-249, 1974.
2. Damon, D: Heterogeneity of distribution of blood and erythrocytes in
   the microcirculation of the hamster. Thesis University of Virginia,
   Charlottesville, VA, USA, 1985.
3. Drake-Holland, AJ, Laird, DJ, Noble, MIM, Spaan, JAE, Vergroesen, I:
   Oxygen and coronary vascular resistance during autoregulation and
   metabolic vasodilation in the dog. J. Phyiol. 348: 285-299, 1984.
4. Duling, BR, Berne, RM: longitudinal gradients in peri arteriolar oxygen
   tension. A possible mechanism for the participation of oxygen in local
   regulation of blood flow. Circ. Res. 27: 669-678, 1970
5. Duvelleroy, MA, Mehel, H, Laver, MB: Hemoglobin-oxygen equilibrium and
   coronary blood flow: an analog model. J. Appl. Physiol. 35(4): 480-484,
   1973
6. Feigl, EO: Coronary physiology, Physiol. Rev. 3: 1-205, 1983.
7. Gorczynski, RJ, Duling, BR: Role of oxygen in arteriolar functional
   vasodilation in hamster striated muscle. Am. J. Physiol. 4(5): H505-
   H515, 1978.
8. Laird, JD, Spaan, JAE: A simple computer model of coronary flow regulation based on interstitial oxygen tension. J. Physiol. 324: 1P, 1981.
9. Krogh, A: The number and the distribution of capillaries in muscles
   with the calculation of the oxygen pressure head necessary for
   supplying the tissue, J. Physiol. 52: 409-415, 1919.
10. Krogh, A: The supply of oxygen to the tissue and the regulation of the
    capillary circulation. J. Physiol. 52: 457-747, 1919.
11. Popel, AS: Analysis of capillary-tissue diffusion in multicapillary
    systems. Math. Bioscienc. 39: 187-211, 1978.
12. Steenbergen, C, Williamson, JR: Heterogeneous coronary perfusion during
    myocardial hypoxia. Adv. Myocard. Vol. 2: 271-284, 1980.
13. Tomanek, RJ, Searls, JC, Lachenbruch, PA: Quantitative changes in the
    capillary bed during developing peak, and stabilized cardiac hyper-
    trophy in the spontaneously hypertensive rat. Circ. Res. 51: 295-304,
    1982.
14. Vergroesen, I: Local regulation of coronary blood flow, Thesis Univer-
    sity of Amsterdam, 1987.
15. Wieringa, PA, Spaan, JAE, Stassen, HG, Laird, JD: Heterogeneous flow
    distribution in a three dimensional capillary network simulation of the
    myocardial microcirculation - A hypothesis. Microcirc. 2(2): 195-216,
    1980.
16. Wieringa, PA: The influence of the coronary capillary network on the
    regulation and control of local blood flow, Thesis Delft University of
    Technology, ISBN 90-9001042-4, 1985.

MYOCARDIAL MICROCIRCULATION IN THE BEATING HEART
- IN VIVO MICROSCOPIC STUDIES

H. Tillmanns, H. Leinberger, F.J. Neumann, M. Steinhausen, N. Parekh,
R. Zimmermann, R. Dussel, W. Kuebler. Med. Univ.-Klinik.

In contrast to other microcirculatory areas, the coronary
microvasculature is continuously exposed to myocardial contraction.
Until recently, methodical difficulties in obtaining quantitative
observations of coronary microvascular blood flow have prevented the
formulation of a clear picture of the hemodynamics in the terminal
vascular bed of the ventricular myocardium. Simultaneous measurements
of pressures, diameters, and blood flow velocities in different parts
of the coronary vascular bed are necessary to identify the variables
which control hymodynamics of the coronary microcirculation, namely
extravascular support and active vaso-motor changes.

METHODS
The in vivo microscopic studies were performed by means of
epiillumination (23) or transillumination (24) of the left
ventricular myocardium. Motion pictures were recorded by a highly
sensitive television camera type system, or by means of high speed
cinematography. Additionally, fluorescence microscopic methods,
intravenous injection of fluorescent dextrans and latex particles
were applied to improve contrast of the microvascular system and to
measure blood flow velocity. Following intravenous bolus injection of
FITC tagged high-molecular dextran, larger cardiac vessels could be
readily distinguished at lower magnifications. Venules could easily
be differentiated from arterioles because of the direction of flow at
areas of bifurcation. At higher magnifications, the proximity and
diameters of capillaries, and the direction of blood flow could be
visualized.
Intraluminal pressures in the microvascular bed were obtained by
micropuncture of arterioles and venules of the beating left
ventricular myocardium. Pressures were continuously recorded by a
resistance servo nulling system according to Wiederhielm (31).

TOPOGRAPHICAL PATTERN OF THE VENTRICULAR MICROCIRCULATION
The capillary arrangement in the left and right ventricle of the
mammalian heart appears to be primarily parallel, with the vessels
lying on either side of the cardiac muscle fibers (2, 16, 23, 24). On
the other hand, several interconnections between capillaries can be
noticed; these intercapillary anastomoses, more often observed near
the confluence to venules, form loops of different lengths (24).
Capillary diameter in the epimyocardium of the beating rat and cat
heart averaged 5.7 μm (25). Similarly, it was shown that during
systole capillary diameter in the superficial layers of the rat and

dog heart declines by about 25% (24). The distances between perfused capillaries in the rat and dog ventricle averaged 18 µm, and the calculated capillary density in the cat, dog and rat heart is in the order of 2480 to 3420/mm². These results are generally consistent with data obtained by other investigators using postmortem injection procedures (2, 7, 20) or stop-motion photomicrographs of the beating rat heart (18).

Regarding flow directions, in the majority of observations, blood flow in adjacent capillaries occurred in the same direction. However, counter-current flow was frequently noted in neighbouring capillaries, particularly in those joined together by large connecting loops (23, 24). Assessment of the extent of co-current and counter-current flow in adjacent capillaries in the rat heart has yielded a ratio of 1.4:1; similar ratios have been reported for the dog and turtle heart (24). These data support the hypothesis that mixed counter-current flow systems provide optimal myocardial oxygen supply (17).

CAPILLARY RECRUITMENT
    The existence of a functional myocardial capillary reserve being recruited during increased cardiac work load, is still disputed. Data showing a considerable recruitment of myocardial capillaries, were predominantly obtained by indicator dilution techniques revealing permeability surface area products of low molecular substances (3, 4, 22). In 1969, Honig et al. reported a marked decrease in intercapillary distances of the rat heart during hypoxia, using stop-motion photomicrographs (18). However, our own in vivo microscopic studies, dealing with the effect of hypoxia on the myocardial microcirculation, did not reveal any significant changes of the distances of plasma-perfused capillaries visualized by fluorescent high-molecular dextran, neither during hypoxia (23) nor during reactive hyperemia or coronary vasodilatation.
    On the other hand, during hypoxia and reactive hyperemia as well as after coronary vasodilatation (dipyridamole, nifedipine), capillary red cell content rose markedly. Thus, during hypoxia (5% O_2 in the breathing mixture) the ratio of capillaries filled with red cells to those containing solely plasma increased from 77% to 95% (28). According to these data, recruitment of myocardial capillaries during hypoxia and reactive hyperemia as well as during coronary vasodilatation occurs only with respect to their red cell content, whereas the distances between plasma-perfused capillaries remain unchanged.

THE EFFECT OF CARDIAC CONTRACTION ON THE MYOCARDIAL
MICROCIRCULATION
    There are numerous reports showing that coronary artery inflow occurs primarily during diastole and that outflow in the coronary sinus takes place mainly during systole (6, 10, 21). The three- to fourfold increase in total coronary resistance during systole is easily to be explained by the increase in compressive resistance of small intramyocardial vessels. This rise of compressive resistance is due to a decline in microvascular diameters. In all species we used in our experiments, arteriolar, capillary, and venular diameters

during systole decreased by 18-27% (24, 27, 29).

In venules (range of diameters 50-100 μm) of the epimyocardium, the pressure curve exhibited a late systolic peak, occurring later than in aorta or coronary arterioles, just before aortic valve closure. Subsequently, venular pressure declined and reached its minimum simultaneously with aortic pressure at end-diastole (27, 29).

In the dog, cat and rat heart, marked variations in red cell velocity between arterioles, capillaries and venules were noticeable (24, 27). In capillaries and venules, peak velocity occurred during systole, but in arterioles it took place during diastole, in the rapid and slow filling period. In deeper epimyocardial layers (300-600 μm below cardiac surface), arteriolar back flow persisted during whole systole, whereas in superficial arterioles back flow was observed only during isovolumic contraction. Capillary and venular red cell velocity in epimyocardial tissue exceeded that in deeper layers; in all regions, peak red cell velocity occurred during rapid and slow ejection and thereby followed the coronary sinus pattern (24, 27, 29).

In coincidence with the late systolic pressure peak, maximal blood flow velocity in coronary venules was noted during slow ejection; in capillaries, however, maximal red cell and particle velocity was observed during rapid ejection. These observations suggest the idea that systolic coronary venular pressure originates from a pressure and volume wave generated by systolic compression of myocardial capillaries (27, 29).

MICROCIRCULATORY CHANGES DURING MYOCARDIAL ISCHEMIA

The structural and functional condition of the microvascular bed in ischemic or infarcting myocardium may be a critical factor in determining the final outcome and reversibility of cellular injury. The microcirculatory consequences of severe or extended myocardial eschemia are quite well documented (1, 8, 9, 12, 13). Thus, after 40 to 60 minutes of uninterrupted ischemia, nuclear pyknosis is to be detected; the increasing endothelial cell swelling leads to the formation of numerous endothelial blebs projecting into the vessel lumen (8). The marked swelling of endothelial cells also causes various degrees of luminal obstruction (1, 8). In the dog heart after 60-90 minutes of coronary artery occlusion, endothelial gaps, stasis of red cells, and the development of platelet and fibrin thrombi are observed (12). The accumulation of platelets in the ischemic tissue is considered to further exacerbate the impairment of microvascular flow (15, 19).

In contrast to permanent ischemia, relatively little is known about the consequences of mild or transient ischemia terminated well within cardiac resuscitation time. According to Kloner and Braunwald, ischemic damage arises first in the myocyte, and this is followed by microvascular injury (12, 13). This claim is based on morphologic data and does not consider disturbances of microvascular function. A study was designed in our laboratory to investigate whether during brief myocardial ischemia of the rat and cat heart - as induced by 10-20 minutes occlusion of the left anterior descending coronary artery with subsequent reperfusion - there are functional microcirculatory disturbances occurring before the onset of detectable morphologic alteration of both the myocyte and the microvasculature.

In considering ischemia-induced changes in the hemodynamics of the microcirculation, we have been particularly interested in determining whether the reduction in coronary blood flow arising from a coronary artery stenosis (5, 11) is a consequence of a decrease in blood flow velocity in individual capillaries or a decrease in the number of capillaries being perfused. As expected, poststenotic myocardial areas exhibited dilatation of smaller coronary arterioles (A_3 and A_4 with diameters of less than 30 μm). In contrast, capillary and venular diameters did not change significantly. Despite arteriolar dilatation, the decline in perfusion pressure resulted in a marked reduction of mean blood flow velocity in the capillaries and venules of both the cat and rat heart (30). Consideration of pulsatile blood flow velocities in small vessels provided additional information, thus severe stenosis of the left anterior descending coronary artery provoked a flattening of the usually marked pulsatile blood flow velocity profile observed under normal conditions (24, 29, 30). In poststenotic capillaries and venules of the cat and rat heart, a marked diminution of systolic red cell velocity profiles was observed in poststenotic arterioles. Thus, severe stenosis of the left anterior descending coronary artery resulted in a reduction of diastolic arteriolar red cell velocity, whereas systolic arteriolar red cell velocity increased slightly. This flattening of microvascular blood flow velocity profiles is probably due to the loss of contractile force induced by myocardial ischemia.

The drop of perfusion pressure in poststenotic arterioles induced by a severe narrowing or temporary occlusion of the supplying artery could also be shown to cause an increase in the distance between plasma-perfused capillaries, as visualized by fluoresceine-tagged high-molecular dextran (30). The increase of functional intercapillary distances in ischemic myocardium results in deterioration of regional myocardial oxygen supply, since, according to the Krogh model (14), a rise of diffusion distances leads to a decline of oxygen supply to the third power.

Ten minutes after coronary artery ligation (in the rate) or severe artery narrowing (in the cat), the red cell content of plasma-perfused capillaries decreased (25, 30). Thus, while under physiological conditions, approximately 78% of plasma-perfused capillaries contain red cells, in myocardial areas supplied by a stenosed vessel the ratio of capillaries filled with red cells to those containing plasma alone was markedly diminished (26). In addition, temporary myocardial ischemia was occasionally found to provoke red cell aggregation in terminal arterioles and capillaries, thereby exaggerating the severity of regional myocardial malperfusion. Futhermore, after 15-20 minutes of ischemia, leukocytes often appeared in slow-flow capillaries of the ischemic zone (26). Due to their lower deformability compared to red cells, during ischemia leukocytes tend to plug capillary branches. Under these circumstances we noted that capillaries down-stream were still filled with fluorescent dextran, i.e. they were still experiencing plasma flow; red cells, however, were not detectable since they could not pass the leukocytes that were trapped at the capillary branch. Thus, leukocyte plugging, in addition to diminished red cell deformability, may be an important contributor to regional malperfusion in the ischemic myocardium.

In addition to the hemodynamic and rheological changes induced by ischemia, impairment of microvascular function may arise as a consequence of changes in capillary permeability. After 10 minutes of myocardial ischemia, a rise of capillary and postcapillary venular permeability was indicated by extravascular clouds of fluorescent dextran (26). This increase in microvascular permeability was quantified using iodine-125-labelled albumin. In these experiments we found that after 10 and 20 minutes of coronary artery ligation, myocardial albumin activity rose to 199% and 372%, respectively, of the value observed in control tissue. Prolongation of the ischemic period to 40 minutes did not result in any further increase of iodine-125 accumulation (25). The rise of microvascular permeability in the ischemic myocardium was not influenced by indomethacin (10 ug/kg i.v.) and the thromboxane A_2 synthetase inhibitor dazoxyben (30 ug/kg i.v.).

Myocardial platelet accumulation after prolonged ischemia is claimed to be an important pathogenic factor contributing to disturbances of microvascular flow (15, 19). After brief myocardial ischemia for 10 minutes, peripheral areas of ischemic myocardial regions showed accumulation of platelets. After varying periods of reperfusion following coronary artery ligation for 10 minutes, Chromium-51 platelet activity in the previously ischemic myocardium rose significantly with a maximum reached after 10 minutes of reperfusion. In contrast to indomethacin which proved to be ineffective, the thromboxane A_2 synthetase inhibitor dazoxyben provoked a marked reduction of chromium-51 platelet activity in the ischemic (and reperfused) myocardium.

The aforementioned data indicate that after brief periods (10-20 minutes) of myocardial ischemia major changes occur in the flow characteristics of red cells and leukocytes, and that platelet trapping and major changes of capillary permeability can also occur. Therefore, microcirculatory disturbances occurring before the onset of detectable structural changes of the microvasculature, may well be the primary cause of myocardial cell death.

REFERENCES

1.   Armiger LC, Gavin JB: Changes in the microvasculature of ischemic and infarcted myocardium. Lab. Invest. 33: 51-56, 1975.
2.   Bassingthwaighte JB, Yipintsoi T, Harvey RB: Microvasculature of the dog left ventricular myocardium. Microvasc. Res. 7: 229, 1974.

3. Duran WN: Effects of muscle contraction and of adenosine on capillary transport and microvascular flow in dog skeletal muscle. Circ. Res. 41: 642-647, 1977.

4. Duran WN, Marsicano TH, Anderson RW: Capillary reserve in isometrically contracting dog heart. Am. J. Physiol. 233: H276-H281, 1977.

5. Gould KL, Lipscomb K, Hamilton GW: Physiologic basis for assessing critical coronary stenosis. Instantaneous flow response and regional distribution during coronary hyperemia as measures of coronary flow reserve. Am. J. Physiol. 33: 87, 1974.

6. Gregg DE, Green HD: Registration and interpretation of normal phasic inflow into a left coronary artery by an improved differential manometric method. Am. J. Physiol. 130: 114-135, 1940.

7. Hort W: Quantitative Untersuchungen ueber die Kapillarisierung des Herzmuskels im Erwachsenen- und Greisenalter bei Hypertrophie und Hyperplasie. Virchows Arch. Pathol. Anat. 327: 560, 1955.

8. Jennings RB, Kloner RA, Ganote CE, Hawkins HK, Reimer KA: Changes in capillary fine structure and function in acute myocardial ischemic injury. In: Microcirculation of the Heart. Theoretical and Clinical Problems, edited by H. Tillmanns, W. Kuebler, H. Zebe, p. 87-96, Springer, Berlin, 1982.

9. Jennings RB, Sommers H, Smyth GA, Flack HA, Linn H: Myocardial necrosis induced by temporary occlusion of a coronary artery in the dog. Arch. Pathol. 70: 68-78, 1960.

10. Johnson JR, Wiggers CJ: Alleged validity of coronary sinus outflow as a criterion of coronary reactions. Am. J. Physiol. 118: 38-51, 1937.

11. Klocke FJ: Coronary blood flow in man. Prog. Cardiovasc. Dis. 19: 117-166, 1976.

12. Kloner RA, Braunwald E: Observations on experimental myocardial ischemia. Cardiovasc. Res. 14: 371-395, 1980.

13. Kloner RA, Ganote CE, Jennings RB, Reimer KA: The "no reflow" phenomenon after temporary coronary occlusion in the dog. J. Clin. Invest. 54: 1496-1508, 1974.

14. Krogh A: The number and distribution of capillaries in muscles with calculations of the oxygen pressure head necessary for supplying the tissue. J. Physiol. (Lond.) 52: 409, 1919.

15. Leinberger H, Suehiro GT, McNamara JJ: Myocardial platelet trapping after coronary ligation in primates. J. Surg. Res. 27: 3-40, 1979.

16. Ludwig G: Capillary pattern of the myocardium. Meth. Achiev. Exp. Pathol. 5: 238-271, 1971.

17. Luebbers DW: Die Bedeutung des Sauerstoffdruckes fuer die O_2-Versorgung des normalen und insuffizienten Herzens. In: Heart Failure: Pathophysiological and Clinical Aspects, edited by H. Reindell, J. Keul, E. Doll, p. 287, G. Thieme-Verlag, Stuttgart, 1968.

18. Martini J, Honig CR: Direct measurement of intercapillary distance in beating rat heart in situ under various conditions of O_2 supply. Microvasc. Res. 1: 244, 1969.

19.   Moschos CB, Lahiri K, Lyons M, Weisse AB, Oldewurtel HA, Regan TJ: Relation of microcirculatory thrombosis to thrombus in the proximal coronary artery: effect of aspirin, dipyridamole and thrombolysis. Am. Heart J. 86: 61-68, 1973.

20.   Rakusan K: Oxygen in the Heart Muscle. Charles C. Thomas, Springfield, Illinois, 1971.

21.   Rebatel F: Recherches experimentales sur la circulation dans les arteres coronaires. These (par. 288), Paris, 1872.

22.   Renkin EM, Hudlicka O, Sheehan RM: Influence of metabolic vasodilation on blood-tissue diffusion in skeletal muscle. Am. J. Physiol. 211: 87-98, 1966.

23.   Steinhausen M, Tillmanns H, Thederan H: Microcirculation of the epimyocardial layer of the heart. I. A method for in vivo observation of the microcirculation of superficial ventricular myocardium of the heart and capillary flow pattern under normal and hypoxic conditions. Pfluegers Arch. 378: 9-14, 1978.

24.   Tillmanns H, Ikeda S, Hansen H, Sarma JSM, Fauvel JM, Bing RJ: Microcirculation in the ventricle of the dog and turtle. Circ. Res. 34: 561-569, 1974.

25.   Tillmanns H, Kuebler W: What happens in the microcirculation? In: Therapeutic Approaches to Myocardial Infarct Size Limitation, D.J. Hearse and D.M. Yellon (eds.), p. 107-124, Raven Press, New York, 1984.

26.   Tillmanns H, Leinberger H, Neumann FJ, Steinhausen M, Parekh N, Zimmermann R: Early microcirculatory changes during brief ischemia - primary events in ischemic myocardial injury? Circulation 70, Suppl. II-88, 1984.

27.   Tillmanns H, Leinberger H, Thederan H, Steinhausen M, Kuebler W: Pressure-velocity-diameter relations in the microvessels of the heart. Biblthca. Anat. 20: 484-489, Karger, Basel, 1981.

28.   Tillmanns H, Steinhausen M, Dart AM, Leinberger H, Kuebler W: New aspects of myocardial capillary recruitment during hypoxia and reactive hyperemia. Circulation 66, Suppl. II-43, 1982.

29.   Tillmanns H, Steinhausen M, Leinberger H, Thederan H, Kuebler W: Pressure measurements in the terminal vascular bed of the epimyocardium of rats and cats. Circ. Res. 49: 1202-1211, 1981.

30.   Tillmanns H, Steinhausen M, Leinberger H, Thederan H, Kuebler W: Hemodynamics of the coronary microcirculation during myocardial ischemia. Circulation 64, Suppl. IV-40, 1981.

31.   Wiederhielm CA, Woodbury JW, Kirk ES, Rushmer RF: Pulsatile pressures in the microcirculation of frog's mesentery. Am. J. Physiol. 207: 173-176, 1964.

CHANGES IN MYOCARDIAL BLOOD FLOW AND MYOCARDIAL FUNCTION ARE NOT NECESSA-
RILY UNAMBIGOUSLY RELATED

ROBERT S. RENEMAN, THEO ARTS, CORNELIS H. AUGUSTIJN, FRITS W. PRINZEN AND
GER J. VAN DER VUSSE

1. INTRODUCTION

It is generally assumed that there is a direct relation between changes
in myocardial blood flow and myocardial function. A severe reduction in
myocardial blood flow, as during ischemia, however, does not necessarily
result in a profound fall in myocardial fiber shortening at all sites in
the region affected. On the contrary, under certain circumstances a limited
decrease in blood flow in the epicardial layers of the left ventricular
wall may result in complete cessation of fiber shortening in these layers.
Important aspects that have to be considered, when studying the relation
between changes in myocardial blood flow and function, are the metabolic
consequences of the flow reduction and the loading conditions of the myocardium. Evenso restoration of myocardial blood flow following ischemia
does not always result in recovery of myocardial function.

In this chapter some situations will be discussed in which there is no
direct relation between changes in myocardial blood flow and function.

2. MAPPING OF EPICARDIAL FIBER SHORTENING AND TRANSMURAL BLOOD FLOW DURING MYOCARDIAL ISCHEMIA

Epicardial fiber shortening can be assessed (09) from the epicardial
deformation parameters circumferential shortening, base-to-apex shortening
and shear deformation which is associated with torsion of the left ventricle around the base-to-apex axis (02). These deformation parameters can
be determined locally by assessing the mutual displacement of a triplet of
markers (01). Recently we have developed a mapping system allowing the
measurement of fiber shortening or area decrease during systole, simultaneously at various sites of the epicardium of the left ventricle (12;
13). In this technique 40-60 white, circular markers (1.5 mm in diameter)
are attached to the epicardium with histoacryl glue at distances of 5-7 mm.
The markers generally cover an area of 15-20 cm^2. The motion of the markers
is recorded by means of a video camera similar to methods used in gait
analysis (14) or to measure strains in cat knee joint capsule (05). One
marker is made larger so that it can be used as a reference in all frames.
After storage on tape, marker positions and displacements are determined by
off-line analysis in a highly automated way. Markers are distinguished from
the background by grey-level detection. The position of the markers is
calculated as the center of gravity, which is depicted as a black pixel in
the original video image. A special program has been developed to trace the
markers from frame to frame (12). To calculate fiber shortening in the
epicardial fiber direction, this direction is assessed in each experiment.

The fiber shortening, as assessed simultaneously at various sites of the left ventricular epicardium, is shown in Figure 1.

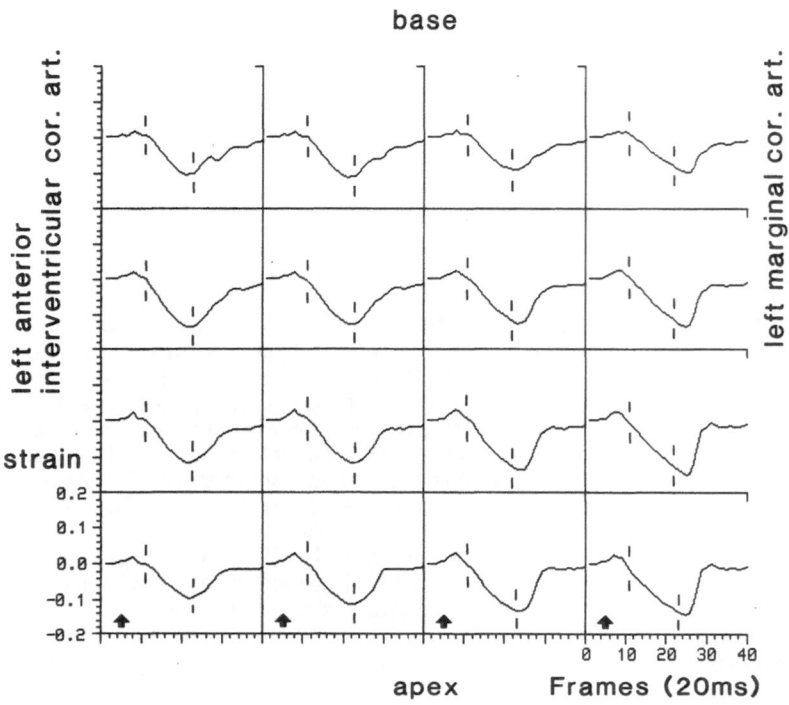

FIGURE 1. Epicardial fiber shortening (i.e. a decrease in strain) during a normal cardiac cycle as recorded in an open-chest dog simultaneously in 16 areas of the left anterior ventricular wall by means of a TV technique. Each frame represents 20 ms. The arrow head indicates the onset of the R-wave of the ECG. The vertical lines in each tracing represent the onset and end of the ejection phase, as determined from the electromagnetically recorded instantaneous ascending aortic flow tracing.

Relatively detailed information about the blood flow distribution in the wall of the left ventricle can be obtained with the use of radioactive microspheres injected into the left atrium and taking a reference sample via a limb artery. After the experiments the left ventricular free wall is divided into 30 to 40 transmural pieces and after weighing the radioactivity in these pieces is determined relative to that in the reference sample, providing transmural myocardial blood flow in ml/min/g tissue (11). If wanted the tissue pieces can be divided into an endocardial and an epicardial part. By using microspheres labelled with different isotopes, myocardial blood flow can be determined at various intervals during the experiments.

By measuring off-line fiber shortening or epicardial area decrease, which is directly related to wall thickening, during systole and myocardial blood

flow in the same regions of the left ventricular free wall, using the white
markers as reference points, the relation between myocardial blood flow and
mechanical function can be investigated under normal and pathological
circumstances. In this way maps of the absolute values of myocardial blood
flow and, for example, area decrease during systole at the epicardium of
the left ventricular free wall can be made during regional myocardial
ischemia. To be able to compare the data obtained in the various experiments both myocardial blood flow and area decrease are normalized by defining the central ischemic values (lowest blood flow and area decrease
values in each experiment) as 0% and the remote normoxic values as 100%. In
Figure 2 maps of transmural blood flow in and epicardial area decrease of
the left ventricular free wall are shown after 5 min regional ischemia, as
induced by total occlusion of the left interventricular coronary artery
(LAICA) in an open-chest dog. In the top illustrations maps of the absolute
values and in the bottom illustrations the contourlines for the 30, 50 and
70% levels of blood flow and area decrease are depicted. When defining
arbitrarily the 50% level of blood flow as the border of the ischemic
region the data presented in Figure 2 show that the region between the 30
and 50% epicardial area decrease contourlines is wider than the region
between these contourlines for transmural blood flow. This indicates that
in this particular case in the ischemic zone the decrease in epicardial
fiber shortening is less pronounced than the fall in transmural blood flow.

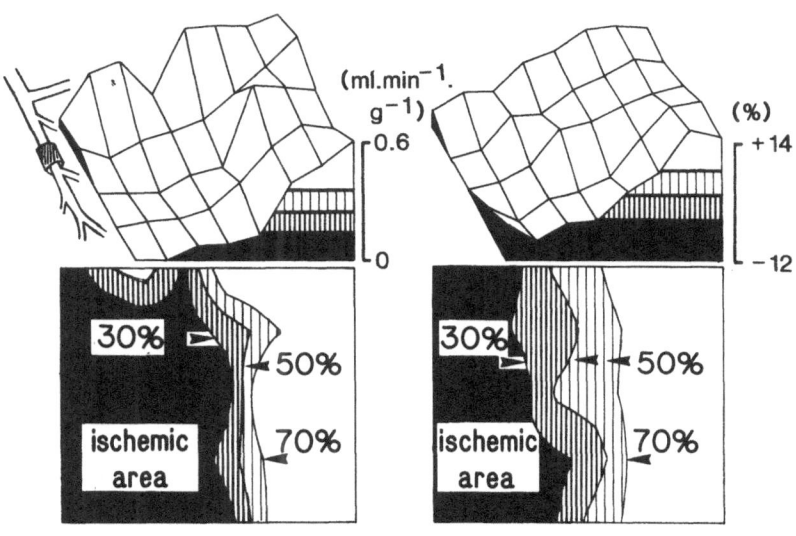

TRANSMURAL BLOOD FLOW   AREA DECREASE

FIGURE 2. Maps of transmural blood flow and epicardial area decrease in
systole during regional myocardial ischemia, as induced by occlusion of the
left interventricular coronary artery. In the top illustrations maps of the
absolute values and in the bottom illustrations the contourlines for the
30, 50 en 70% levels of blood flow and area decrease are depicted. The
central ischemic values of these parameters are defined as 0% (black areas)
and the remote normoxic values as 100%. The 50% level of blood flow is
arbitrarily taken as the border of the ischemic area.

3. MYOCARDIAL BLOOD FLOW, FIBER SHORTENING AND METABOLISM ACROSS THE ISCHEMIC LEFT VENTRICULAR WALL

As discussed in section 2 epicardial fiber shortening can be assessed from epicardial deformation parameters. From these parameters it is also possible to estimate fiber shortening in the inner layers. The latter is based on the experimental observation that epicardial shortening in the direction of the fibers in the inner layers is closely related to fiber shortening in these layers (10; 09). Myocardial blood flow can be determined as described in section 2. Information about myocardial metabolism can be obtained by measuring the myocardial content of such substances, as glycogen, creatine phosphate (CP) and ATP, through biopsies, and the concentration of, for example, lactate, hydrogen ions and inorganic phosphate (Pi) in the local venous effluent.

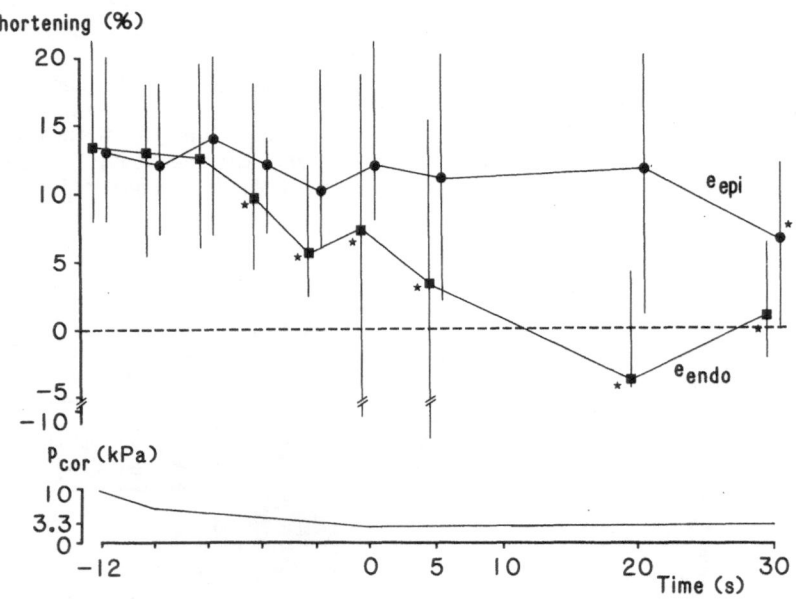

FIGURE 3. Fiber shortening in the endo (e_{endo}) and epicardial layers (e_{epi}) of the area of the left ventricular wall perfused by the left interventricular coronary artery (LAICA) before and during 30 s regional, low flow myocardial ischemia, as induced by partial occlusion (stenosis) of the LAICA. In the bottom tracing the pressure, as measured in the LAICA distal to the site of stenosis, is depicted. The median values and 95% confidence limits are shown. * = significantly lower (P<0.05) than the value before induction of ischemia. (After Prinzen et al, 1986a; with permission of the American Physiological Society).

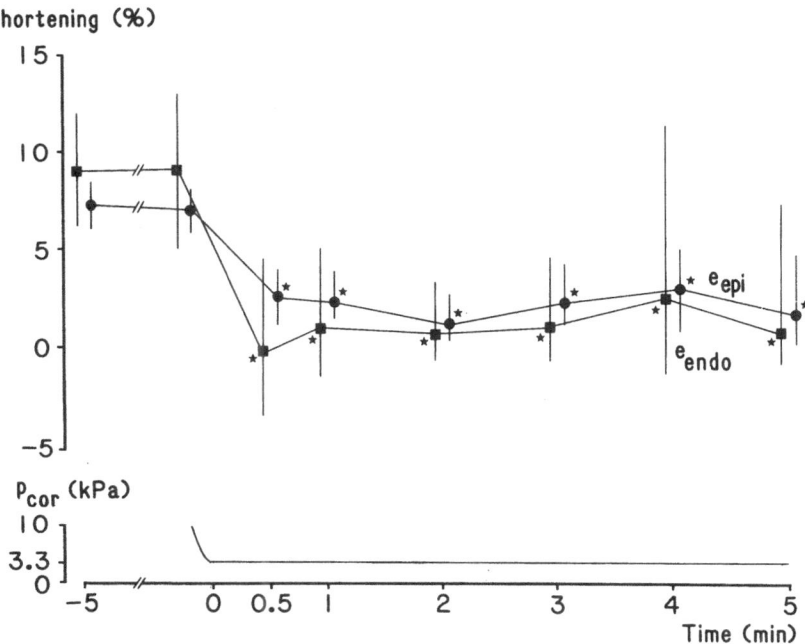

FIGURE 4. Fiber shortening in the endo (e_{endo}) and epicardial layers (e_{epi}) of the area of the left ventricular wall perfused by the left interventricular coronary artery (LAICA) before and during 5 min regional, low flow myocardial ischemia, as induced by partial occlusion (stenosis) of the LAICA. In the bottom tracing the pressure, as measured in the LAICA distal to the site of stenosis is depicted. The median values and 95% confidence limits are shown. * = significantly lower (P<0.05) than the value before induction of ischemia. (After Prinzen et al, 1986a; with permission of the American Physiological Society).

Experiments on open-chest dogs reveal that during low flow regional myocardial ischemia, as induced by partial occlusion (stenosis) of the LAICA, in the ischemic area endocardial fiber shortening during the ejection phase decreases within a few seconds after onset of stenosis, whereas epicardial fiber shortening starts to decrease about 30 sec later. Fiber shortening in the endocardial layers of the ischemic area stops between 10 to 20 sec of ischemia (Figure 3). Fiber shortening in the epicardial layers of the ischemic area falls to about 25% of the initial value after 1 min of ischemia and remains at this level thereafter (Figure 4). In these experiments local epicardial deformation in the ischemic area is measured with three inductive coils, one transmitter coil and two sensor coils, as described in detail before (01). After 1 min of ischemia in the endocardial layers the cessation of fiber shortening is associated with a reduction of myocardial blood flow of 68% (Figure 5) and of CP of 46%. In contrast a 60% reduction of fiber shortening in the epicardial layers is associated with a decrease in myocardial blood flow of only 32% (Figure 5) and no significant decrease in CP in those layers. Hydrogen ions, Pi and lactate are released simultaneously into the venous blood draining the ischemic area, starting within 1 min of ischemia. The content of ATP and glycogen in the ischemic myocardial tissue does not change significantly during the first minutes of ischemia (09). These observations indicate that the decrease in fiber shortening in the endocardial layers during myocardial ischemia results from metabolic dearrangements, as reflected by the depletion of CP. The impaired fiber shortening in the epicardial layers under these circumstances cannot be explained by metabolic disturbances and is likely a consequence of the failing mechanical performance of the endocardial layers. In this situation the entire stress in the left ventricular wall has to be carried by the epicardial layers, resulting in diminished fiber shortening in these layers.

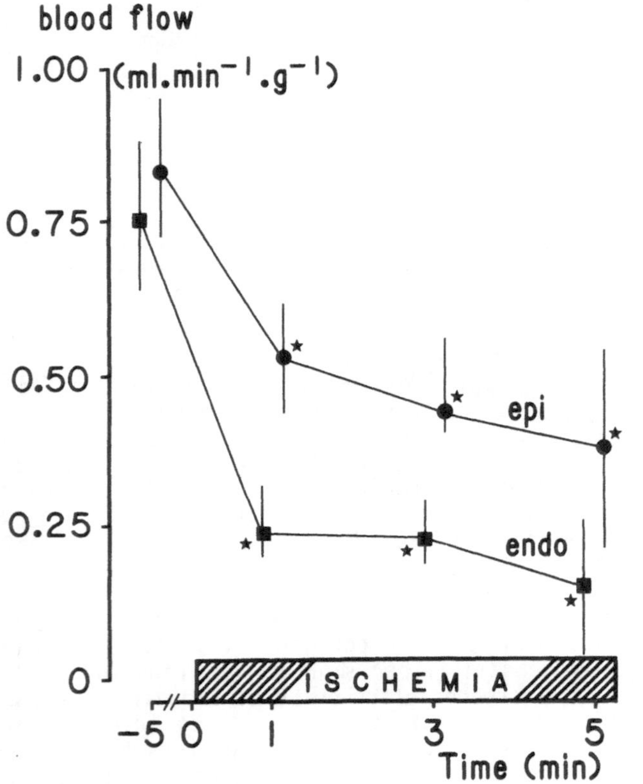

FIGURE 5. Time course of regional myocardial blood flow in the endo and epicardial layers of the ischemic part of the anterior left ventricular wall. Median values and 95% confidence limits are shown. * = significantly lower (P<0.05) than the value before induction of ischemia. (After Prinzen et al, 1986a; with permission of the American Physiological Society).

Several mechanisms have been proposed to explain the relation between CP and mechanical function. In in vitro preparations the important role of CP as a transporter of energy from the mitochondria to the myofibrils has been established (03; 08). According to this theory, a decrease in CP could directly affect the phosphorylation of the myofibril-bound ADP, and therefore contraction. Directly related to the decrease in CP content is the increase in inorganic phosphate content (06). An increase in the latter content could also cause contractile failure by decreasing the phosphorylation potential and hence the free energy change of ATP hydrolysis to a level below which no reaction with sarcoplasmatic reticular ATP-ase can occur. Acidosis has also been suggested as a trigger for early contractile failure (04; 07). In our studies no measurements of tissue pH have been performed, but the finding that release of hydrogen ions into the blood starts within 1 min of ischemia is in agreement with the observations of other investigators employing direct measurement of myocardial pH (16). Therefore, myocardial acidosis may occur rapidly enough to be responsible for the impairment of fiber shortening in the inner layers immediately after onset of ischemia. It is still a matter of debate, however, whether the degree of acidosis is severe enough to explain complete cessation of contractile function.

The observation that during regional, low flow ischemia fiber shortening in the epicardial fibers stops, despite the fact that myocardial blood flow diminishes only to a limited extent, demonstrates that there is not always an unambiguous relation between myocardial flow and function. In this particular situation extreme loading of the fibers prevents them from shortening notwithstanding significant blood supply.

4. REPERFUSION FOLLOWING MYOCARDIAL ISCHEMIA - A COMPARISON BETWEEN RESTORATION OF MYOCARDIAL FUNCTION AND FLOW

It is obvious that the core of an ischemic myocardial region can only survive when blood flow will be restored. However, there is increasing evidence that acute restoration of flow, and, hence, of oxygen delivery, to the area at risk may be deleterious to the myocardium. Therefore, it is

TABLE 1. Regional myocardial blood flow in the centre of the ischemic and reperfused LAICA area. Diltiazem adminstration was started at -30 min and lasted throughout the experiment. Flow data are expressed as ml/min/g wet weight of tissue. Data shown are median values and 95% confidence limits. a and b indicate $P<0.05$ and $0.05<P<0.10$, respectively as compared with corresponding values at time -10 min. c indicates $0.05<P<0.10$ as compared with corresponding value in control group.

	Time (min)			
	Pre-ischemic	Ischemic	Reperfused	
	-10	55	65	120
Subepicardium				
Control	0.53	0.06[a]	2.12[a]	0.63
	0.28-1.34	0.03-0.32	1.16-4.02	0.21-1.08
Diltiazem	0.56	0.04[a]	1.49[a,c]	0.57
	0.46-0.88	0.01-0.23	1.24-3.07	0.38-0.70
Subendocardium				
Control	0.42	0.03[a]	2.01[a]	1.02[a]
	0.36-0.63	0.00-0.16	0.20-3.75	0.47-1.42
Diltiazem	0.56	0.00[a]	1.26[b]	0.82
	0.42-0.91	0.00-0.11	0.39-4.13	0.49-1.35

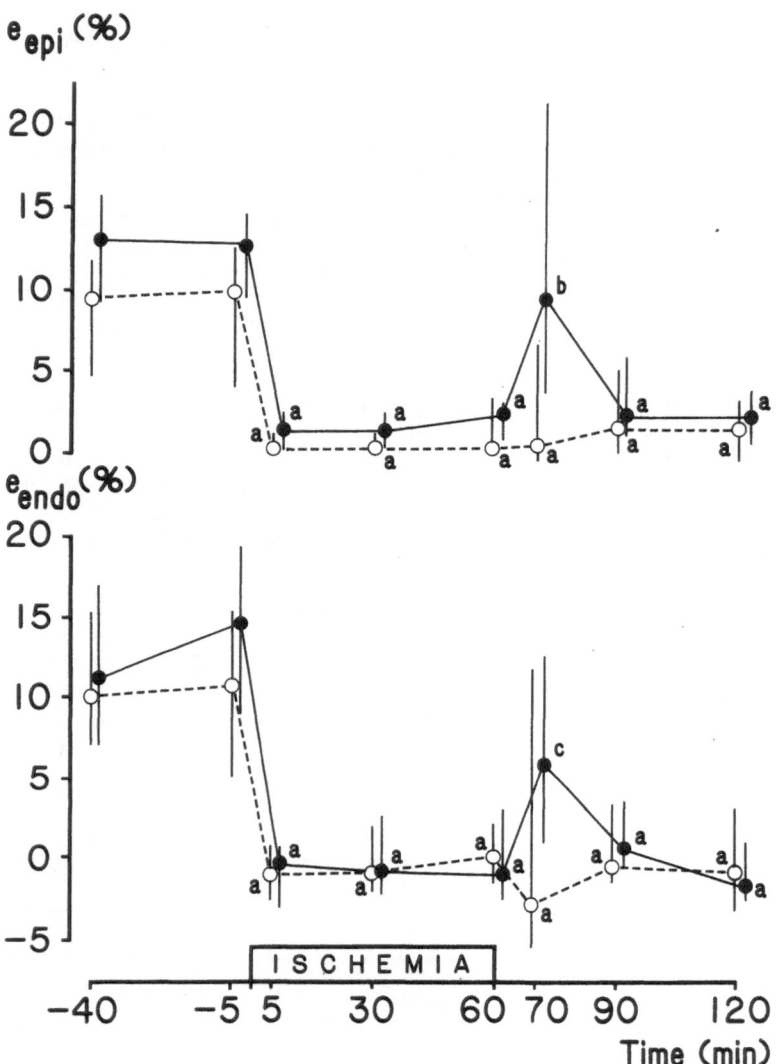

FIGURE 6. Fiber shortening in the epi (e_{epi}) and endocardial layers (e_{endo}) of the area of the left ventricular free wall perfused by the left inter-ventricular coronary artery (LAICA) before and during 1 hour of regional myocardial ischemia (total occlusion of the LAICA), and during reperfusion. Open circles refer to control animals, closed circles to diltiazem treated animals. The data are presented as median values and 95% confidence limits. a indicates $P<0.05$ as compared with the values at time -5 min, b and c indicate $P<0.05$ and $0.05<P<0.10$ for postischemic values, respectively as compared with the values at time 60 min within the same group. (After Van der Vusse et al, 1986; with permission).

still matter of debate whether reinstallation of blood flow to ischemic myocardium will cause the affected tissue to regain its contractile function.

In experiments on open-chest dogs, we have investigated the effect of 60 min reperfusion on the functional and metabolic recovery of myocardium subjected to 60 min of ischemia. In these experiments fiber shortening in the endo and epicardial layers is estimated and the metabolic status of the myocardium is determined as described in section 3. Myocardial blood flow is assessed with radioactively labeled microspheres (section 2) and regional myocardial ischemia is induced by occlusion of the LAICA. Restoration of blood flow (Table 1) to the area at risk does not result in recovery of myocardial function in both the endo and epicardial layers during the period of observation (Figure 6). This can likely be explained by the depletion of ATP and glycogen stores, still present at the end of the reperfusion period. It should be kept in mind that the myocardial CP content is generally restored within 1 hour of reperfusion, reaching values not significantly different from the control values anymore (15). Although the administration of diltiazem (bolus injection of 0.1 mg/kg/body weight prior to ischemia, followed by a continuous infusion of 0.1 mg/kg/h) diminishes the depletion of ATP and glycogen stores in the endocardial layers of the previously ischemic tissue (15), the compound does not permanently improve mechanical function of the reperfused area. Only during the first 10 min of reperfusion fiber shortening in the endo and epicardial layers temporarily increases (Figure 6). It is interesting to note that the reactive hyperemia response during early restoration of flow is less pronounced in the animals treated with diltiazem, as compared to the control animals (Table 1).

These observations demonstrate that restoration of blood flow to ischemic areas does not necessarily result in recovery of mechanical function of these areas. This does not exclude the possibility that mechanical function improves when blood flow to the region at risk is restored for longer periodes of time.

5. CONCLUSION

The experimental data, as discussed in this chapter, show that there is not always an unambigeous relation between myocardial blood flow and mechanical function. For example, myocardial fiber shortening may stop completely, despite the fact that blood flow to the area under investigation is diminished only to a limited extent. Also restoration of blood flow to ischemic myocardium does not necessarily result in recovery of mechanical function.

ACKNOWLEDGEMENTS

The authors are indebted to Jos Heemskerk, Karin van Brussel and Lucienne de Boer for their help in preparing the manuscript. Supported by Medigon/ZWO grant number 900-516-091.

REFERENCES

01. Arts T, Reneman RS: Measurement of deformation of canine epicardium in vivo during cardiac cycle. Am J Physiol 239: H432-H437, 1980.
02. Arts T, Veenstra PC, Reneman RS: Epicardial deformation and left ventricular wall machanics during ejection in the dog. Am J Physiol 243: H379-H390, 1982.

03. Bessman SP, Geiger PJ: Transport of energy in muscle: the phosphoryl-creatine shuttle. Science Wash DC 211: 448-452, 1981.
04. Cobbe SM, Poole-Wilson PA: Tissue acidosis in myocaridal hypoxia. J Mol Cell Cardiol 12: 761-771, 1981.
05. Hoffman AH, Grigg P: A method for measuring strains in soft tissue. J Biomech 17: 795-800, 1984.
06. Kammermeier H, Schmidt P, Juengling E: Free energy change of ATP-hydrolysis: a causal factor of early hypoxic failure of the myocardium. J Mol Cell Cardiol 14: 267-277, 1982.
07. Katz AM, Hecht HH: The early "pump" failure of the ischemic heart. Am J Med 47: 1497-1502, 1969.
08. McClellan G, Weisberg A, Winegrad S: Energy transport from mitochondria to myofibril by a creatine phosphate shuttle in cardiac cells. Am J Physiol 245: C423-C427, 1983.
09. Prinzen FW, Arts T, Van der Vusse GJ, Coumans WA, Reneman RS: Gradients in fiber shortening and metabolism across ischemic left ventricular wall. Am J Physiol 250: H255-H264, 1986a.
10. Prinzen FW, Arts T, Van der Vusse GJ, Reneman RS: Fiber shortening in the inner layers of the left ventricular wall as assessed from epicardial deformation during normoxia and ischemia. J Biomech 17: 801-811, 1984.
11. Prinzen FW, Van der Vusse GJ, Reneman RS: Blood flow distribution in the left ventricular free wall in open-chest dogs. Basic Res Cardiol 76: 431-437, 1981.
12. Prinzen TT, Arts T, Prinzen FW, Reneman RS: Mapping of epicardial deformation using a video precessing technique. J Biomech 19: 263-274, 1986b.
13. Reneman RS, Allessie MA, Arts T, Augustijn CH, Leerssen HM, Prinzen FW: Electrical and mechanical mapping of the left ventricular free wall during normoxia and regional myocardial ischemia - The effect of electrical stimulation. Analysis and simulation of mechanics, perfusion and electrical performance in ischemic heart disease. Sideman S(ed): Boca Raton: CRC Press, in press.
14. Taylor KD, Moittier FM, Simmons DW, Cohen W, Pavlak R, Cornell DP, Hanking GB: An automated motion measurement system for clinical gait analysis. J Biomech 15: 505-516, 1982.
15. Van der Vusse GJ, Van der Veen FH, Prinzen FW, Coumans WA, Van Bilsen M, Reneman RS: The effect of diltiazem on myocardial recovery after regional ischemia in dogs. Europ J Pharmacol 125: 383-394, 1986.
16. Watson RM, Markle DR, Ro YM, Goldstein SR, McGuire DA, Peterson JI, Patterson RE: Transmural pH gradient in canine myocardial ischemia. Am J Physiol 246: H232-H238, 1984.

LOCAL MYOCARDIAL PERFUSION MONITORED BY ELECTRICAL RESISTIVITY
-AN EXPLORATORY TECHNIQUE-

P. STEENDIJK, A.D. VAN DIJK, J. BAAN

1. INTRODUCTION

Abnormal conduction and electrocardiographic patterns following myocardial ischemia are related to changes in electrical properties of the myocardium. The local electrical resistivity of the myocardium influences the shape and velocity of the excitation wave [1-3]. The anatomical structure of the myocardium reveals inhomogeneities which may be reflected in its electrical properties. At microscopic level (10-100 μm), the intracellular medium, the extracellular medium, the muscle fiber membrane and the blood containing capillaries all possess distinct electrical properties. At a larger scale (100-1000 μm) the muscle fibers and vasculature are organized such that anisotropic properties can be anticipated. It has indeed been known since Rush's work [4] that macroscopic (i.e. scale 1-10 mm) resistivity in the muscle fiber direction (ρ_l, longitudinal resistivity) is lower than resistivity perpendicular to that direction (ρ_t, transverse). Many investigators confirmed this finding, but the reported values for ρ_l and ρ_t vary considerably among authors. First, this variation may be due to different conditions of the preparations. Van Oosterom [5] showed that myocardial resistivity measured transmurally changes dramatically when local ischemia is induced. Wojtczak [6] demonstrated changes in passive electrical properties of cow ventricular muscle with hypoxia. Second, resistivities were studied at different frequencies. Recent model studies as well as experimental results in skeletal muscle show that the effective resistivities are dependent on the frequency of the excitation current [7,8]. At low frequencies, the major conduction pathways are probably through the extracellular fluid and blood, whereas at higher frequencies the effective membrane impedance is reduced allowing current to flow more uniformly throughout the tissue resulting in a lower effective resistivity. Third, the myocardium is generally modelled as an infinite or semi-infinite homogeneous anisotropic volume conductor, with resistivity ρ_l in one direction (representing the muscle fiber direction) and resistivity ρ_t in the other two directions. The validity of this model, however, is limited in particular because fiber direction is not uniform throughout the myocardium, but changes from -60° (with respect to circumferential direction) at the epicardium through 0° at midwall to +60° at the endocardium [9]. Therefore, the interpretation of measured electrical data in terms of resistivities depends on the applicability of the volume conductor model in a specific experimental preparation.

An important omission in the majority of the models used appears to be the neglected presence of blood(vessels) in the myocardium. Ten to 15% of the heart wall is occupied by blood [10,11], which is less resistive than muscle tissue as a whole, and capillary vessels run largely parallel to the muscle fibers [12]. Thus, myocardial blood content and perfusion may have a sizeable influence on the (passive) electrical properties of the heart wall. Based on this hypothesis, perfusion-related changes in the myocardium would have a measurable effect on, and conversely may be monitored by, local myocardial resistivity. To test this hypothesis we developed a small epicardial sensor to measure local myocardial resistivities in the open chest preparation. We studied myocardial resistivity in 9 dogs both during normal flow and during conditions of changes in flow. In the present paper the results from these experiments are given, preceded by a theoretical analysis of the measurement of myocardial resistivity with the four electrode technique.

2. THE FOUR ELECTRODE TECHNIQUE
2.1. Principle

Resistivity of biological tissues and fluids is usually measured with the four electrode technique. Basically this method employs one pair of electrodes to apply a current and another pair to sense the resulting voltage in a medium. By using non current-carrying sensing electrodes problems with electrode polarization are avoided. To evaluate the resistivity of a medium from applied current and measured voltage, an assumption has to be made about the current distribution. In many cases the medium can be readily approximated as either infinite or semi-infinite or as a thin slab and the current distribution is easily calculated. In some cases, however, neither of these models is appropriate. We therefore set up a more general model describing the application of the four electrode technique to a layer of finite thickness, enclosed between two semi-infinite media, all three media having different resistivities. This model covers all approximations mentioned above and offers the flexibility of describing some of the more complicated configurations frequently encountered.

2.2. Volume conductor models

Using a linear array of four equidistant electrodes with electrode separation a, the relation between a current injected via the outer two electrodes (I), the resulting voltage on the inner pair of electrodes (V) and resistivity (ρ) in an isotropic, uniform, infinite medium is:

$$V_{inf} = \frac{I \rho}{4 \pi a} \tag{1}$$

If the electrode array is applied on the flat surface of a semi-infinite medium bounded by another semi-infinite medium with $\rho=\infty$ (such as air) then:

$$V_{semi-inf} = \frac{I \rho}{2 \pi a} \tag{2}$$

The solution for a slab, a thin layer of medium bounded by air on both sides, only holds if the thickness of the slab (δ) is small compared to the electrode separation ($\delta<<a$):

$$V_{slab} = \frac{I \rho \ln 2}{\pi \delta} \tag{3}$$

By applying appropriate coordinate transformations, these results can be extended to uniform anisotropic media [13]. In figure 1, a more general model is illustrated. The electrode array is applied on the top surface of a layer of finite thickness (d) with resistivity ρ_2, which is enclosed by two semi-infinite media with resistivities ρ_1 and ρ_3. The potential distribution for the configuration is calculated using the image technique. In analogy with light phenomena, from an observation point not only the primary current source is "seen", but also its partial reflections from the two boundaries. The strength of these images depend on the reflection

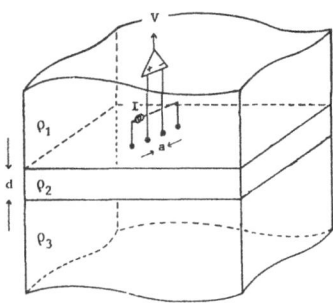

Figure 1: The four electrode array applied to a layer-formed medium
with thickness d, enclosed by two semi-infinite media.

coefficients K_1 and K_3 (see below). As there are two boundaries there will
be multiple reflections that must be taken into account. The result is that
the voltage difference between the sensing electrodes is:

$$V_{layer} = \frac{I \rho_2}{4 \pi a} (1+K_1) (1+\tau) \tag{4}$$

with:

$$\tau = 2(1+K_1) \sum_{n=1}^{\infty} K_1^{n-1} K_3^n \left(\frac{1}{\sqrt{(2nd/a)^2 + 1}} - \frac{1}{\sqrt{(2nd/a)^2 + 4}} \right) ,$$

$$K_1 = \frac{(\rho_1-\rho_2)}{(\rho_1+\rho_2)} \quad \text{and} \quad K_3 = \frac{(\rho_3-\rho_2)}{(\rho_3+\rho_2)}$$

2.3. Penetration depth

If the medium of interest has a finite depth, application of the semi-
infinite medium approximation (equation (2)) leads to an over- or underestimation, depending on the geometry and resistivities of the surrounding
media [14]. The effective area or penetration depth of the four electrode
system primarily depends on the distance between the current electrodes.
With a larger spacing the current spreads deeper into the medium and deeper
layers will contribute to the resistivity measurement. Equation (4) allows
to quantify this effect as illustrated in figure 2. The four electrode
array is applied to the medium of interest (with resistivity ρ_2), which
forms a layer of finite thickness (d) and is enclosed by air ($\rho_1=\infty$, thus
$K_1=1$) and a medium with resistivity ρ_3. The apparent resistivity, defined
as $\rho'=2\pi aV/I$ (equation (2)), deviates from the actual resistivity ρ_2
because the presence of a medium with a different resistivity (ρ_3) causes a
distortion of the assumed "semi-infinite" current distribution:

$$\rho' = \rho_2 (1 + \tau) \tag{5}$$

$$\text{with } \tau = 4 \sum_{n=1}^{\infty} K_3^n \left(\frac{1}{\sqrt{(2nd/a)^2 + 1}} - \frac{1}{\sqrt{(2nd/a)^2 + 4}} \right)$$

Figure 2 shows that the influence on the measured voltage of media located
deeper than twice the electrode spacing is less than 10%. If the resistivities of the media are comparable in magnitude ($0.5<\rho_3/\rho_2<2$) an electrode
spacing equal to the layer thickness is already small enough to limit this
effect to about 10%.

108

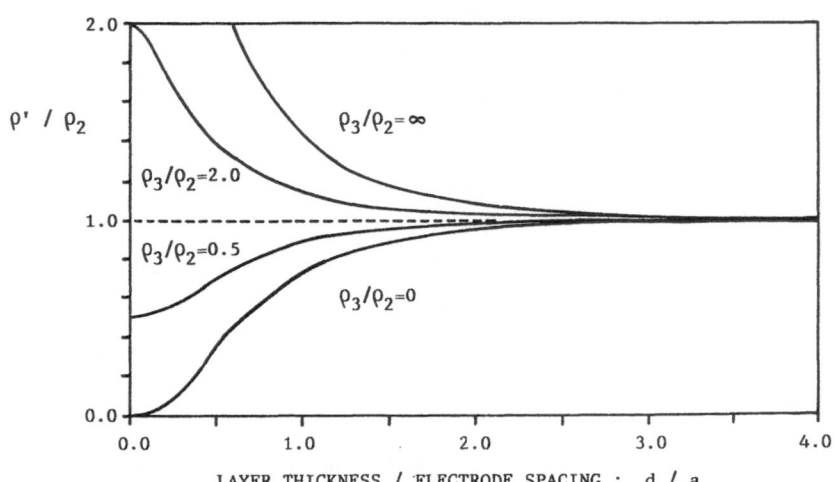

LAYER THICKNESS / ELECTRODE SPACING : d / a

Figure 2: The apparent resistivity ρ', (i.e. calculated from measured voltage using the semi-infinite medium approximation), of a medium forming a layer on top of a semi-infinite medium, divided by its actual resistivity ρ_2, as a function of the relative thickness of the layer for four values of ρ_3/ρ_2.

2.4. Application to cardiac muscle

The fiber structure of cardiac muscle results in an anisotropic macroscopic resistivity. When all fibers are assumed to run parallel, the myocardium can be modelled electrically as an anisotropic volume conductor with resistivity ρ_l in one direction (representing the fiber direction) and resistivities ρ_t in the two transverse directions. With a four electrode system applied to the surface of such a medium, assumed semi-infinite, the voltage difference becomes dependent on the orientation (determined by the angle α) of the electrode array with respect to the fiber direction [4]:

$$V_{aniso}(\alpha, \rho_l, \rho_t) = \frac{I}{2 \pi a} \left(\frac{\cos^2\alpha}{\rho_l \rho_t} + \frac{\sin^2\alpha}{\rho_t^2} \right)^{-\frac{1}{2}} \tag{6}$$

If the four electrode array is aligned along the fiber direction ($\alpha=\pi/2$) equation 6 reduces to:

$$V_l = \frac{I \rho_t}{2 \pi a} \tag{7}$$

while with $\alpha=0$ (i.e. perpendicular to fiber direction):

$$V_t = \frac{I \sqrt{(\rho_l \rho_t)}}{2 \pi a} \tag{8}$$

Therefore the two resistivities can be obtained as:

$$\rho_t = V_l \frac{2 \pi a}{I} \tag{9}$$

$$\rho_l = \frac{V_t^2}{V_l} \frac{2 \pi a}{I} \tag{10}$$

This approach is obviously meaningful only if the assumption of parallel fibers is valid in the effective area of the array, while on the other hand the electrode distance should be large enough to overcome the inhomogeneities at microscopic cellular level. The latter constraint leads to a lower limit for a of about 100 μm. Streeter's data on the transmural orientation of fiber direction [9] indicate a change in fiber direction of about 20° over the first 10% of wall thickness. Thus, to approximate uniform fiber direction, measurements should be limited to a thin epicardial layer. According to figure 2 an electrode distance of 1 mm is appropriate to limit the influence of layers deeper than about 1 mm to less than 10%. These considerations led to the development of a sensor with 1 mm electrode separation (see below). Analyzing the same situation as leading to equation (5), but for anisotropic media, it follows that analogous to equations (7) and (8):

$$V_\ell = \frac{I \; \rho_t}{2 \; \pi \; a} \; (1 + \tau_\ell)$$ (11)

$$V_t = \frac{I \; \sqrt{(\rho_t \; \rho_\ell)}}{2 \; \pi \; a} \; (1 + \tau_t)$$ (12)

with:

$$\tau_\ell = 4 \sum_{n=1}^{\infty} K_3{}^n \; (\frac{1}{\sqrt{(\rho_t/\rho_\ell} \; (2nd/a)^2+1)} - \frac{1}{\sqrt{(\rho_t/\rho_\ell} \; (2nd/a)^2+4)})$$

$$\tau_t = 4 \sum_{n=1}^{\infty} K_3{}^n \; (\frac{1}{\sqrt{((2nd/a)^2+1)}} - \frac{1}{\sqrt{((2nd/a)^2+4)}})$$

Thus, for the measurement of the voltage in transverse direction V_t, equation (12) is similar to equation (5) since $\tau_t = \tau$. But in the longitudinal direction (measurement of V_ℓ to obtain ρ_t) the correction factor, τ_ℓ, becomes dependent on the anisotropy, expressed by the ratio ρ_t/ρ_ℓ. If the ratio exceeds unity, as in cardiac muscle, this leads to a lesser influence of the deeper layers, because τ_ℓ is smaller than τ. Using the same model one can easily show that the presence of a relatively insulating thin layer (d/a<0.1) as formed by the epicardial membrane does not influence the measurements, but a similar layer consisting of blood or saline (if present) would have a sizeable disturbing effect.

3. TECHNIQUE

Based on the four electrode method we developed an epicardial sensor to measure myocardial resistivities. To obtain local resistivity in two perpendicular directions (parallel and perpendicular to epicardial muscle fiber direction) two linear arrays of 4 equidistant platinum electrodes are mounted crosswise on a perspex holder. The diameter of the electrodes is 0.4 mm and the inter-electrode distance is 1 mm. The eight electrode system is incorporated in a small flexible silicone suction cup with a 16 mm outer diameter (figure 3). Using a slight vacuum, maintained with a pump via a suction tube, the sensor is easily affixed to the beating heart. Gross visual inspection showed no migration of the sensor.

Resistivities were measured with the four electrode method using an analog signal conditioner-processor (Leycom, model Sigma-5, Oegstgeest, The Netherlands) developed for intraventricular volume-conductance measurement [15]. Basically a 10 μA, 15 kHz sinusoidal excitation current is applied to the outer electrodes of one of the four electrode arrays and the voltages on the inner two electrodes of that array are fed into a high input impedance (>1 $M\Omega$) differential amplifier. The system is calibrated by submerging the sensor in a large container filled with a saline solution of

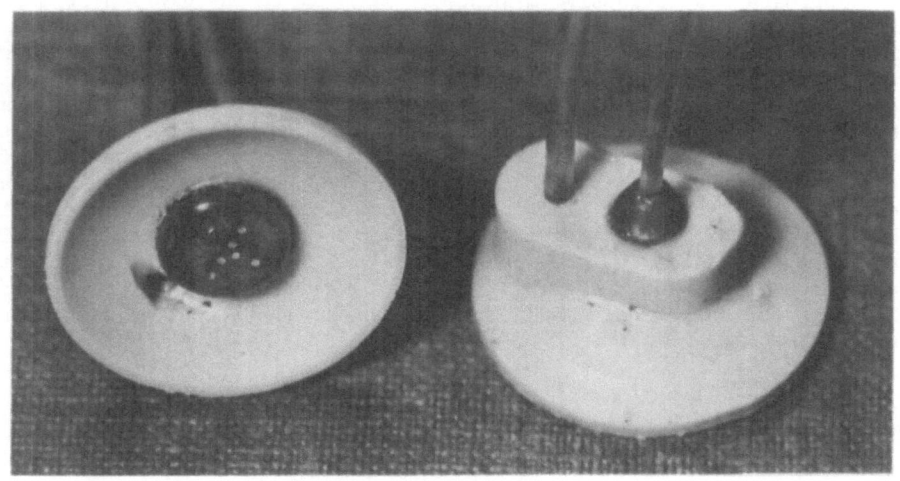

Figure 3: The sensor, an eight electrode transducer consisting of two arrays of 4 platinum electrodes (inter-electrode distance 1 mm) mounted crosswise on a perspex holder, incorporated in a small flexible suction cup.

known resistivity. During most experiments we switched from one four electrode array to the other every 5 s, but it proved possible to have continuous simultaneous recordings from both arrays by using two measurement systems working at different frequencies.

4. EXPERIMENTAL PREPARATION AND PROTOCOL

We performed experiments in 9 open chest mongrel dogs (20-25 kg) to study the effects of increased and decreased coronary blood flow on local myocardial resistivity.

After premedication with 5 ml of Hypnorm (10 mg fluanison and 0.2 mg of fentanyl per ml) intramuscularly and 1 ml of atropine subcutaneously the dogs were anesthetized with 9 mg/kg sodiumpentobarbital (Nembutal) and 2 ml methadone (i.v.) and intubated. The dogs were ventilated by a fixed-volume positive-pressure respirator (Dräger-Pulmonat) with a 3:1 mixture of N_2O and O_2. Anesthesia was maintained with an intravenous infusion of methadone (2.5 mg/hr) and droperidol (12.5 mg/hr). Blood volume and pressure were controlled by intravenous infusion of dextran (Macrodex). After thoracotomy, the pericardium was opened, the left anterior descending coronary artery (LAD) exposed and a snare occluder placed around it. In 6 dogs a perivascular electromagnetic flow probe (Skalar, Delft, The Netherlands) was placed on the LAD proximal to the occluder. A dual micromanometer catheter (Honeywell MTC) was inserted into the left ventricle via the right carotid artery with the proximal pressure transducer above the aortic valve and the distal transducer in the left ventricle. Via the right femoral artery a latex balloon occluder catheter was placed in the descending aorta. Continuous recordings of standard lead II ECG, left ventricular pressure, arterial blood pressure and pulsatile and mean coronary blood flow were made on an eight-channel paper recorder.

To create transient changes in myocardial perfusion we applied two interventions: 1) Inflation of the latex balloon positioned in the descending aorta to increase perfusion pressure and thereby increase global coronary flow. 2) Occlusion of the left anterior descending coronary artery with the snare to produce a decrease in local myocardial perfusion. To measure myocardial resistivities the sensor was placed in the perfusion region of the LAD with one of the electrode arrays along the epicardial muscle fiber direction, as it was estimated by direct visual inspection. After inspection of the measured resistance values from both arrays the sensor was rotated slightly as necessary to maximize the difference between the two signals. In the resulting position the higher resistance value was taken to represent ρ_t and the lower value to represent $\sqrt{(\rho_t \rho_l)}$ as indicated in equations (7) and (8). Resistivities were monitored semi-continuously by switching from one electrode array to the other every 5 s. Recordings were obtained during periods of about 10 min: preceded by a control period of 1-2 min, either the LAD or the aorta descendens was occluded for about 2 min, followed by a relaxation period of at least 5 min after release of the occlusion.

5. RESULTS

We monitored myocardial electrical resistivities both during normal and modified flow conditions. Mean control values for myocardial resistivities during normal flow conditions were measured in 9 dogs. Mean values for each dog obtained from roughly 5 measurements at slightly different sites on the anterior free wall of the left ventricle, resulted in a standard deviation typically amounting to 10% of the mean value. The variation in mean resistivities between dogs was about 20%. Averaging a total of 55 measurements in all 9 dogs we found a mean value and standard deviation of 250±50 Ωcm (n=55) for the longitudinal resistivity, ρ_l, and 370±60 Ωcm (n=55) for the transverse resistivity, ρ_t. The effects following occlusion of the descending aorta in a typical experiment are shown in figure 4. The first tracing shows the alternated measurement of myocardial resistivities. The upper level gives ρ_t, the lower level the square root of the product of ρ_t and ρ_l. Both levels are going down although at different rates, during the occlusion and increase upon release of the occlusion. From these two levels ρ_t and ρ_l are obtained and plotted as shown in figure 5. Figure 6 shows a similar plot from a typical experiment where the LAD coronary artery was occluded to produce a local reduction in myocardial blood flow. Both ρ_t and ρ_l increase during the intervention, and decrease upon release albeit to a different extent.

The results were analyzed by calculating the relative maximal increases or decreases in longitudinal and transverse resistivities during the interventions with respect to the preceding control values. The relative changes in the resistivities following aortic occlusion were not statistically significant. Longitudinal resistivity, ρ_l, showed a tendency to increase, 5±15% (n=24, NS), and ρ_t tended to decrease slightly, -2±7%, (n=24, NS). For both resistivities we occasionally saw opposite changes upon repeating the experiment after replacing the sensor at a slightly different position in the same dog. In contrast, the relative changes in resistivities with decreased local flow conditions were more pronounced and consistent with a single exception as shown in figure 7. Reducing local perfusion by occluding the LAD coronary artery resulted in a significant increase in both ρ_l and ρ_t. Longitudinal resistivity increased 14±15% (mean±s.d., n=15, p<0.005), while transverse resistivity increased 9±7% (mean±s.d., n=16, p<0.001). Resistivities tended to return to control after the intervention, but often remained slightly elevated with respect to the initial values.

112

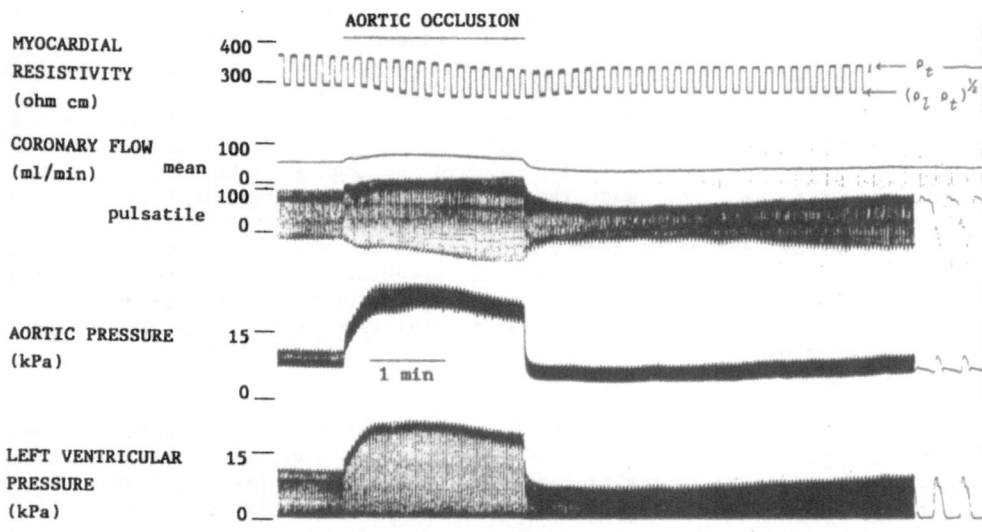

AORTIC OCCLUSION

MYOCARDIAL RESISTIVITY (ohm cm)

CORONARY FLOW (ml/min)   mean
                         pulsatile

AORTIC PRESSURE (kPa)   1 min

LEFT VENTRICULAR PRESSURE (kPa)

Figure 4: Effects of a transient occlusion of the descending aorta. The upper tracing shows the measurement of myocardial resistivities with the sensor, alternatively 5 s parallel (upper level) and 5 s perpendicular (lower level) to fiber direction.

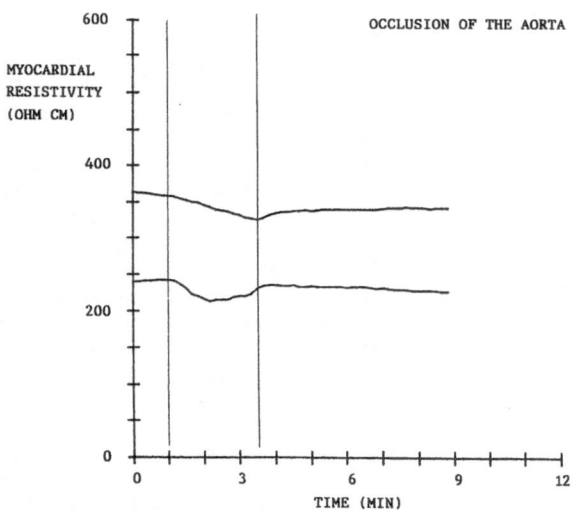

Figure 5: Same experiment as depicted in figure 4, showing the calculated values for transverse (top) and longitudinal (bottom) myocardial resistivities as a function of time. Occlusion period is indicated by vertical lines.

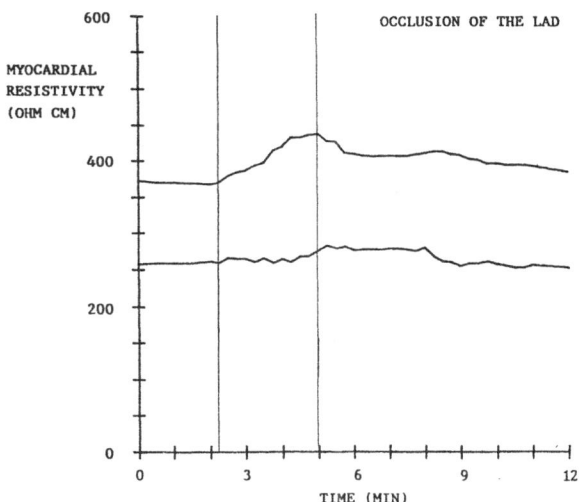

Figure 6: Transverse (top) and longitudinal (bottom) resistivities during transient occlusion of the left anterior descending coronary artery as a function of time. Occlusion period is indicated by vertical lines.

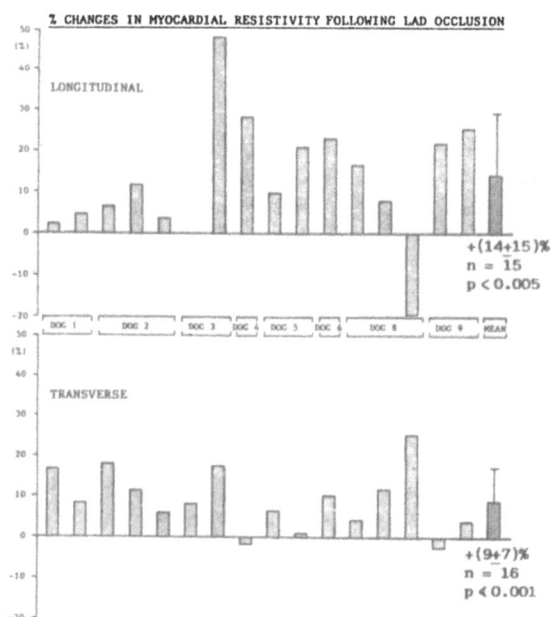

Figure 7: Relative changes in longitudinal and transverse myocardial resistivities during transient occlusion of the left anterior descending coronary artery, measured in 8 open chest dogs.

6. DISCUSSION

6.1. Mathematical model

To quantify the penetration depth of a four electrode system in the myocardium we set up a multi-layered mathematical model. The theoretical results indicate that in general the influence of layers deeper than twice the inter-electrode spacing of the four electrode array is less than 10% and in the specific case of myocardium, where anisotropy (ratio ρ_t/ρ_l) is about 2, this effect will be limited to less than 5%. The sensor developed and used by us is theoretically estimated to be sensing an epicardial layer of 1-2 mm thickness. We tested the penetration depth of the system by placing the sensor in a container with a saline solution with known resistivity and measuring the apparent resistivity of the saline solution while advancing the sensor towards the surface of a block of non-conductive perspex. The measurements were in accordance with the theoretical results (upper curve figure 2) and we found that the overestimation of saline resistivity was limited to 10% as long as the distance between the sensor and the non-conducting boundary was more than 1.9±0.2 mm. Other potential problems are the presence of the epicardial membrane or a possible thin fluid layer on the epicardium. The mathematical model shows that the influence of a very thin and relatively insulating layer such as the epicardial membrane may be neglected. A layer formed by saline or blood, media which are less resistive than the myocardium, may lead to a serious underestimation of myocardial resistivity. Such a shunting layer with a thickness only one tenth of the electrode spacing already decreases measured resistivity by 10-30%.

6.2. Sensor

The present sensor was developed to measure myocardial resistivities non traumatically and continuously in the open chest preparation. Therefore a non penetrating electrode system was used, applied to the epicardium by means of a suction cup. Migration and especially rotation of the sensor would hamper the interpretation of the data since determination of the longitudinal and transverse resistivities from the measured voltages depends on the proper alignment of the arrays with muscle fiber direction, and any misalignment results in an underestimation of the anisotropy. Although movement of the sensor with respect to the epicardium has not been assessed quantitatively it was absent on direct visual inspection. In some cases when the sensor had been applied a long time the vacuum used for fixation of the sensor caused a small rim of hematomic tissue at the borderzone of the transducer, but since this rim falls outside the region measured we do not expect it to pose a problem.

6.3. Resistivity measurements

Values of the resistivities of myocardial tissue reported in the literature range from 390 to 705 ohm cm for the transverse and from 125 to 265 ohm cm for the longitudinal direction [2,3,4,6,16], whereas we found 370±60 and 250±50 ohm cm respectively. A number of factors may explain the wide range of values reported. Most reported values were obtained at frequencies of about 1 kHz or less whereas we measured at 15 kHz. Although a frequency dependence has not yet been demonstrated experimentally in heart muscle, recent model studies and data from skeletal muscle show a substantial decrease in the transverse resistivity above 10 kHz [7,8], which may explain our relatively low values for the transverse resistivity. Furthermore, our results as well as those in literature indicate that the resistivities strongly depend on the condition of the preparation. Thus, results obtained from isolated trabeculae and the heart in situ may not be comparable. A third factor may be that the extent of applicability of the volume conductor models used is different in the various preparations presented in the literature, e.g. none of the models takes into account the change in fiber direction.

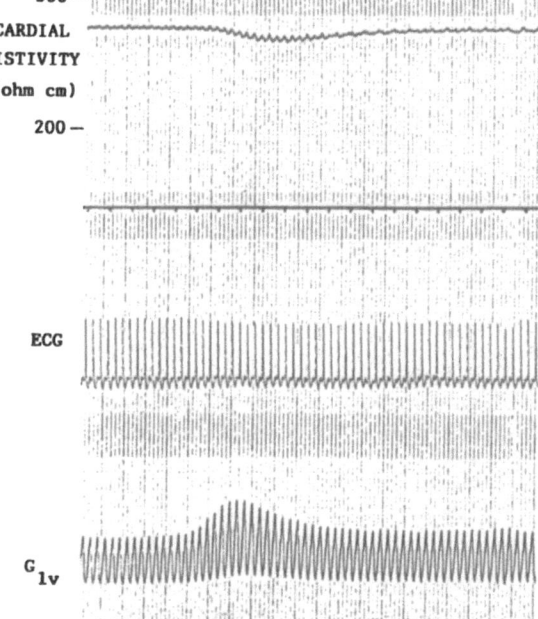

Figure 8: The subsequent passage of low resistive blood, due to a 2 ml bolus of hypertonic saline injected in the pulmonary artery, monitored by the conductance, G, of blood in the left ventricle measured with an eight electrode catheter (lower tracing) and myocardial resistivity measured with the epicardial sensor (upper tracing).

6.4. Changes in myocardial resistivities

The present measurements in the superficial myocardial layer reveal that changes in myocardial perfusion and concomitant changes in blood content are reflected by changes in the electrical properties, especially during conditions of flow reduction and ischemia. Our hypothesis is that with the present technique, major current pathways run through the interstitial fluid and the vasculature and the observed changes in resistivities reflect changes in geometry and effective resistivities of these media. In figure 8 a direct effect of a change in the resistivity of blood on myocardial resistivity is seen. The resistivity of the blood was made transiently less resistive (more conductive) by injecting a 2 ml bolus of hypertonic saline in the pulmonary artery. The lower tracing shows the conductance of blood in the left ventricle measured with an eight electrode catheter [15], the upper tracing the resistivity of the myocardium measured with the epicardial sensor. The tracings reveal the subsequent passage of the bolus through the left ventricle and the myocardium. Further research is required to gain insight in the physiological and anatomical factors causing the behavior observed during the interventions in perfusion. E.g., we do not know whether the increased global coronary flow is reflected in an increased blood content in the epicardial layer in which we measure nor do we know the influence of a possible redistribution of red blood cells and plasma containing capillaries (Tillmans, this volume). Neither do we know how much of the observed effects on resistivities upon local flow reduction are caused by a decrease in blood volume and how much by an absence of erythrocyte motion or perhaps by swelling of the mitochondria. But the developed simple, non-traumatic, on-line technique appears to hold a promise to study perfusion-related changes in the myocardium. Different electrode configurations and excitation frequencies than those used so far will permit us to study electrical properties at different wall depths and to make a better distinction between different tissue components. The significant changes following occlusion of the LAD coronary artery indicate that the present technique may be successfully applied to monitor local ischemia in the open chest preparation, or clinically e.g. during coronary artery bypass grafting surgery.

ACKNOWLEDGEMENT
The authors gratefully acknowledge J. Karsdon and A.E. Marcus for their assistance during the experiments. This research was supported by grants from the Netherlands Heart Foundation and the Foundation for Technical Sciences.

REFERENCES
1. Spach M.S., P.C. Dolber: Relating extracellular potentials and their derivatives to anisotropic propagation at a microscopic level in human cardiac muscle. Circ. Res. 58: 356, 1986.
2. Clerc L.: Directional differences of impulse spread in trabecular muscle from mammalian heart. J. Physiology 255: 335, 1976.
3. Roberts D.E., A.M. Scher: Effect of tissue anisotropy on extracellular potential fields in canine myocardium in situ. Circ. Res. 50: 342, 1982.
4. Rush S., J.A. Abildskov, McFee R.: Resistivities of body tissues at low frequencies. Circ. Res. 12: 40, 1963.
5. Oosterom A. van, R.W. de Boer, R.Th. van Dam: Intramural resistivity of cardiac tissue. Med. & Biol. Eng. & Comput. 17: 337, 1979.
6. Wojtczak J.: Contractures and increase in internal longitudinal resistance of cow ventricular muscle induced by hypoxia. Circ. Res. 44, 88, 1979.
7. Gielen F.L.H., H.E.P. Cruts, B.A. Albers, K.L. Boon, W. Wallinga- de Jonge, H.B.K. Boom: Model of electrical conductivity of. skeletal muscle based on tissue structure. Med. & Biol. Eng. & Comput. 24, 34, 1986.
8. Zheng E., S. Shao, J.G. Webster: Impedance of skeletal muscle from 1 Hz to 1 MHz. IEEE Trans. BME-31/6: 477, 1984.
9. Streeter D.D., H.M. Spotnitz. D.P. Patel. J. Ross, E.H. Sonnenblick: Fiber orientation in the canine left ventricle during diastole and systole. Circ. Res. 24: 339, 1969.
10. Morgenstern C., U. Holjes, G. Arnold, W. Lochner: The influence of coronary pressure and coronary flow on intracoronary blood volume and geometry of the left ventricle. Pflugers Arch. 340: 101, 1973.
11. Hoffman E.A., E.L. Ritman: Intramyocardial blood volume - implications for analysis of myocardial mechanical characteristics via in vivo imaging of the heart. (in press).
12. Bassingthwaighte J.B., T. Yipintsoi, R.B. Harvey: Microvasculature of the dog left ventricular myocardium. Microvasc. Res. 7: 229, 1974.
13. Plonsey R.: Bioelectric phenomena. McGraw-Hill Book Co., New York, 1969.
14. Robillard, P.N., D. Poussart: Spatial resolution of four electrode array. IEEE Trans. BME-26/8: 465, 1979.
15. Baan J., E.T. van der Velde, H. de Bruin, G. Smeenk, J. Koops, A.D. van Dijk, D. Temmerman, J. Senden, B. Buis: Continuous measurement of left ventricular volume in animals and man by conductance catheter. Circ. 70: 812, 1984.
16. Weidman S.: Electrical constants of trabecular muscle from mammalian heart. J. Physiol. 210: 1041, 1970.

III

Clinical assessment of myocardial perfusion

QUANTITATIVE DIGITAL ANGIOGRAPHIC TECHNIQUES

JOHAN H.C. REIBER, PH.D., CORNELIS J. KOOIJMAN, M.SC., CORNELIS J. SLAGER, M.SC., JAN J. GERBRANDS, M.SC., AD DEN BOER, B.SC., JAN VAN OMMEREN, M.SC., FELIX ZIJLSTRA, M.D., PATRICK SERRUYS, M.D.

1. SUMMARY

There is an increasing demand for the objective and reproducible assessment of coronary arterial dimensions and for the functional significance of coronary obstructions to study the efficacy of new recanalization techniques in the catheterization laboratory, to evaluate new approaches to achieve regression or no-growth of coronary atherosclerosis and also as a means for diagnostic and therapeutic decision making during the cardiac catheterization procedure. This last application requires the use of digital cardiac imaging systems with the capability to store the images on-line on real-time disks; at the present time, the other applications are usually evaluated off-line from 35mm cinefilm.

In this chapter an overview will be presented on the different techniques that have been developed for the quantitative analysis of the size and shape of coronary arterial segments, and of the functional significance of coronary obstructions. The first approaches towards the quantitative anatomic description have been based on the (semi)-automated boundary detection of the arterial segments and the subsequent computation of the relative and absolute length and width dimensions; later approaches have attempted to determine the cross-sectional narrowing of obstructions from a single angiographic view by densitometry. Different techniques have been developed to assess the functional significance of an obstruction: 1) calculation of pressure-flow characteristics; 2) generation of parametric images to determine regional coronary flow reserve. In general, all algorithms are applicable to both digitized cineframes and the on-line acquired digital images, possibly requiring slight modifications from the one medium to the other.

2. INTRODUCTION

The limitations in the visual interpretation of the morphology of coronary obstructions have been well documented in the literature. These are: the large intra- and interobserver variabilities, the fact that visually only relative percent diameter and/or area stenosis can be estimated, and thirdly that the functional or physiologic significance is very difficult, if not impossible, to assess. Moreover, the ever increasing application of recanalization techniques in the catheterization laboratory, such as PTCA (1), the use of thrombolytic agents (2), the introduction of the stent (3), and possibly in the near future laser (4) and/or spark erosion (5) techniques, the need to study the effects of vasoactive drugs (6) and the interest in finding ways to achieve regression or no-growth of coronary atherosclerosis (7), have stimulated the research and development towards computer-based techniques for the objective and reproducible quantitative analysis of the coronary morphology. Such techniques should provide, among others, absolute measurements on the minimal diameter, extent and asymmetry of the obstructions, relative percent diameter and area stenosis, the roughness of the coronary arterial segment, as well as data on the mean diameters of nonobstructed coronary segments, assessed from multiple angiographic views. By combining all stenosis measurements, the functional pressure-flow effects of the stenosis, as well as coronary flow reserve can be assessed (8). In those situations, where the obstructions are very asymmetric, such as post-PTCA where dissections frequently occur, the computation of relative and absolute cross-sectional narrowing by densitometry seems the ultimate goal to achieve. In addition, techniques have been developed to study the regional coronary flow reserve by measuring the contrast arrival times and density in the myocardium at hyperemic and basal states (9).

In general, the quantitative analysis of coronary obstructions is performed from 35 mm cinefilm. However, recent developments in digital cardiac imaging systems have been directed towards obtaining such measurements on-line during the catheterization procedure from video digitized images. With the present limitations in spatial resolution of these on-line digitized images, this approach is particularly of interest as a tool for diagnostic and/or therapeutic decision making during the catheterization procedure. However, with the use of modern small field-of-view (FOV) image intensifiers (4" and 5" FOV) and the increase in data transfer rates such that 1024^2 images at 30 frames/sec will become feasible, it may be possible in the near future to assess the effects of long-term interventions on-line using the diameter and densitometric cross-sectional area measures mentioned above.

In this chapter an overview will be given of the different techniques that are now available for the quantitative morphologic, densitometric and functional computer-aided analysis of the coronary obstructions (10).

3. IMAGE DIGITIZATION

Because of its inherently high resolution, 35 mm cinefilm has continued to be the medium of choice for the registration of interventional coronary angiograms. For the digitization of selected cineframes, basically two approaches have been taken: 1) a video camera-based system with optical magnification (10,11); and 2) a CCD camera with a high resolution linear CCD-array that is mechanically scanned over the projected image (10).

The CCD-camera cinefilm digitizer is a standard cineprojector (Tagarno 35 CX) with a field-installable modification package for high resolution digitization of a selected cineframe. This modification package consists of a film guiding system, a specially developed optical chain and a linear array (1728 elements) CCD camera; the array can be moved mechanically over a total of 2846 positions. The monochromatic light source consists of an array of LED's optimally suitable for densitometric analysis of the cinefilm. Any area of 6.9 x 6.9 mm in a selected cineframe (size 18 x 24 mm) can be digitized by the CCD-camera with a resolution of 512 x 512 pixels with 8 bits of grey levels. Effectively, this means that the entire cineframe of size 18 x24 mm can be digitized at a resolution of 1329 x 1772 pixels. A homogeneity in the brightness distribution over the entire digitized image of better than 5% has been achieved (12).

The currently commercially available digital cardiac imaging systems allow 512 x 512 matrix acquisitions at 30 frames/sec and 1024 x 1024 matrix acquisitions at max. 7 frames/sec, although the 30 frames/sec 1024^2 acquisitions have been announced already by a number of companies. In general, plumbicon video tubes with a gamma=1, with either interlaced or noninterlaced scanning systems have been used. For high resolution digitization noninterlaced (progressive) scanning should be used with preferably 10 bits of density resolution.

4. CALIBRATION

To compute absolute sizes of the arterial segment analyzed, a calibration factor needs to be determined. Basically, two different approaches have been in use for the coronary arteries: (1) analytically from geometric X-ray system parameters; (2) on the basis of the known diameter of the contrast catheter. Following the first approach, the size of an object in the plane through the center of rotation of the X-ray system (isocenter) and parallel to the image intensifier input screen can be determined from simple geometric principles from the height levels of X-ray tube and image intensifier. Wollschlaeger et al. have developed a method to calculate the exact radiological magnification factors for each point in the fields of view of biplane multidirectional isocentric X-ray equipment (13). By this approach they avoid two error sources: contour detection of the catheter segment, and the differential magnification of the scaling device and the arterial segment.

If the catheter is used as a scaling device, the contours of a short segment of the tip or shaft may either be defined manually with a writing tablet, or contour detection techniques similar to those used for the coronary segments may be applied.

If the known size of the catheter in a single angiographic view is used for calibration purposes, the computed calibration factor is only applicable to objects in the plane of the catheter parallel to the image intensifier input screen. The change in magnification for two objects located at different points along the X-ray beam axis is about 1.5% for each centimeter that separates the objects axially with the commonly used focus-image intensifier distances. For coronary segments lying in other planes corrections to the calibration factor can be assessed from other views.

From the above it is clear, that for the measurement of truly absolute sizes of coronary segments, two views, preferably but not necessarily orthogonal to each other, are required. However, if one is only interested in the changes in sizes of coronary segments as a result of long- or short-term interventions, excellent results can be achieved from single plane views. For these situations one must make sure that for the repeat angiogram the X-ray system is positioned in exactly the same geometry as during the first angiogram. This requires registration of the angles and height levels of the X-ray system, preferably on-line with a microprocessor-based geometry read-out system (14). Although the calibration factor used for a particular coronary arterial segment is then only an approximation of the true calibration factor, the same systematic error will be present for the first and repeat angiograms.

5. PINCUSHION DISTORTION AND CORRECTION

It is well-known that particularly the older types of image intensifiers introduce a geometric distortion, the socalled pincushion distortion. This results in selective magnification of an object near the edges of the image as compared to its size in the center of the field. These differences need to be corrected for, if absolute diameter measurements are to be derived from coronary angiograms. The standard procedure to assess the degree of distortion present is to film a cm-grid, which is positioned against the input screen of the image intensifier. This needs to be done only once for a given image intensifier tube at each of the available magnification modes.

We have developed a procedure that allows the fully automated detection of the wires and intersection points in the 1:1 projected cineframe. For a given point in the image which does not coincide with one of the displayed intersection positions, the correction vector is determined by means of bilinear interpolation between the correction vectors of the four neighboring intersection points. The contour positions of the catheter and coronary segments can be corrected for the pincushion distortion by means of these correction vectors.

6. CONTOUR DETECTION CORONARY ARTERIAL SEGMENT

For the computer-assisted definition of the boundaries of a selected coronary segment, in general, the following steps can be distinguished: 1) definition global centerline of coronary segment; 2) edge enhancement; 3) contour definition. The different implementations of these steps will be discussed in some more detail in the following paragraphs.

6.1 Definition global centerline

Edge positions of coronary segments in the digitized images can best be detected along scanlines perpendicular to the local centerline direction of the segment. For these purposes the first step in the contour detection algorithm requires the definition of the global trajectory of the centerline. In general, two approaches have been advocated: 1) the user-definition of the global centerline; and 2) automated tracking of the centerline.

The user-interactive approach requires that the operator defines a midline estimate for the arterial segment to be analyzed by indicating a few center points along the vessel by means of a sonic pen or writing tablet (10,15). This centerline is then smoothed and defines the scanlines perpendicular to the local centerline directions for the computation of the edge positions. Several groups have advocated to update this centerline by a new centerline computed from the contour positions once these have been detected and to repeat the contour detection procedure. By means of this iterative approach the influence of the user definition of the center points on the detected contour positions can be minimized.

Barth et al. and Le Free et al. have developed automated tracking procedures for the centerline (16,17).

6.2 Edge enhancement

Edge enhancement of the digitized data is usually based on the application of first or second derivative functions or a combination of these two. In general, these derivative functions are applied to the individual scanlines perpendicular to the local centerline directions and the edge positions are subsequently defined on the basis of a given contour definition criterion.

6.3 Contour definition

To date there does not seem to be a generally accepted contour detection technique; each research group has developed and used their own algorithm. In general, one can distinguish between local and global edge definition procedures. With the local procedure the edge points are defined on a scanline by scanline basis, possibly using expectation windows or the like to limit the search regions (11,15-18). With the global procedures, all the intensity and/or derivative information along the arterial segment are taken into account in the definition of the arterial contour (10).

This global approach is less sensitive to intervening structures such as branches and overlying structures than the local approach. In our laboratory, the global contour detection procedure is performed iteratively: following the first iteration of the contour detection procedure and if necessary, the manual correction of erroneous contour points, a new centerline is computed as the midline of the detected points and the contour detection procedure is repeated, resulting in the final arterial boundaries (10).

Following contour definition, by whatever technique, a smoothing procedure is usually applied to each of the detected contour paths, which may consist of a least-squares error first degree polynomial fit through a number of nearest points on each side of the edge point under consideration. On the basis of these smoothed contours, quantitative data about the arterial dimensions can be obtained in the contour analysis phase. An example of automatically detected contours along the middle portion of an LAD-segment is shown in Fig. 1.

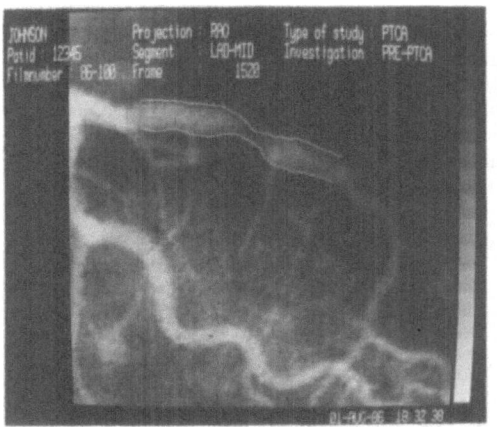 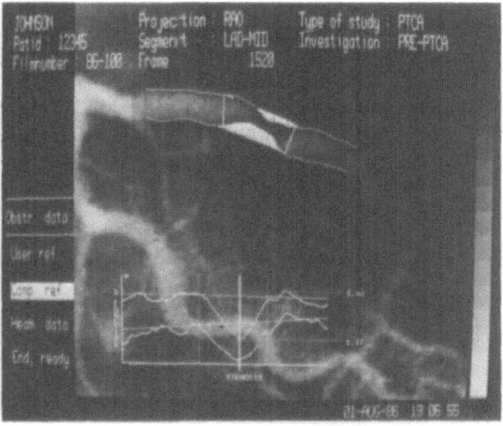

FIGURE 1. Example of magnified portion of a mid LAD-segment in the RAO-view, with automatically detected boundaries.

FIGURE 2. For the example of Fig. 1 the estimated pre-disease dimensions of the vessel at the site of the obstruction (reference edges) have been calculated. The upper function is the diameter function with the straight line through it being the reference diameter function; the lower function is the densitometric area function.

7. CONTOUR ANALYSIS

From the contours of the analyzed arterial segment, following pincushion correction and calibration, a diameter function can be determined by computing the distances between the left and right edges. Particularly the minimal obstruction diameter is of great importance as it is present to the inverse fourth power in the formulas describing the pressure loss over a coronary obstruction. Moreover, to determine the effect of interventions on the severity of coronary obstructions, one should compute the changes in minimal obstruction diameter and not those in percentage diameter narrowing, as the reference position in general will also be affected by the intervention.

The usual way to determine percentage diameter (D) stenosis of a coronary obstruction, requires the user to indicate a reference position in the arterial segment. It is clear that this computed %-D narrowing of an obstruction depends heavily on the selected reference position. In arteries with a focal obstructive lesion and a clearly normal proximal arterial segment, the choice of the reference region is straightforward and simple. However, in cases where the proximal part of the arterial segment shows combinations of stenotic and ectatic areas, the choice may be very difficult. To minimize these variations, the interpolated or computer-defined reference technique has been developed (10). By this method an estimate of the normal or pre-disease arterial size and luminal wall location is obtained; tapering of the vessel to account for a decrease in arterial caliber associated with branches is taken care of. The reference diameter is now taken as the value of the reference diameter function at the location of the minimal obstruction diameter. An example of this technique is shown in Fig. 2 for the obstruction of Fig. 1. The actual luminal contours of the arterial segment (inner contours) are superimposed in the image as well as the estimated pre-disease reference contours (outer contours). The difference in area between the reference and the detected luminal contours is marked over the obstructive lesion; this area is a measure for the atherosclerotic plaque in this particular angiographic view. The upper function is the diameter function with the straight line being the reference diameter function; the lower function is the densitometric area function (see section Densitometry).

In addition, this interpolated or computer defined reference diameter technique allows the assessment of the symmetry or asymmetry of the lesion in a given view. The symmetry measure is given as a value between 0 and 1, with 1 representing a concentric lesion and 0 the most severe case of asymmetry or eccentricity.

From the available morphological data of the obstruction, the Poisseuille and turbulent resistances at different flows and thus the resulting transstenotic pressure gradients can be computed on the basis of the well-known fluid-dynamic equations (8,10).

For the example of Fig. 2, the following quantitative measurements were obtained:

extent obstruction	:	7.51 mm	symmetry measure	:	0.53
reference diameter	:	3.16 mm	diameter stenosis	:	63.1 %
obstruction diameter	:	1.17 mm	area stenosis (densito-		
reference area (assuming			metric)	:	89.4 %
circular cross section)	:	7.86 mm^2	transstenotic pressure		
obstruction area (densi-			gradient at mean flow		
tometric)	:	0.84 mm^2	of 1 ml/s	:	3.04 mmHg
area atherosclerotic					
plaque	:	9.90 mm^2			

Information about the "roughness" of the arterial segment and thus about diffuse coronary artery disease may be obtained by subdividing the coronary segment into an integer number of subsegments with a length of approximately 5 mm and calculating for each subsegment the minimal, maximal, mean diameter and the standard deviation of the diameter values. The standard deviation is possibly a measure for diffuse atherosclerosis; clinical validation procedures need to be carried out to determine the true value of this parameter. On the basis of the ratio of the standard deviation value and the difference between minimal and maximal diameter, it can be determined whether a subsegment is focally or diffusely diseased, or normal. Fig. 3 shows the four subsegments for the example of Fig. 1; the derived subsegmental data are given in Table I.

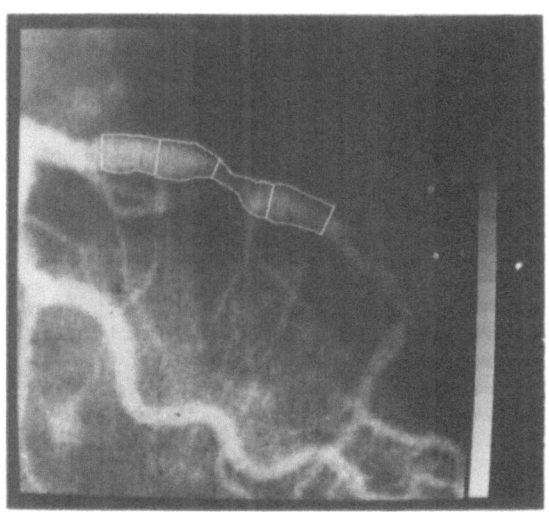

FIGURE 3. To obtain information about the "roughness" (irregularities) of the arterial segment, the segment is subdivided into a integer number of subsegments with lengths of approximately 5 mm and for each subsegment the ratio of the standard deviation and the difference between minimal and maximal diameter is computed. The subsegmental data for this example are presented in Table I.

TABLE I. Subsegmental data for the example of Fig. 3. Segment no. 1 is the most proximal segment.

Segment	1	2	3	4
Length (mm)	5.51	5.51	5.51	5.51
Minimal diam. (mm)	2.92	1.74	1.17	2.68
Maximal diam. (mm)	3.29	3.27	3.03	3.40
Mean diam. (mm)	3.04	2.85	2.02	2.99
Stand. dev. (mm)	0.12	0.48	0.69	0.24
Focal or Diffuse Disease	NO	YES	YES	NO

8. DENSITOMETRY

Since the luminal cross section at a coronary obstruction is frequently irregular in shape, percentage diameter reduction measured in a single angiographic view is of limited diagnostic value. The hemodynamic resistance of an obstruction is determined to a great extent by the minimal cross-sectional area. Computation of this cross-sectional area reduction from the percentage diameter reduction measured in a single view requires the assumption of, e.g., circular cross sections, an assumption which hardly ever holds. The resulting error may be reduced by incorporating two orthogonal projections and computing elliptical cross sections. However, with the often occurring eccentric lesions even this last approach may yield inaccurate results.

Several groups have attempted to derive relationships between the path lengths of the X-rays through the artery and the absolute brightness values in the digitized image; by such densitometric approach one would obtain the information required to compute the cross-sectional areas from a single angiographic view (10,19-22). It is clear that a homogeneous mixing of the contrast agent with the blood must be assumed for the measurement to have any meaning.

Most authors assume that the X-ray absorption process, comprising the first part of the imaging chain from X-ray source to the image intensifier input screen, can be described by the Lambert-Beer law. In general, for the remaining subsystems of the cinefilm imaging chain comprising the image intensifier, the cinefilm exposure and development process, and the film sampling process which may be achieved via video A/D conversion, with a CCD camera or other device, simplified transfer functions are used neglecting the influence of spatially nonhomogeneous responses. By this approach the response of film exposure, the density D versus log (exposure) curve, is being linearized (linear transfer function).

On the other hand, Doriot et al. have developed a physical model which takes the polychromasy and scattered X-ray radiation into account and have shown that this relation can be approximated by a 2nd order polynomial (20). The coefficients of this polynomial depend primarily on the voltage applied to the X-ray tube and on the iodine concentration of the injected contrast medium. For a particular X-ray system the coefficients of the polynomial can simply be obtained once by means of a linear wedge filled with contrast material.

We have attempted to correct for the nonlinearities in the D versus log (E) plot and for the daily variations in the cinefilm processing (10,19). For this purpose, a special sensitometer has been developed which allows 21 full cineframes covering the entire densitometric range of the film to be exposed on each film cassette before it is mounted on the image intensifier of the X-ray system immediately prior to the angiographic procedure (Fig. 4). The color temperature of the light source in the sensitometer is approximately equal to that of the output screen of the image intensifier. The analysis procedure of a coronary cineangiogram therefore starts with the digitization of these 21 sensitometric frames, allowing the assessment of a nonlinear transfer function.

By means of this calibration procedure many nonlinear, both temporally and spatially variant effects in the film-processing and the film-video or film-CCD camera system are taken into account. It has indeed been shown that this sensitometric approach improves the accuracy of measurement of cross-sectional area measurements as compared to the linear approach (23).

In a digital cardiac system, the transfer function from the output of the image intensifier up to the digitized image can be assumed to be a linear function.

The basic steps in the densitometric procedure to compute percentage cross-sectional area reduction of a selected lesion can be summarized as follows (Fig. 5). The contours of a selected arterial segment are detected as described before. On each scanline perpendicular to the centerline, a profile of brightness values is measured. This profile is transformed into

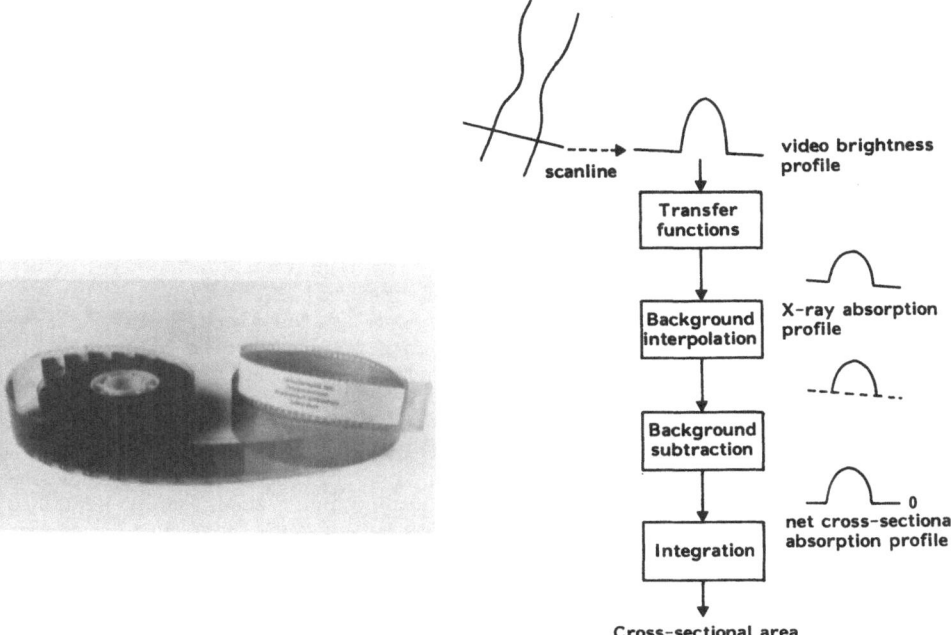

FIGURE 4. Example of cinefilm with
sensitometric strip of 21 homoge-
neously exposed cineframes.

FIGURE 5. Flow diagram of the densitometric analysis procedure.

an absorption profile by means of the computed transfer functions (linear
or nonlinear depending on the technique used). The background contribution
is estimated by computing the linear regression line through the background points directly left and right of the detected contours. Subtraction of this background portion from the absorption profile within the
arterial contours yields the net cross-sectional absorption profile. Integration of this function results in a measure for the cross-sectional
area at the particular scanline. By repeating this procedure for all the
scanlines, the cross-sectional area function A(i) is obtained. Percentage
area reduction of an obstruction is determined by comparing the minimal
area value at the obstruction with the mean value at a selected reference
position. The earlier mentioned interpolated approach can also be applied
for the estimation of the pre-disease area values. If we assume that the
cross section at the reference position is circular, absolute cross sectional values (in mm^2) along the arterial segment and thus for the minimal
cross section can be obtained.

The lower function in the example of Fig. 2 is the densitometric area
function for this segment. A percentage densitometric cross sectional area
reduction of 89.4% was found, indicating that the obstruction is slightly
more severe than one would estimate by assuming a circular obstruction
cross-sectional area (86% area reduction).

It will be clear that the densitometric analysis of coronary arterial
segments is a complex problem because of all the potential problems that

may arise. In addition to all the possible error sources mentioned above, another important aspect is the orientation of the vessel of interest with respect to the X-ray beam. In addition, sidebranches or branches lying very close to the arterial segment to be analyzed will cause errors in the background correction technique. Although various phantom studies have been published on the densitometric analysis of obstructions, until to date not a single technique has been validated in a well-designed in-vivo study.

9. APPROACHES TOWARDS STANDARDIZATION IN ANGIOGRAPHIC DATA ACQUISITION AND ANALYSIS

Our quantitative analysis approach has been validated extensively (10, 24). The accuracy and precision of the edge detection procedure as assessed from cinefilms of contrast-filled acrylate models were found to be -30 m and 90 m, respectively. The variability of the quantitative analysis procedure itself determined by repeatedly analyzing a set of clinical coronary cineangiograms was less than 0.12 mm for absolute arterial dimensions and 3.94% for the interpolated percentage diameter stenosis measurement. The variabilities in the measurements with repeated cineangiographies and analyses depend heavily on the number of precautions taken. For the best-controlled study, the variability in minimal obstruction diameters was found to be 0.22 mm and 7.23% for the interpolated percentage diameter stenosis. The absolute variability measures will increase dramatically if the angiographic technique is not carried out properly.

Therefore, the following approaches towards standardization in the angiographic data acquisition procedure have been proposed:

- Precise registration of the angulations of the X-ray system for the different angiographic views, so that the repeat angiographies can be performed in the same views as used in the first angiographic investigation.
- Administration of a vasodilative drug immediately prior to angiographic investigations.
- Use of modern isoviscous and iso-osmolar contrast agents.
- Administration of contrast medium preferably by ECG-triggered injector.
- Selection of contrast catheter constructed of such material that high quality image results (high angiographic image contrast and edge gradient).
- Measurement of actual size catheter with micrometer following the catheterization procedure.

10. FUNCTIONAL SIGNIFICANCE OF A CORONARY OBSTRUCTION

In the previous sections different techniques have been described for the assessment of the anatomic severity of a coronary obstruction. These approaches are well suited to determine the morphologic effects of interventions. However, from a clinical or physiologic point of view it is of great interest to know to what extent a coronary obstruction limits the blood flow to the perfused area of the myocardial muscle, i.e. the question is raised: what is the functional significance of the obstruction.

An essential concept relating stenosis anatomy to its functional effects is that of coronary flow reserve. It is defined as the ratio of maximum coronary flow after a maximal vasodilatory stimulus to resting flow. Under resting conditions, coronary blood flow in an artery does not change until a relatively tight stenosis of 80-85% diameter narrowing. However, coronary flow reserve is impaired at 40-50% diameter narrowing, whereas flow in a normal artery increases three to four times in response to a vasodilatory stimulus such as pharmacologic coronary vasodilators, a brief coronary occlusion or physical stress.

Poor correlations have been found between coronary flow reserve and percent diameter narrowing in human coronary artery disease. Absolute cross-sectional area has been suggested as a better parameter; however, for the individual patient this parameter does not seem to have sufficient predictive accuracy either. Therefore, other approaches have been developed to determine the functional significance more reliably.

Gould et al. have derived a relation between coronary perfusion pressure, coronary flow reserve and the severity of stenosis (8,25). By accounting for all stenosis dimensions of length, absolute diameter, relative percent narrowing and asymmetry, the relation between the pressure gradient across the stenosis and coronary flow can be derived on the basis of standard fluid-dynamic equations. As a result, the distal coronary perfusion pressure-flow relation can be predicted from the stenosis dimensions for any given aortic pressure.

In a graph relating normalized coronary perfusion pressure and coronary flow times the base-line control value, the intersection of this coronary perfusion pressure-flow relation with a straight line denoting the normal, experimentally observed relation between coronary perfusion pressure and flow under conditions of maximal coronary vasodilation in the absence of a stenosis, gives the coronary flow reserve for a given stenosis (8,25). This interesting approach still requires further validation in human coronary artery disease.

Another approach to determine the coronary flow reserve is based on the determination of contrast medium appearance time in myocardial regions of

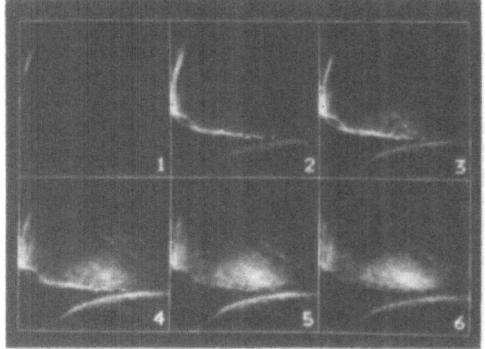 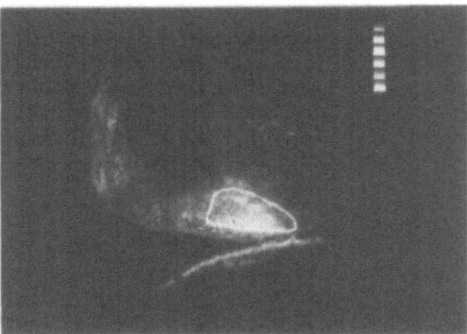

FIGURE 6. End-diastolic cineframes, digitized in 512 x 512 eight-bit matrices from 6 consecutive heart beats following contrast injection. Stationary background structures were eliminated by means of logarithmic mask-mode background subtraction using the ED-cineframe acquired prior to contrast administration as a mask.

FIGURE 7. Contrast Medium Appearance Picture (CMAP) in hyperemic state with user-defined ROI. (Black/white reproduction of color coded functional image.)

interest and of the corresponding vascular volume at baseline and after hyperemia. The timing and density of a selectively injected contrast medium bolus as it traverses the coronary circulation can be depicted in dual parameter color coded functional images. This technique has been advocated by R.A. Vogel et al. (9). Although it is usually applied to digitally acquired images, we have used the technique on 35 mm cineframes (26).

The parametric imaging technique uses atrial pacing to regularize cycle length to provide optimal interframe registration and selective, ECG-gated, power contrast medium injection to standardize the timing and flow rates of the contrast bolus. Five to eight end-diastolic (ED) cineframes are selected for digitization from successive cardiac cycles. These cineframes are digitized at a resolution of 512x512 pixels and 256 grey levels. The digitized images are corrected for the dark current of the video-camera. Logarithmic mask-mode background subtraction is applied to the unique subset to eliminate non-contrast medium densities. The last ED-cineframe prior to the contrast administration is chosen as a mask. An example of a series of 6 consecutive background subtracted ED-cineframes is shown in Fig. 6.

From the sequence of background subtracted cineframes, an appearance time picture is generated using a fixed threshold (12%) in pixel brightness level. The individual pixels in this image are color coded, based on the sequence number of the heart cycle in which the pixel intensity for the first time exceeds the threshold, starting from the beginning of the ECG-triggered contrast injection.

The relative regional vascular volume is calculated from a maximum intensity image, which is also generated from the sequence of background subtracted cineangiograms. Each picture element in this regional volume image represents the maximal pixel intensity level found within the series of images.

From the appearance time picture and the maximum intensity image a dual parameter Contrast Medium Appearance Picture (CMAP) can be generated, in which the color denotes the appearance time and the intensity of the color the vascular volume. Within a user-defined Region-of-Interest (ROI) mean contrast intensity and appearance time can be computed (Fig. 7).

Such CMAP's are generated in the basal and hyperemic states. To compute the hyperemic CMAP, the coronary angiogram is repeated 30 sec. after a bolus injection of 10 mg papaverine into the coronary artery. The coronary flow reserve (CFR) is then calculated by the following equation:

$$ CFR = \frac{\text{vascular volume}_h}{\text{appearance-time}_h} \cdot \cdot \frac{\text{vascular volume}_b}{\text{appearance-time}_b} \text{ , with} $$

h= hyperemia and b= baseline.

11. CLINICAL RESULTS CFR-MEASUREMENTS FROM PARAMETRIC IMAGES

The CMAP technique was applied to seventeen coronary arteries of patients with single vessel coronary artery disease (CAD) and 6 coronary arteries of patients without CAD. The 17 coronary artery lesions were all single discrete stenoses in the proximal parts of the vessels before any sidebranch occurred. The anatomic severity of the coronary obstructions was determined with our Cardiovascular Angiography Analysis System (CAAS); the minimal cross-sectional area (MLCA, mm^2) and the area stenosis (AS,%) were assessed for each stenosis from an average of 2.3 angiographic projections. The relation between CFR and MLCA was best described by the quadratic equation:

$$CFR = 0.28 + 0.91 \text{ MLCA} - 0.039 \text{ (MLCA)}^2, \quad r = 0.92,$$

and the relation between CFR and AS by:

$$CFR = 5.0 - 3.3(AS \times 10^{-2}) - 1.3(AS \times 10^{-2})^2, \quad r = 0.92.$$

The investigated vessels were divided into three categories on the basis of both AS and MLCA (Table II). The 6 normal coronary arteries were compared with the 6 coronary arteries with an AS between 50% and 70% and a MLCA between 2 and 4.5 mm^2 (moderate CAD) and with the 11 coronary arteries with an AS in excess of 70% and a MLCA less than 2 mm^2 (severe CAD). The vessels with severe CAD had a mean CFR of 1.0 (s.d. ± 0.3) and differed highly significantly (p= 0.001) from the CFR of the vessels with moderate CAD, who had a mean CFR of 2.6 (s.d. ± 0.7). The difference between the normal vessels (CFR = 5.0 ± 1.0) and the vessels with moderate CAD was also highly significant (p $< 10^{-4}$).

TABLE II. Relation between quantitative assessed coronary artery dimensions and CFR.

	CAD		normals
	severe N = 11	moderate N = 6	N = 6
MLCA	< 2 mm^2	2-4.5 mm^2	> 4.5 mm^2
AS	> 70%	50-70%	0%
CFR (mean ± SD)	1.0 ± 0.3	2.6 ± 0.7	5.0 ± 1.0
		p = 0.001	p $< 10^{-4}$

Although these results look very promising, it must be realized that in the two-dimensional images there does not exist a one-to-one relation between a coronary segment and the corresponding myocardial region that is perfused by that segment. Overprojections with other regions may occur. Therefore, at the present time we are studying the possibilities of three-dimensional reconstruction of the myocardium from two orthogonal projections to overcome such problems.

ACKNOWLEDGEMENTS

The author wishes to thank Elfrieda van den Ende and Ria Kanters-Stam for their secretarial assistance in the preparation of this manuscript.

REFERENCES

1. Serruys PW, Reiber JHC, Wijns W, Brand M van den, Kooijman CJ, Katen HJ ten, Hugenholtz PG: Assessment of percutaneous transluminal coronary angioplasty by quantitative coronary angiography: diameter versus densitometric area measurements. Amer J Cardiol 54, 1984: 482-488.
2. Serruys PW, Arnold AER, Brower RW, Bono DP de, Bokslag M, Lubsen J, Reiber JHC, Rutsch W, Uebis R, Vahanian A, Verstraete M: Effect of continued rt-PA administration on the residual stenosis after initially successful recanalization in acute myocardial infarction - a quantitative coronary angiography study of a randomized trial. (Submitted to Eur Heart J)

132

3. Puel J, Sigwart U, Joffre F, Rousseau H, Courtault A, Bounhoure JP, Wallstén H: Percutaneously implantable endo-coronary prosthesis: preliminary results in the treatment of post-dilatation re-stenosis. JACC 9, 1987: 106A (abstract).
4. Isner JM, Clarke RH: Laser angioplasty: unraveling the Gordian Knot. JACC 7, 1986: 705-708.
5. Slager CJ, Essed CA, Schuurbiers JCH, Bom N, Serruys PW, Meester GT: Vaporization of atherosclerotic plaques by spark erosion. J Am Coll Cardiol 5, 1985: 1382-1386.
6. Serruys PW, Lablanche JM, Reiber JHC, Bertrand ME, Hugenholtz PG: Contribution of dynamic vascular wall thickening to luminal narrowing during coronary arterial vasomotion. Z Kardiol 72, 1983: 116-123.
7. Arntzenius AC, Kromhout D, Barth JD, Reiber JHC, Bruschke AVG, Buis B, Gent CM van, Kempen-Voogd N, Strikwerda S, Velde EA van der: Diet, lipoproteins, and the progression of coronary atherosclerosis. The Leiden Intervention Trial. N Engl J Med 312, 1985: 805-811.
8. Gould KL, Kirkeeide RL: Assessment of stenosis severity. In: State of the Art in Quantitative Coronary Arteriography. JHC Reiber, PW Serruys (Eds), Martinus Nijhoff Publishers, Dordrecht/Boston/Lancaster, 1986: 209-228.
9. Vogel RA: The radiographic assessment of coronary blood flow parameters. Circulation 72, 1985: 460-465.
10. Reiber JHC, Serruys PW, Slager CJ: Quantitative coronary and left ventricular cineangiography; methodology and clinical applications. Martinus Nijhoff Publishers, Boston/Dordrecht/Lancaster, 1986.
11. Sanders WJ, Alderman EL, Harrison DC: Coronary artery quantitation using digital image processing techniques. Comp Cardiol 1979: 15-20.
12. Kooijman CJ, Kalberg R, Slager CJ, Tijdens FO, Plas van der J, Reiber JHC: Densitometric analysis of coronary arteries. In: Signal Processing III: Theories and Applications. IT Young, J Biemond, RPW Duin, JJ Gerbrands (Eds), North-Holland, Amsterdam/New York/Oxford/Tokyo, 1986: 1405-1408.
13. Wollschlaeger H, Lee P, Zeiher A, Solzbach U, Bonzel T, Just H: Improvement of quantitative angiography by exact calculation of radiological magnification factors. Comp Cardiol 1985: 483-486.
14. Reiber JHC, Serruys PW, Kooijman CJ, Slager CJ, Schuurbiers JCH, Boer A den: Approaches towards standardization in acquisition and quantitation of arterial dimensions from cineangiograms. In: State of the Art in Quantitative Coronary Arteriography. JHC Reiber, PW Serruys (Eds), Martinus Nijhoff Publishers, Dordrecht/Boston/Lancaster, 1986: 145-172.
15. Selzer RH, Shircore A, Lee PL, Hemphill DH, Blankenhorn DH: A second look at quantitative coronary angiography: some unexpected problems. In: State of the Art in Quantitative Coronary Arteriography. JHC Reiber, PW Serruys (Eds), Martinus Nijhoff Publishers, Dordrecht/Boston/Lancaster, 1986: 125-144.
16. Barth K, Epple E, Irion KM, Faust U, Decker D: Quantifizierung von Stenosen der Herzkranzgefässe durch Digitale Bildauswertung. Erg Bd Biomed Technik 26, 1981.
17. LeFree M, Simon SB, Lewis RJ, Bates ER, Vogel RA: Digital radiographic coronary artery quantification. Comp Cardiol 1985: 99-102.
18. Kirkeeide RL, Fung P, Smalling RW, Gould KL: Automated evaluation of vessel diameter from arteriograms. Comp Cardiol 1982: 215-218.

19. Reiber JHC, Slager CJ, Schurrbiers JCH, Boer A den, Gerbrands JJ, Troost GJ, Scholts B, Kooijman CJ, Serruyw PW: Transfer functions of the X-ray-cine-video chain applied to digital processing of coronary cineangiograms. In: Digital Imaging in Cardiovascular Radiology. PH Heintzen, R Brennecke (Eds), Georg Thieme Verlag, Stuttgart, 1983: 89-104.
20. Doriot P-A, Pochon Y, Rasoamanambelo L, Chatelain P, Welz R, Rutishauser W: Densitometry of coronary arteries - an improved physical model. Comp Cardiol 1985: 91-94.
21. Sandor T, Als AV, Paulin S: Cine-densitometric measurement of coronary arterial stenoses. Cath Cardiovasc Diagn 5, 1979: 229-245.
22. Nichols AB, Gabrieli CFO, Fenoglio JJ, Esser P: Quantification of relative coronary arterial stenosis by cinevideodensitometric analysis of coronary arteriograms. Circ 69, 1984: 512-522.
23. Reiber JHC, Kooijman CJ, Slager CJ, Boer A den, Serruys PW: Improved densitometric assessment % area-stenosis from coronary cineangiograms. X World Congress of Cardiology, Washington, 1986: 39 (Abstract).
24. Reiber JHC, Serruys PW, Kooijman CJ, Wijns W, Slager CJ, Gerbrands JJ, Schuurbiers JCH, Boer A den, Hugeholtz PG: Assessment of short-, medium- and long-term variations in arterial dimensions from computer-assisted quantitation of coronary cineangiograms. Circ 71, 1985: 280-288.
25. Kirkeeide RL, Gould KL, Parsel L: Assessment of coronary stenoses by myocardial perfusion imaging during pharmacologic coronary vasodilation. VII. Validation of coronary flow reserve as a single integrated functional measure of stenosis severity reflecting all its geometric dimensions. JACC 7, 1986: 103-113.
26. Zijlstra F, Ommeren J van, Reiber JHC, Serruys PW: Does quantitative assessment of coronary artery dimensions predict the physiological significance of a coronary stenosis? Circulation (accepted for publication).

METABOLIC CONSEQUENCES OF MYOCARDIAL UNDERPERFUSION

A. VAN DER LAARSE

INTRODUCTION

In the healthy heart myocardial perfusion adapts itself to the work the heart exerts and the metabolic rate associated herewith. Under resting conditions myocardial blood flow is about 20% of the maximal value which is reached under maximal work load. The remaining 80% is often referred to as "reserve capacity". Several abnormal or pathological conditions diminish this "reserve capacity", either by reducing the maximal blood flow or by increasing the resting blood flow (Hoffman, 1984). To these conditions belong anemia, arterial hypoxia, myocardial hypertrophy and coronary artery stenosis. The present contribution deals with the metabolic consequences of myocardial ischemia. The methods to study specific ischemia-induced alterations of metabolic pathways are presented. Their value in diagnosis and therapy of ischemic heart disease is evaluated and discussed with emphasis to (future) use in a modern cardiology department.

Myocardial metabolic pathways
Normally, the main source of metabolic energy is free fatty acid (FFA). FFA is taken up by the myocyte, shuttled into the mitochondria and oxidized in a pathway often referred to as β-oxidation. In this pathway NAD^+ and FAD are cofactors receiving reducing equivalents. In the respiratory chain the reduced cofactors ($NADH + H^+$ and $FADH_2$) are oxidized again and the electrons are passed through Coenzyme Q and several cytochromes to oxygen, which is converted to H_2O. The free energy liberated in the chain of redox reactions is conserved by the phosphorylation of ADP to ATP. A high (or low) mitochondrial ATP/ADP ratio has an inhibitory (or stimulating) effect on the turnover of the respiratory chain.
Another metabolic substrate, not as important as FFA normally, is glucose which is converted to pyruvate in a pathway called glycolysis. Glucose moieties can also be stored within the myocyte as glycogen, which is an endogenous fuel store to be called upon under several circumstances like β-adrenoceptor stimulation (via an intracellular cAMP concentration rise), hypoxia and ischemia. In the conversion of glucose (a C6-sugar) to pyruvate (a C3-sugar) NAD^+ is the acceptor of reducing equivalents. Normally, glycolysis and glycogenolysis are partly inhibited, predominantly due to a high cytoplasmic ATP/ADP ratio.

Effects of ischemia on β-oxidation and glycolysis
One of the first consequences of myocardial metabolism under ischemic conditions is the rise of the $NADH/NAD^+$ ratio, probably due to a shortage of oxygen as a electron acceptor in the respiratory chain. The involvement of NAD^+ and FAD in the β-oxidation causes this pathway to slow down. Via con-

version of pyruvate to lactate, which produces 1 molecule of NAD$^+$ per molecule of pyruvate, glyco(geno)lysis can proceed. Mild ischemia even stimula-
tes glyco(geno)lysis by removing the partial inhibition by a high ATP/ADP
ratio. Therefore, under conditions of mild ischemia a slowed β-oxidation in
combination with a stimulated glyco(geno)lysis may produce sufficient ATP
to maintain vital functions of the myocardium involved, although contractile function may be depressed to some degree.
Severe ischemia brings β-oxidation to a stop and causes only a transient
stimulation of glyco(geno)lysis. The inhibition of glyco(geno)lysis after a
short period of stimulation is caused by two factors mainly: glycogen depletion and intracellular acidosis. Acidosis is the outcome of severe ATP
hydrolysis and massive lactate formation. Glycogen depletion and massive
lactate formation are also responsible for the increase of intracellular
osmolarity and intracellular edema. Cell swelling may be the factor responsible for ischemia-induced progressive increase of coronary vascular
resistance, presumably at the capillary level. Fig. 1 gives a schematic
representation of the derangement of several metabolic processes induced by
myocardial underperfusion.

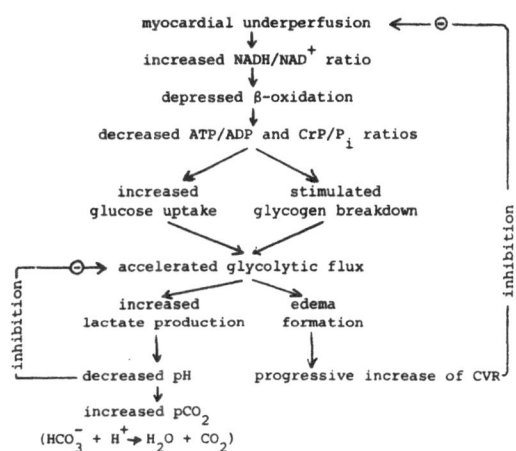

FIGURE 1. Schematic representation of the effects of myocardial underperfusion on myocardial metabolism. Abbreviations: ATP: adenosine triphosphate;
ADP: adenosine diphosphate; CrP: creatine phosphate; P_i: anorganic phosphate; CVR: coronary vascular resistance; pCO_2: partial pressure of carbon
dioxide. NADH/NAD$^+$ is the ratio of reduced and oxidized nicotinamide
dinucleotide concentrations.

Table 1 gives a survey of the metabolic compounds that can be monitored in
a heart perfused in vitro, or in the in vivo heart. The techniques involved
are mentioned for each compound listed.

ATP, CrP, H$^+$

^{31}P-NMR spectroscopy is usually carried out in hearts perfused in vitro. Three ATP peaks and one CrP peak can be obtained. Peak areas are measures of their respective intracellular concentrations. From the splicing of the anorganic phosphate (P$_i$) peak, often referred to as chemical shift, intracellular pH* can be calculated. A future application of in vivo myocardial pH measurement may be the diagnosis of rejection of the transplanted heart. Takach et al. (1986) recently published that rejection of transplanted cat hearts was associated with depression of myocardial pH. They reported a fall of 0.2 pH unit and 0.6 pH unit in mild rejection and severe rejection cases, respectively.

Table 1. Key compounds that can be followed during impairment of regional myocardial blood flow

compound	in vitro=1 in vivo=2	technique
ATP, CrP	1,2	^{31}P-NMR spectroscopy
H$^+$	1	^{31}P-NMR spectroscopy
H$_2$O	1,2	T2-relaxation time in MRI
FFA	1,2	^{11}C-label in PET
Glucose	1,2	^{18}F-DOG in PET
NADH	1	Fluorimetry
Lactate	1,2	Cardiac catheterisation,
	1	^{1}H-NMR spectroscopy
Pyruvate	1	^{14}C-label counter

Abbreviations: ATP: adenosine triphosphate; CrP: creatine phosphate; FFA: free fatty acid; NADH: reduced nicotinamide adenine dinucleotide; NMR: nuclear magnetic resonance; MRI: magnetic resonance imaging; PET: positron emission tomography; DOG: 2-deoxyglucose

A recent breakthrough is ^{31}P-NMR spectroscopy in canine and human hearts in vivo using a surface radiofrequency coil laid over the thorax. Chance et al. (1985) analyzed the relation between work load and CrP/P$_i$ ratio. While in the normal canine heart the CrP/P$_i$ ratio fell from 5 at normal work load to about 4 at ventricular tachycardia, the heart compromised by hypoxia or ischemia operates under reduced CrP/P$_i$ (about 2) at normal work load and falls to extremely low levels (0.6) during ventricular tachycardia. In children normally a CrP/P$_i$ ratio of 2.0 is found, whereas in a child with cardiomyopathy this ratio is around 1.0 (Whitman et al., 1985). By administration of glucose i.v. or after a meal enriched with glucose, the CrP/P$_i$ ratio in the child with cardiomyopathy increased to near-normal values of about 1.8. This technique will become of great importance in diagnosis and therapy of a wide variety of abnormalities in a number of organs, such as heart and liver.

Edema

Recently developed imaging facilities connected to the ^{1}H-NMR apparatus have been employed to distinguish normal from acutely infarcted myocardium. The increases of spin-echo signal intensity, as well as the increase of the T2-relaxation time in infarcted canine myocardium compared to non-infarcted areas of the same heart are considerable, and even much greater than the

*negative logarithm of H$^+$ concentration

increase in water content (Wesbey et al., 1984). Probably within some years this technique may enable the distinction between normal myocardium (normal water content), ischemic, and acutely infarcted myocardium (increased water content) and chronically infarcted myocardium (subnormal water content).

Free fatty acids, 2-deoxyglucose

Two extremely useful substrates have been tested extensively in hearts using the positron emission tomograph: ^{11}C-palmitate, a free fatty acid (FFA) and ^{18}F-deoxyglucose (DOG), a glucose analogon. Many efforts in the development and the evaluation of this technique have been made by Schelbert and coworkers. After i.v. administration of ^{11}C-palmitate myocardium takes up this substrate to reach maximum levels after about 4 min. In normal myocardium a higher maximum of label is observed than in ischemic myocardium. In the following 20 min label is cleared faster in normal than in ischemic myocardium. The fraction that is rapidly cleared is high (about 60%) in normal myocardium and much smaller (about 25%) in ischemic myocardium (Schelbert et al., 1983).

Long-lasting derangements of uptake and clearance of label after transient regional ischemia of the canine heart were detected using ^{11}C-palmitate (Schwaiger et al., 1985).

The group of Sobel and coworkers demonstrated that revascularization of an acutely occluded coronary artery in canine hearts by i.c. streptokinase infusion was associated with an increase of ^{11}C-palmitate uptake by the affected myocardium (Bergmann et al., 1982). The more the uptake increased to normal levels, the smaller was the infarct size: recanalization of the infarct-related coronary artery at 12-14 h after onset of infarction neither resulted in any increase of label uptake, nor was it associated with any limitation of infarct size.

2-Deoxyglucose is taken up by the myocyte, and phosphorylated to 2-deoxyglucose-6-phosphate (DOG-6-P) by the enzyme hexokinase, just like glucose. Contrary to glucose, DOG-6-P is not converted to DOG-1-P nor to 2-deoxyfructose-6-P. The intact sarcolemma, as present in normal and ischemic myocytes, is impermeable to DOG-6-P and other phosphorylated substances. So, once formed, DOG-6-P remains trapped within the myocyte. As glycolysis plays a minor role in normally functioning myocardium, glucose and DOG uptake rates are normally small. Ischemia is a strong stimulus for glucose and 2-deoxyglucose uptake, at least initially. But if prolonged underperfusion has turned ischemic myocardium into infarcted myocardium, glucose and DOG are not longer taken up.

With ^{18}F-labeled DOG Schelbert and coworkers demonstrated that ischemic human myocardium reveals underperfusion (visualized by ^{13}N-ammonia) associated with increased DOG uptake (Schelbert, 1986). The simulateneous presence of increased ^{18}F-DOG uptake and reduced perfusion is usually called a "mismatch". In infarcted myocardium underperfusion is associated with very low DOG-uptake, or no DOG-uptake at all ("match"). A fascinating observation is that in 34 myocardial segments of which infarction is diagnosed by the development of typical Q-waves, 22 segments show ^{18}F-DOG uptake. Of these 22 segments, 7 segments revealed a "mismatch" while in the remaining 15 segments the ^{18}F- DOG uptake was associated with the presence of perfusion. In the 12 segments showing no ^{18}F-DOG uptake no perfusion was observed (Schelbert, 1986). These results strongly suggest the presence of still viable myocardium in the infarcted area.

These diagnostic methods using labeled metabolites are very useful in diagnosing cardiac ischemia and infarction, and in evaluating the effects of early interventions like PTCA and thrombolysis. The costs of PET appara-

138

tus will, at least in the near future confine this technique to specialized centers.

Lactate

A valuable and relatively inexpensive technique to diagnose myocardial ischemia is the measurement of the plasma lactate concentration difference in aorta and sinus coronarius (Δ(A-CS)lactate). Lactate extraction and lactate production are presented by a positive or a negative value of the ratio Δ(A-CS)lactate/(A)lactate. By drawing blood from the great cardiac vein and from the aorta in patients whose infarct-related coronary artery was the left anterior descending artery, Hattori et al. (1985) demonstrated that local lactate extraction decreased, and lactate production increased with the extent of regional contractile impairment. Goldstein et al. (1980) who administered ^{14}C-pyruvate to isolated perfused rabbit hearts, showed that lactate accumulation (measured biochemically) in ischemic regions of the heart correlated with accumulation of label (measured in a radioactivity counter) in these segments.

Quite recently, myocardial lactate accumulation was measured by ^{1}H-NMR spectroscopy. Although in this spectrum many peaks are present which can not simply be ascribed to known compounds, the lactate peak can be recorded with Hahn spin-echo pulse sequences (Ugurbil et al., 1984). Using surface coils, it is theoretically possible to obtain ^{1}H-NMR spectra from in vivo human hearts. In the near future one may even expect the development of "lactate imaging" of the heart.

NADH

Some decades ago surface fluorimetry of exposed organs of living experimental animals was developed to measure intracellular NADH. Excited at a wavelength of 340 nm NADH emits light of a wavelength of 480 nm. With surface fluorimetry Mills et al. (1977) observed that coronary artery ligation induces an immediate increase of intracellular NADH concentration which decreases to a preischemic value after reperfusion.

The group of Renault and coworkers (1984) developed an optical fiber catheter through which light from a nitrogen laser (wavelength 337 nm) is introduced and through which the NADH fluorescence is conducted outward, and fed to a photomultiplier via a band-pass filter of 480 nm. The results published apply to epicardial NADH fluorescence of isolated buffer-perfused and blood-perfused rat hearts, but one may expect that in the near future results of in vivo applications, such as measurement of endocardial NADH fluorescence in in vivo hearts, will be published.

SUMMARY

The metabolic consequences of myocardial underperfusion have been studied extensively in experimental animals using in vitro biochemical methods. Recently, progress in technological developments allows measurement of ischemia-induced metabolic changes in hearts in vivo. Although at high costs, systems such as positron emission tomography (PET) and nuclear magnetic resonance (NMR) are currently available for these purposes. These methods will lead to a further change in the way the cardiologist approaches the abnormal heart: after the anatomic (localization and severity of stenosis) and dynamic approach (coronary flow and left ventricular function parameters) cardiology will become expanded with the biochemical approach. As biochemistry provides for the vital link between perfusion and contraction a "biochemical" diagnosis will add to the understanding of the pathological state of the heart, and "biochemical" monitoring will contribute to the evaluation of therapy.

REFERENCES

1. Bergmann SR, Lerch RA, Fox KAA, Ludbrook PA, Welch MJ, Ter-Pogossian MM, Sobel BE: Temporal dependence of beneficial effects of coronary thrombolysis characterized by positron tomography. Am. J. Med. 73:573-581, 1982.

2. Chance B, Clark BJ, Nioka S, Subramanian H, Maris JM, Argov Z, Bode H: Phosphorus nuclear magnetic resonance spectroscopy in vivo. Circulation 72 (suppl. IV): IV-103-IV-110, 1985.

3. Goldstein RA, Klein MS, Sobel BE: Detection of myocardial ischemia before infarction, based on accumulation of labeled pyruvate. J. Nucl. Med. 21:1101-1104, 1980.

4. Hattori R, Takatsu Y, Yui Y, Sakaguchi K, Susawa T, Murakami T, Tamaki S, Kawai C: Lactate metabolism in acute myocardial infarction and its relation to regional ventricular performance. J. Am. Coll. Cardiol. 5:1283-1291, 1985.

5. Hoffman JIE: Maximal coronary flow and the concept of coronary vascular reserve. Circulation 70:153-159, 1984.

6. Mills SA, Jöbsis FF, Seaber AV: A fluorometric study of oxidative metabolism in the in vivo canine heart during acute ischemia and hypoxia. Ann. Surg. 186:193-200, 1977.

7. Renault G, Raynal E, Sinet M, Muffat-Joly M, Berthier JP, Cornillault J, Godard B, Pocidalo JJ: In situ double-beam NADH laser fluorimetry: Choice of a reference wavelength. Am. J. Physiol 246:H491-H499, 1984.

8. Schelbert HR: Probing the heart's biochemistry with positron emission tomography. Jpn. Circ. J. 50:1-29, 1986.

9. Schelbert HR, Henze E, Keen R, Schon HR, Hansen H, Selin C, Huang SC, Barrio JR, Phelps ME: C-11 palmitate for the noninvasive evaluation of regional myocardial fatty acid metabolism with positron-computed tomography. IV. In vivo evaluation of acute demand-induced ischemia in dogs. Am. Heart J. 106:736-750, 1983.

10. Schwaiger M, Schelbert HR, Keen R, Vinten-Johansen J, Hansen H, Selin C, Barrio J, Huang SC, Phelps ME: Retention and clearance of C-11 palmitic acid in ischemica and reperfused canine myocardium. J. Am. Coll. Cardiol. 6:311-320, 1985.

11. Takach TJ, Glassman LR, Rodriguez ER, Falcone JT; Ferrans VJ, Clark RE: Acute rejection after cardiac transplantation: Detection by interstitial myocardial pH. Ann. Thorac. Surg. 42:619-626, 1986.

12. Ugurbil K, Petein M, Maidan R, Michurski S, Cohn JN, From AH: High resolution proton NMR studies of perfused rat hearts. FEBS Lett. 167:73-78, 1984.

13. Wesbey G, Higgings CB, Lanzer P, Botvinick E, Lipton MJ: Imaging and characterization of acute myocardial perfusion in vivo by gated nuclear magnetic resonance. Circulation 69:125-130, 1984.

14. Whitman GJR, Chance B, Bode H, Maris J, Haselgrove J, Kelley R, Clark BJ, Harken AH: Diagnosis and therapeutic evaluation of a pediatric case of cardiomyopathy using phosphorus-31 nuclear magnetic resonance spectroscopy. J. Am. Coll. Cardiol. 5:745-749, 1985.

EVALUATION OF MYOCARDIAL BLOOD FLOW WITH RADIONUCLIDE TECHNIQUES

E.E. van der Wall, E.K.J. Pauwels, A.V.G. Bruschke

Introduction

In recent years the use of radioactive tracers in clinical cardiology has become a routine procedure in the diagnosis and management of patients of cardiac disease. Radionuclide techniques have achieved a role equal in importance to electrocardiography, echocardiography, and cardiac catheterization. Broadly speaking, radionuclide techniques fall into two major categories: those concerned with the heart as a muscle and those concerned with the heart as a pump. Since this review regards the scintigraphic aspects of coronary artery perfusion, attention will mainly be focused on the techniques that deal with the heart as a muscle. Before entering these issues, some necessary technical information will be provided.

Cardiac instrumentation

Radionuclide imaging is performed with a gamma camera connected with a computer. The function of the gamma camera is to convert radioactivity into a pictorial representation. After uptake of a radioactive tracer in a specific organ, the gamma rays (photons) of the tracer are detected by the gamma camera, which finally produces electronic signals. The electronic signals are computed as X,Y signals and visualized on an oscilloscope on the camera console as well as sent to a computer for subsequent data analysis. The currently used gamma cameras can grosso modo be divided into 1) the conventional gamma camera, and 2) the positron camera. The conventional gamma camera is a stationary or mobile system with a field of view of 40 cm, which can easily be positioned over the chest cage of the patient. This type of camera is very well suited for routine procedures in large number of patients, because of the wide availability of gamma-emitting radioactive tracers and its relative low cost. A drawback is the difficulty of exactly quantitating radionuclide concentrations in tissue because of attenuation of radioactivity as a function of the distance between organ and camera.

The positron camera is a less widely available and rather expensive type of camera, and is therefore mostly used as a research tool. It employs one or multiple rings of detectors arranged in opposing pairs around the patient. Only positron-emitting radioactive tracers can be detected on the basis of positron-electron annihilation. Positrons are positively charged electrons which travel only a very short distance (less than 1 mm) to encounter an electron. When the positron and the electron combine, both are annihilated and the energy of the two particles is converted to two high energy photons (511 kiloelectronVolt) that are emitted 180° apart in opposite directions. Major advantages of this approach include accurate tomographic localization of regional events in organs, adequate correction for photon attenuation and therefore more reliable reflection of the quantity of activity within the heart than is obtained with conventional camera systems.

Radiopharmaceuticals

Radionuclides have three main characteristics:
(1) type of emission, i.e. radiation of alpha, beta, gamma or positron rays, (2) level of energy expressed in kiloelectronVolt (keV), and (3) physical and biological half-life. The ideal radionuclide for cardiac evaluation should have the following properties: (1) a pure gamma-(or positron) emitting tracer with a photon energy of 100-200 keV (positron, 511 keV), (2) a physical half-life of several minutes or hours to permit serial measurements over a short time period, (3) no pharmacologic effects which might affect physiological conditions, and 4) wide availability and low cost. So far, no currently used cardiac imaging agent meets all these requirements.

Methods for measuring blood flow

Many methods for assessing myocardial blood flow have been reported. Most techniques are based on the Fick principle which states that blood flow to an organ is equal to the uptake of any substance divided by the arteriovenous concentration difference of that substance. The principle can be rephrased as:

change of amount/time = flow concentration in - flow concentration out.
In formula:

$$\frac{dq(t)}{dt} = F.(A(t) - B(t)),$$

where the change of quantity in the organ with time dq/dt is related to the flow (F) times the difference in concentration of the input A and output B. Inherent to this principle are the following assumptions: (1) adequate mixing of the substance with the blood, (2) steady state of the system during measurement, (3) no influence of the amount of the substance on transit time, (4) no recirculation of the substance, and (5) unidirectional and steady flow. Myocardial blood flow measurements with radioactive tracers are based on assumptions on tracer kinetics, and these measurements are all directly or indirectly related to the Fick principle. In the following section the evaluation of myocardial blood flow with the use of radioactive tracers will be discussed.

Radionuclide agents for evaluation of blood flow

Radioactive tracers which are extracted from the input network in proportion to flow are known as flow-limited tracers i.e. the amount of tracer which diffuses through the tissue is limited only by the amount delivered. Such tracers are labeled <u>microspheres</u> or labeled macroaggregates. Tracers which are not flow-limited are diffusion-limited i.e. the capillary endothelium or the cellular membranes acts like diffusion barriers. Substances like potassium, thallium, rubidium, ammonia (all monovalent cations) and also inert gases are diffusion-limited tracers. The differences between flow- and diffusion-limited tracers have major consequences for the extraction fraction and net tissue tracer uptake. The extraction fraction is defined as the fraction of activity that is removed by the myocardial tissue between input and output. The net tissue tracer uptake is the product of extraction fraction times flow. For flow-limited tracers the extraction fraction is one (complete extraction) and the net tracer uptake shows a linear response. In case of diffusion-limited tracers the extraction fraction decreases as flow increases and the net tissue tracer uptake shows a nonlinear response (Fig. 1).

142

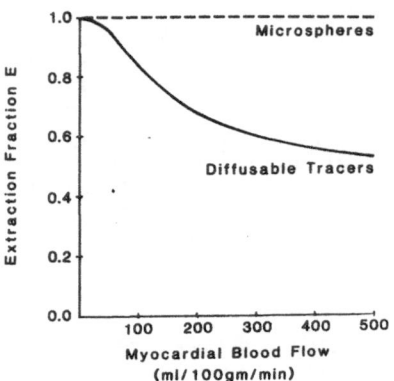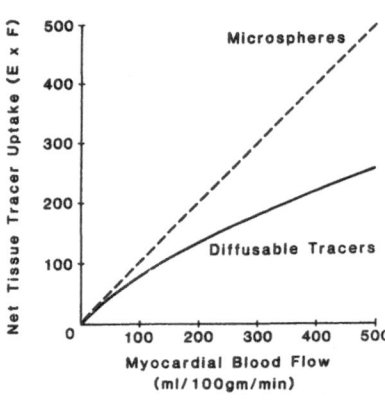

FIGURE 1. Initial capillary transit extraction fraction (E) and net tissue tracer uptake for microspheres and diffusible tracers of blood flow (F). Extraction fraction and the relationship to blood flow is shown in the left panel. Microspheres are completely extracted during a single capillary transit and the extraction fraction is one. This, however, does not apply to diffusible tracers. Their extraction fraction declines with increasing blood flows because of decreasing capillary residence times with less time for transmembraneous exhange. The right panel shows the net tissue tracer uptake as the product of extraction fraction and blood flow. Note the linear response for microspheres and the nonlinear response for diffusible tracers. The latter response is cause by the flow-dependent decrease in extraction fraction.
From Schelbert HR; Evaluation and quantification of regional myocardial blood flow with positron emission tomography. In: new concepts of cardiac imaging, Eds, Pohost GM, Higgins CB, Morganroth J, Ritchie JL, Schelbert HR, 197, 1987 (with permission).

In practice, however, diffusion-limited tracers can adequately be used for evaluation of relative myocardial perfusion in normal myocardium and in ischemic or infarcted myocardial areas.

A number of agents have been used or investigated for the evaluation of myocardial blood flow. They can be categorized into three different groups, each of which is governed by a different set of tracer kinetic assumptions. The extent to which the assumptions concerning the behaviour of a tracer satisfy the mathematical modeling requirements varies between the various classes. The three classes are:
(1) Monovalent cations,
(2) Inert gases,
(3) Particulate agents such as microspheres or macroaggregates.

(1) *Monovalent cations*
The initial distribution of radiopharmaceuticals which have a high

extraction will be proportional to relative perfusion. This principle was first described by Leon Sapirstein and provides estimates of flow from the relation:

$$q(t) = F.E \int_{0}^{t} C(t)dt,$$

which means:
amount present in organ = flow x extraction x concentration.

It is based on the assumption that an intravenously administered tracer is taken up and released by cells throughout the organism in a consistent fashion independent of regional blood flow or metabolic status of the tissue. If a tracer meets these criteria, it will be distributed in proportion to regional perfusion. Most radiopharmaceuticals employed for determinations based on this type of analysis are monovalent cations, which are predominantly potassium analogs. They can be divided into gamma- and positron-emitting agents.

a. *Gamma-emitting agents*
Thallium-201 is the most common gamma-emitting agent for assessment of myocardial perfusion scintigraphically, although also potassium-43 and rubidium-81 have been used. These agents enter the myocardium by the energy requiring sodium-potassium-ATPase pump mechanisms. They differ in their physical half-lives, gamma emissions, and in myocardial extraction and washout. In a single transit through the coronary bed, the extraction of thallium is 88%, and of potassium and rubidium between 65 and 75%.
Since the myocardial extraction and total body extraction are usually similar, the time course of blood clearance and myocardial concentration will differ for each agent. The most rapid concentration rise in the myocardium occurs with thallium, followed by that of potassium and rubidium. The importance of the time needed for localization stems from the need to maintain a 'steady-state' during the interval of radionuclide concentration rise in the myocardium. Within three circulatory periods, the majority of monovalent cationic myocardial tracer with high extraction fraction (thallium-201, rubidium-81, and potassium-43) has concentrated in the myocardium.
The uptake and distribution of the monovalent cations correlates well with the distribution of myocardial blood flow, whereby uptake is the product of blood flow and extraction fraction. For thallium-201 the extraction fraction is inversely related to flow when coronary flow is in the normal range. At high and low flows, however, the extraction is respectively much less and greater, resulting in underestimation of true flow in high flow states and overestimation of true flow in low flow states. Still thallium-201 is at present the prime radiopharmaceutical for myocardial perfusion imaging in clinical cardiology.
After intravenous injection of 2 milliCurie (mCi) or 74 MegaBequerel (MBq) thallium-201 about 4 percent of tracer localizes in the myocardium and within 10 minutes a myocardial image with a count density of about 2000 counts/cm^2 can be recorded (Fig. 2).

Myocardial infarction or ischemia may be diagnosed by the visually estimated findings of absent or diminished tracer uptake in regional myocardial areas (Fig. 3).

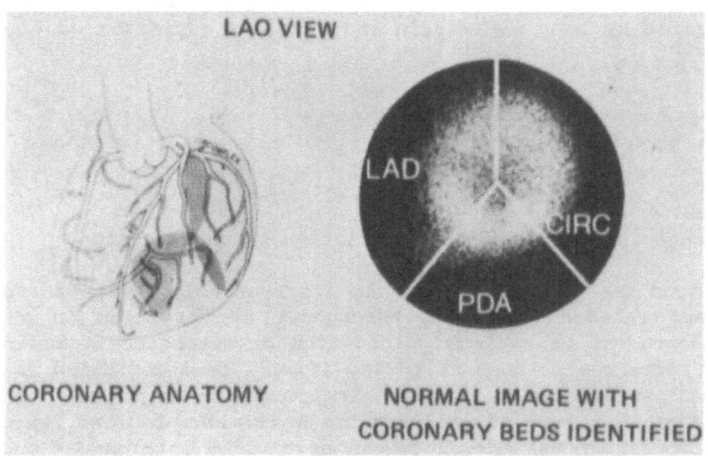

FIGURE 2. *The LAO view best differentiates the major coronary arterial beds, as shown schematically on the left: the LAD supplies the anteroseptal myocardium, the CIRC supplies the posterolateral myocardium, and the PDA supplies the inferior myocardium. In the LAO myocardial image, as shown in a normal study on the right, the anteroseptal myocardium is represented by an anteroseptal wedge of activity, the posterolateral myocardium by a posterolateral wedge, and the inferior myocardium by an inferior wedge.*
From Ritchie JL, Hamilton GW, Williams DL, et al: Myocardial imaging with radionuclide-labeled particles: Analysis of the normal image, abnormal image, and technical considerations, Radiology 121:131, 1976, with permisson).
CIRC = left circumflex; PDA = posterior descending artery; LAD = left anterior descending.

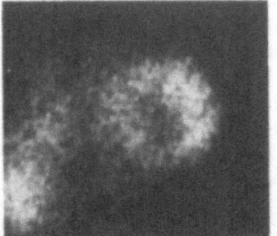 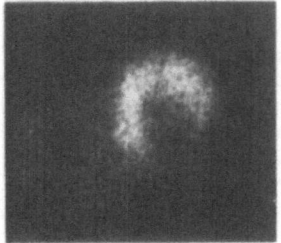

FIGURE 3. *Thallium-201 scintigrams in a patient with anteroseptal myocardial infarction (left) and inferior myocardial infarction (right).*

Thallium-201 is particularly useful in conjunction with the electrocardiogram during a standard exercise stress test for the detection of suspected coronary artery disease. The exercise scintigrams may show perfusion defects that are resolved on the rest images taken 4 hours after exercise, indicating reversible ischemia based on a hemodynamic significant stenosis in one of the major coronary arteries. If both the exercise and rest scintigrams have similar defects i.e. show persistence of defects, then this finding is consistent with the presence of tissue necrosis based on a previous myocardial infarction. These observations of reduced myocardial perfusion visualized by thallium-201 have made this tracer a valuable tool in the diagnosis of coronary artery disease. However, thallium-201 has several important shortcomings as an adequate perfusion marker: (1) the low-level gamma emission of 80 keV is not ideal for in vivo imaging since a fair amount of photons will be attenuated by absorption in the body, (2) the extraction of thallium-201 is decreased in high blood flow states, and (3) the physical half-life of 72 hours precludes rapid sequential imaging and may give a relatively high total body exposure. From these observations it can be concluded that absolute measurements of coronary blood flow can not be made with the gamma-emitting monovalent cations. The findings on the thallium-201 scintigrams have to be readed as relative intensities of distribution on the images. Since thallium-201 has been used for over 10 years in clinical cardiology, it may be mentioned that absolute measurements of coronary flow may not be required for clinical decision making and that relative determinations of regional distribution may suffice for clinical purposes.

b. *Positron emitting radionuclides*

Positron-emitting potassium analogs used for tomographic assessment of myocardial perfusion include isotopes of rubidium (^{82}Rb), nitrogen-13-labeled ammonia (employed in the form of $^{13}NH_4^+$), and labeled water ($H_2^{15}O$).

Table 1. Myocardial perfusion agents

	Half-life	keV	Intra-venous	Intra-coronary
1. *Monovalent cations*				
a. Gamma				
Thallium-201 ($^{201}_{43}$Tl)	74 h	69, 83	+	
Potassium-43 (^{43}K)	22.4 h	373, 619	+	
Rubidium-81 (^{81}Rb)	4.7 h	511, 190	+	
b. Positron				
Rubidium-82 (^{82}Rb)	75 s	511	+	
Nitrogen-13-ammonia ($^{13}NH_4^+$)	10 min	511	+	
$H_2^{15}O$ (labeled water)	2 min	511	+	
2. *Inert gases*				
Xenon-133 (^{133}Xe)	5.3 days	81, 204		+
Krypton-81m (^{81m}Kr)	13 s	190		+
3. *Particulate agents*				
Carbon-11(^{11}C)-microspheres	20 min	511		+
Technetium-99m(^{99m}Tc)-macroaggregates	6 h	140		+
Gallium-68 (^{68}Ga)-macroaggregates or albumin	68 min	511		+
4. *New agents*				
^{99m}Tc-Diars	6 h	140	+	
^{99m}Tc-isonitriles	6 h	140	+	

Diars = diarsenical complex

146

Although positron-emitting agents can be imaged with a conventional Anger camera or a modified multicrystal camera, the best images are recorded with positron ring devices. The positron instruments combine high sensitivity and high resolution for myocardial imaging. Recent studies by Gould et al. (1) suggest that reductions of luminal diameter of less than 50% can be detected when these radionuclides are administered in conjunction with dipyridamole vasodilatation. The regional distribution of both ammonia and rubidium have excellent correlations with that of microspheres although they share the limitations of being diffusion-limited tracers (Fig. 4).

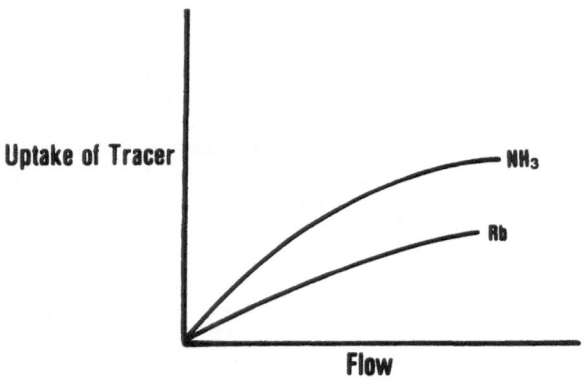

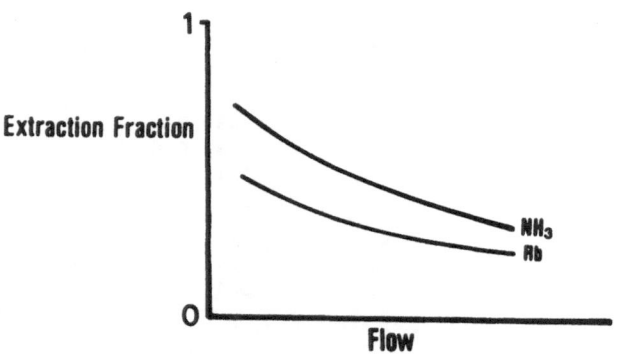

FIGURE 4. Uptake and extraction fraction of two partially extracted tracers, N-13-ammonia and rubidium-82, are shown as a function of flow. Extraction of these and similar tracers falls off at higher flows because shortened residence time in the capillary bed reduces uptake across capillary membranes.
From Gould KL, Mullani N, Wong W, Goldstein RA: Positron emission tomography. In: Cardiac imaging and image processing, Eds, Collins SE, Skorton DJ, 330-360, 1986 (with permission).

Rubidium-82
Rubidium-82 (half-life 75 seconds) is daughter of cyclotron-produced strontium-82 (half-life 25 days). The production of the parent strontium-82 requires a high-energy cyclotron, and is accompanied by the production of small quantities of strontium-85 as a radiocontaminant. Since strontium

radionuclides localize in bone and have a long biological half-life, the generator system has been refined to minimize the 'breakthrough' of the parent in the eluate. Rubidium-82 (30 to 40 mCi) is eluted from the generator as a monovalent cation and, with a continuous supply from a bedside generator, an intravenous infusion results in an equilibrium in the arterial blood within four half-lives because of the dynamic equilibrium that develops between delivery and decay. The regional myocardial activity can be measured 30 seconds after turning off the intravenous infusion when the arterial activity has dropped to less than 50% of the maximum value in the myocardium. Myocardial imaging with rubidium-82 requires fast acquisition of data. The images recorded during the first 1-2 minutes after intravenous administration depict the blood pool distribution of the radionuclide (if images are recored with gating, ejection fraction and regional wall motion can be determined), while images recorded after 2 minutes depict regional perfusion. Reasonable quality images can be recorded for 4 to 6 half-lives after infusion, i.e. 1 to 2 half-lives consumed with blood clearance and the remainder for myocardial perfusion.

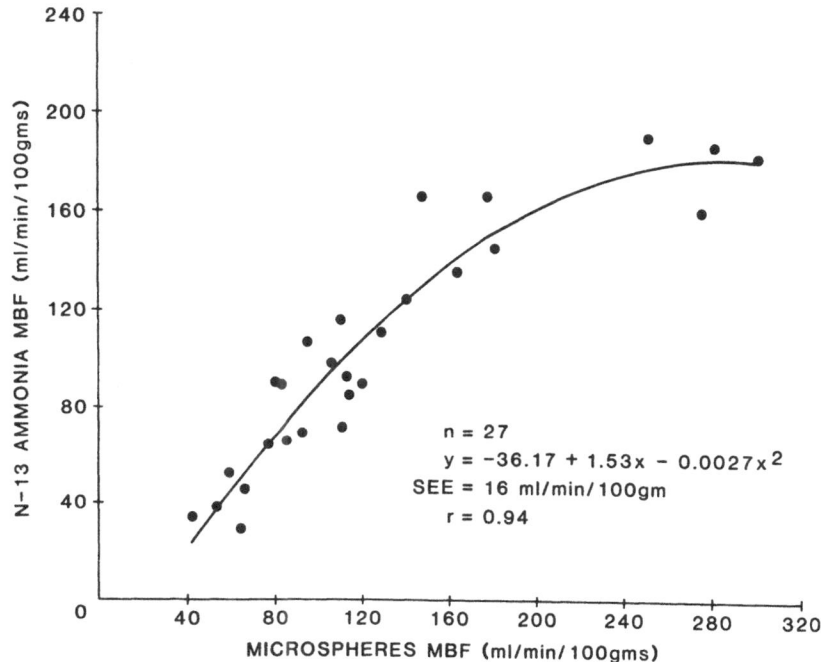

$$n = 27$$
$$y = -36.17 + 1.53x - 0.0027x^2$$
$$SEE = 16 \text{ ml/min/100gm}$$
$$r = 0.94$$

FIGURE 5. Relation between regional myocardial blood flow (MBF) determined with the microspheres technique and with Nitrogen-13 labeled-positron emission tomography in 27 dog experiments.
From Shah A, et al: J Am Coll Cardiol 5:92, 1985 (with permission).

Rubidium-82 imaging provides a repeatable and noninvasive measure of regional myocardial perfusion since each patient can be used as his own control. This is a considerable advantage when evaluating the responses of the coronary circulation in various physiologic states. Several studies have shown the value of rubidium-82 for the detection of coronary artery disease by the measurement of coronary flow reserve after dipyridamole-induced vasodilation (1,2). In this way performed, clinical decisions are not only based on arteriographic data but mainly on functional degrees of coronary artery abnormality. Relative disadvantages are 1) the remaining blood activity during the measurement after the infusion, 2) the inverse relation between flow and extraction, which may result in underestimation of increases in regional perfusion, and 3) the independent changes in rubidium uptake that can occur during metabolic abnormalities. However, all the experimental and clinical evidence to date indicates that regional decreases in coronary flow are reflected by changes in uptake of rubidium-82.

Nitrogen-13 ammonia
Nitrogen-13 labeled ammonia serves as a flow marker which concentrates in the myocardium with an extraction fraction of approximately 70%. Similar to rubidium-82, the net uptake of the tracer is related to blood flow in a curvilinear fashion (Fig. 5).

This means that the relation between blood flow and myocardial nitrogen-ammonia is relatively linear over the physiological range of blood flow, but falls off at higher flows. Moreover, the uptake of nitrogen-13 ammonia by the myocardium is also dependent on metabolic trapping catalysed by glutamine synthetase. However, changes in myocardial blood flow can adequately be recorded by positron emission tomography, since ammonia activity concentrations measured by positron emission tomography have been shown to correlate very well with the standard microsphere technique (3). Accurate quantitation of regional myocardial perfusion with labeled ammonia (and also with rubidium-82) has been elusive, although valuable clinical information has been obtained including determination of extraction of labeled metabolic substrates (labeled glucose) with reference to estimates of perfusion.
In addition, like rubidium-82, alterations of perfusion and regional myocardial metabolism in response to pharmacological vasodilator stress may be used to assess severity of coronary artery disease. The relationship between abnormalities of ammonia extraction and changes in accumulation of labeled glucose may provide a description of viable but transiently ischemic myocardium.
The detection of coronary artery disease by both rubidium-82 and labeled ammonia during exercise or after dipyridamole administration has been improved compared to conventional planar thallium-201 scintigraphy; sensitivity as well as specificity approach 95%.

Radiolabeled water
A third short-lived cyclotron-produced positron emitting radionuclide, oxygen-15, can be used for measurement of coronary blood flow. The tracer can be administered by inhalation of oxygen-15 labeled carbon dioxide, which results in the distribution of oxygen-15 labeled water. It has also been shown that labeled water can be administered as an intravenous bolus. The myocardial transit is recorded by positron emission tomography, separate blood pool subtraction can be performed with oxygen-15 labeled carbon monoxide, and measurements can then be made of regional myocardial perfusion. This provides another approach to the evaluation of coronary blood flow with negligible contribution from metabolic variables. The utility of this approach has been demonstrated in experimental canine preparations (4). In open chest dogs the single pass extraction of labeled water by the heart averaged 96±5% at flows of 80 to 100 ml/100g/min and did not differ significantly over a wide range of flows (from 12 to 300 ml/100 g/min).

Because the extraction fraction was high and consistent, the extraction of tracer appeared to be flow-limited rather than diffusion-limited over the ranges of flow studied. Thus, the tracer should provide a good index of flow in vivo. The underlying assumptions were tested initially in open chest dogs given a 60 seconds intravenous infusion of oxygen-15 labeled water. Labeled water content was measured directly by analysis of tissue. Regional flow was calculated by direct application of the tissue autoradiographic method. Flows determined in this way correlated closely with flows measured with the radiolabeled microsphere technique (Fig. 6).

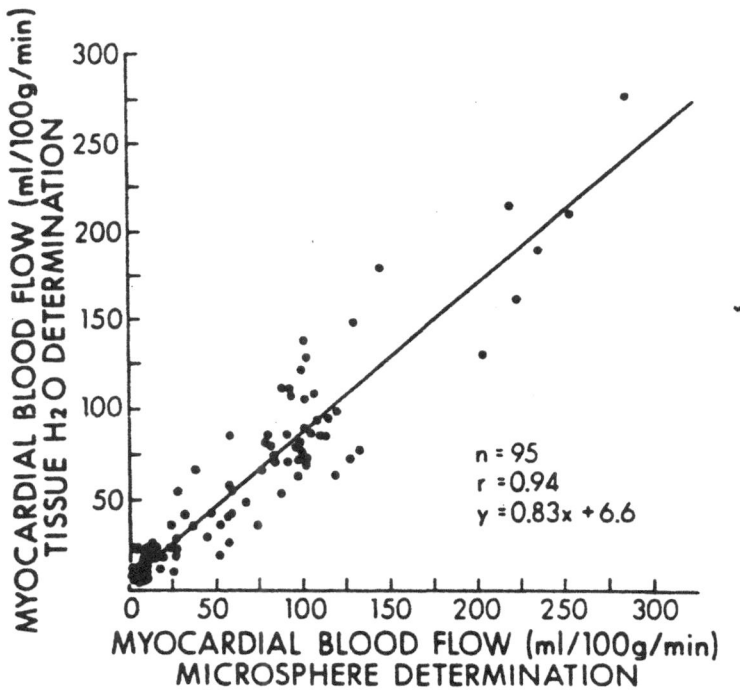

FIGURE 6. Correspondence between myocardial blood flow assessed with oxygen-15 water and radiolabeled microspheres determined invasively. The data, obtained from nine dogs pertain to normal and infarcted myocardium. In four animals flow was augmented with dipyridamole. A close correlation is demonstrated between flow measurements obtained with labeled water and with the microsphere technique.
From Bergman SR et al., Circulation 70; 724, 1984 (by permission of the American Heart Association, Inc.).

The short physical half-life of oxygen-15 (2 minutes) allows sequential collection of the labeled water and labeled carbon monoxide images within approximately ten minutes because counts from the first oxygen-15 study approach background after five half-lives.
Results obtained with positron emission tomography indicated that the labeled water determinations of flow correlated closely with those obtained tomographically with gallium-68 macroaggregated albumin microspheres. In subsequent studies, Huang et al. (5) demonstrated the feasibility of determination of myocardial blood flow with a more prolonged infusion of

oxygen-15 labeled water tracer. Tomographic determinations of flow in vivo correlated closely with measurements with microspheres. A disadvantage of the labeled water technique is the high tracer activity in blood and lungs, which leads to activity cross-contamination. Nevertheless, it provides another approach for assessment of regional myocardial blood flow and represents therefore an interesting application of positron imaging.

(2) *Inert gases*

At times it is desirable to define myocardial perfusion in the catheterization laboratory by direct intracoronary injection. Under these circumstances, either the inert gases such as xenon-133 and krypton-81, or particulate agents such as macroaggregated albumin, can be employed. The use of radioactive inert gases to measure myocardial blood flow requires intracoronary infusion of the gas or inhalation of gas with external detection of the emitted radiation during clearance of dilution of the radioactive gas from the circulation.

Xenon-133

Following intra-arterial administration xenon-133 (half-life 5.3 days) leaves the capillaries and enters tissue in direct proportion to its relative solubility in the tissue compared to that in blood (partition coefficient). Thereafter, the clearance of the tracer from the tissue is dependent on the rate of perfusion. Measurement of coronary perfusion is based upon an approach developed by Kety and Schmidt described first in 1955 and applied initially to measurement of cerebral blood flow. The mathematical model employed describes the exchange of an inert diffusible tracer across the capillary tissue interface and between vascular and tissue compartments. It represents an extension of the Fick principle. Myocardial blood flow can be calculated from analysis of the clearance of radioactivity from the heart with a corollary of the Kety-Schmidt model.

$$F = K\lambda W/D$$

where: F = *myocardial blood flow (ml/100g/min)*
K = *myocardial tracer disappearance rate constant*
λ = *tracer tissue: blood partition coefficient*
W = *weight of the myocardium*
D = *specific gravity of myocardium*

Since the myocardial clearance of xenon-133 usually has a half-time of less than 1 minute, a scintillation camera must be present in the catheterization laboratory to measure the myocardial clearance. The rapid clearance of xenon makes it possible to record myocardial perfusion under several different circumstances in rapid succession, with an extremely low radiation burden to the patient (radiation burden of less than 0.1 rads to the myocardium per 0.5 mCi intracoronary injection, usual dose 20 to 30 mCi). Serial measurements can be performed before, during and after interventions in the catherisation laboratory. Several studies (6,7) have shown the value of xenon-133 in quantitatively determining local perfusion rates in patients with stable angina during atrial pacing or in patients after myocardial infarction or after venous bypass surgery (Fig. 7).

Although the use of xenon-133 allows the measurement of absolute regional flow rates in ml/100g/minute, several limitations have to be mentioned. Xenon-133 suffers from significant soft tissue attenuation because of its low gamma-emmission of 81 keV, which results in variable count statistics depending on uneven thickness of overlying muscle and breast tissue. More-over and more important, xenon-133 shows a high fat solubility in subepi-cardial myocardial muscle which obscures the myocardial signal and slows the clearance of the tracer from the myocardium. Being a diffusable tra-cer, xenon-133 also shows a nonlinear correlation between net tissue tracer uptake and myocardial blood flow. Also problems related to streaming of the tracer from the left main stem to one or the other coronary arteries have to be taken into consideration. Despite these drawbacks, recent studies have shown that proper use and interpretation of the xenon technique may allow rapid and accurate assessment of regional myocardial perfusion.

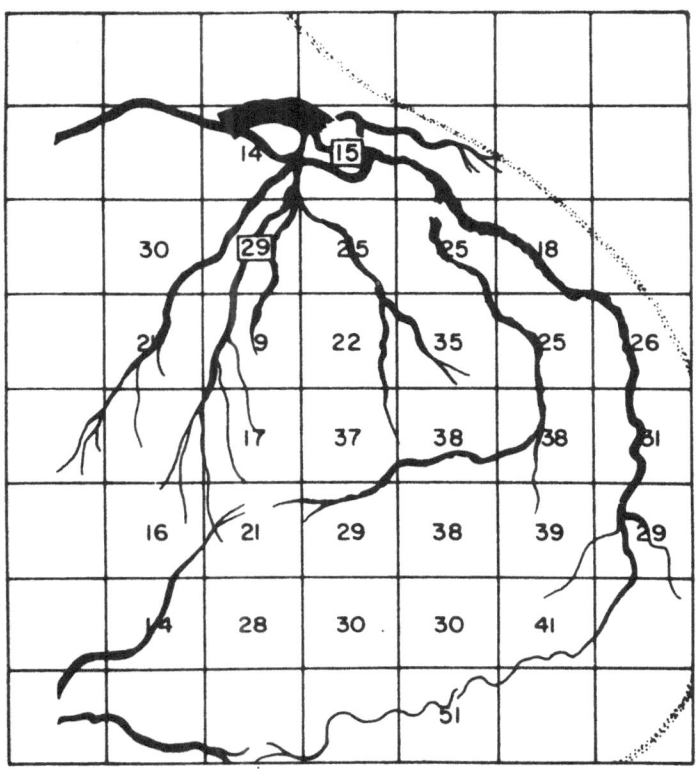

FIGURE 7. Diffuse reductions of myocardial perfusion are apparent in the left ventricular myocardium of a patient with marked disease of the diagonal and circumflex branches and complete occlusion of the anterior descending branch of the left coronary artery.
From Cannon et al. J. Clin. Invest 51: 964, 1972 (by copyright permission of the American Society for Clinical Investigation).

Krypton-81m
Ultrashort-lived nuclides have been suggested for the determination of regional myocardial perfusion. After the introduction of the rubidium-81/krypton-81m generator, it was subsequently shown in animal experiments that krypton-81m (half-life 13 seconds) also had the potential to indicate re-gional myocardial flow changes. The parent rubidium-81 has a half-life of 4.6 hours, which is unfortunately relatively short.

After administration of 20 mCi krypton-81m by continuous infusion directly into the coronary bed, it achieves the highest concentration in areas of greatest perfusion. Static images of the distribution of radionuclide are related to the regional distribution. Following an intervention such as pacing, the radionuclide will reequilibrate in the myocardium dependent on the redistribution of regional perfusion. Approximately three half-lives are required to obtain a new equilibrium state which reflects the regional distribution of perfusion. A second static image recorded under this circumstance can be compared to the image recorded at baseline to identify the change in regional perfusion.

Similar to other diffusable tracers, the relationship of regional perfusion to radionuclide distribution with these agents is not linear. The krypton-81m enters the tissue as a result of its high permeability. The combination of short physical half-life and regional perfusion both contribute to the clearance of the radionuclide from the myocardium. As a result, the changes in regional perfusion contribute relatively little to the effective half-life of this agent (e.g., the effective half-life in normal myocardium is approximately 9 seconds, and if flow is doubled, the half-life decreases to 7 seconds, while if flow is halved the half-life increases to 10 seconds).

Recent clinical studies (8) in 25 patients with coronary artery disease have shown that pacing-induced decrease in krypton-81m perfusion was found in all myocardial areas supplied by coronary arteries with more than 70% luminal narrowing. Also, all areas with more than 90% diameter reduction showed early perfusion defects before general signs of ischemia were noticed. Moreover, flow abnormalities persisted after discontinuation of pacing-induced ischemia, indicating an ongoing decrease in regional myocardial blood flow. These findings suggest that the krypton-81m technique has a greater sensitivity for detecting hemodynamically significant lesions than planar thallium-201 imaging.

Limitations of the technique are that only distributional changes can be assessed and not coronary flow changes in absolute quantities. Whether the observed changes really represent a regional decrease in coronary blood flow is impossible to know. A redistribution of radioactivity from areas with limited vasodilatory reserve and diminished increase in flow during pacing to normal areas can result in changes in krypton-81m perfusion as well. Similar to xenon-133, streaming may occur because of improper mixing of the tracer with blood in the left main stem. This may lead to an uneven and unstable distribution pattern. Advantages over xenon-133 are the high energy spectrum, absence of recirculation, and lack of affinity for fat tissue. In conclusion, the krypton-81m technique allows frequent and rapid determination of regional myocardial blood flow changes in patient with coronary artery disease.

(3) *Particulate agents*

The direct intracoronary administration of particulate radiopharmaceuticals in small quantities (<50,000 particles) is safe, and can be particularly useful for defining the amount and the source of collateral perfusion. In this technique either a single radiolabeled microsphere is administered directly into one coronary artery and a second labeled particulate into the other, or the two radiopharmaceuticals can be administered through the same coronary bed before and after an intervention to define the change in myocardial perfusion (dual isotope technique).

Since the particulate radiopharmaceuticals remain in situ following administration, imaging can be performed for several hours after injection. The radiation burden to the myocardium is low, since only 0.1-0.2 mCi of the radiolabel is required to provide a very high quality image in a short interval of imaging.

Both gamma- and positron-emitting particles have been used. For instance, macroaggregated albumin particles with a size of 30 μ are usually labeled with technetium-99m. Also the positron-emitter gallium-68 has been used to label macroaggregates of albumin somewhat analogous to microspheres for quantification of regional myocardial blood flow in experimental animals. Tomographic measurements of flow corresponds closely with results obtained by quantification of conventional gamma emitting microspheres in samples of tissue assayed in vivo. Recently, carbon-11 has been covalently bound to albumin microspheres and used to measure regional myocardial blood flow tomographically in animals and in man. The limitations of this approach include the need for administration of tracer via left atrium or left ventricle and the potential hazards of administration of particulate material into the coronary circulation supplying myocardium in which perfusion may be compromised already. Nevertheless, adverse effects of such administration have not been evident clinically. Additional potential constraints relate to alterations in the distribution of microspheres with ischemia or when microvascular damage is present as may pertain with ischemia followed by reperfusion.

Direct patient applications have been twofold, 1) to evaluate of the perioperative status of the myocardium, and 2) to assess the physiologic significance of a coronary artery stenosis (9). By injection of different isotopes in each coronary artery, the two coronary beds can be separated which may be useful in preoperative planning. Specifically, the identification of collateral flow from the right coronary artery to the left system, in the presence of prior infarction of the right system, might argue for coronary artery bypass grafting to this artery which would otherwise not be considered since its native bed was infarcted. The second major application of the particle imaging technique is to assess the hemodynamical significance of a given coronary artery stenosis. Particle studies are likely more sensitive than thallium-201 exercise scintigraphy in identifying patients with significant coronary artery disease.

Important limitations are the invasive nature of the technique and the ability to detect only relative differences in flow, reason why the long-range clinical utility of the particle technique is uncertain and still no routine procedure in clinical practice.

(4) *New agents*

The relatively poor resolution of thallium-201 has led to a search for a technetium-99m labeled perfusion agent. Efforts to combine technetium-99m into a lipid soluble charged complex appeared to offer the best opportunity for achieving successful myocardial concentration. Several technetium-99m labeled compounds, such as the diarsenical complex of technetium-99m (DiARS) and a dimethyl phospheno-ethane complex (DMPE), and a hexakis complex of technetium were tested in animals and found to have high myocardial uptake. The rapid myocardial concentration of these compounds fulfilled the criteria of Sapirstein tracers and a high correlation with regional perfusion was found. However, when DiARS and DMPE were administered to human subjects, their myocardial concentration was extremely disappointing.

When human studies with the technetium-99m labeled hexakis-isonitrile compound were performed, however, sufficient concentration was observed in the human myocardium to permit high quality planar and tomographic images to be recorded. This agent combines the properties of high lipid solubility and technetium chelation. This agent achieves a localization of up to 2% of the injected dose in the human myocardium. The model of entry of this agent to the myocardium is not fully understood, but may depend primarily on solubility, rather than specific transport, as is the case with the monovalent cations. Following intravenous administration, the isonitrile localizes in the lungs to a sufficient degree that the myocardium cannot be visualized. The clearance from the lungs is more rapid than that from the heart, which permits myocardial visualization about 1 hour after injection. Serial images recorded after the first hour indicate that myocardial clearance is slow and approximates the physical half-life of technetium-99m. The metabolic fate and the relationship of the distribution of this agent to regional perfusion are under investigation. Recent observations have shown that, unlike thallium-201, the labeled isonitrile does not redistribute after exercise-induced ischemia (10). This means that an additional injection at rest is necessary for the assessment of transient ischemia. Comparison with thallium-201 did show good correlation in detecting normal and ischemic myocardium in patients with coronary artery disease.

Summary

Blood flow measurements are useful in the following clinical situations: detection of coronary artery disease, assessment of pathology after coronary arteriography, pre- and postoperative assessment of coronary artery disease, and detection of acute myocardial infarction. Recent data have demonstrated the utility of applying gamma- and positron-emission tracers for delineation of myocardial ischemia and reperfusion in acute and chronic derangements. In addition, the functional impact of subcritical coronary arterial stenose on myocardial perfusion is definable with the radionuclide approach before and after pharmacologically induced vasodilatory stress.

In contrast to radionuclide techniques, angiographic criteria only define the distribution of the coronary stenoses and collaterals without directly characterizing the functional impact of the summation of these phenomena on myocardial perfusion. Accordingly, clinical assessment of the significance of coronary arterial abnormalities are likely to ultimately require consideration not only of angiographic data but also functional estimates or regional perfusion and factors which potentially modify extraction or clearance of radiolabeled tracers.

It is clear nowadays that the use of radioactive tracers for functional assessment of coronary artery flow have gained a definite role in experimental and clinical cardiology.

REFERENCES

1. Gould KL, Goldstein RA, Mullani NA, Kirkeeide RL, Wong W-H, Tewson TJ, Berridge MS, Bolomey LA, Hartz RK, Smalling RW, Fuentes F: Noninvasive assessment of coronary stenoses by myocardial perfusion imaging during pharmacologic coronary vasodilation. VIII. Clinical feasibility of positron cardiac imaging without a cyclotron using generator-produced rubidium-82. J Am Coll Cardiol 4:775, 1986.
2. Goldstein RA, Mullani NA, Wong W-H, Hartz RK, Hicks, CH, Fuentes F, Smalling RW, Gould KL: Positron imaging of myocardial infarction with rubidium-82. J Nucl Med 27:1824, 1986.
3. Gould KL, Schelbert HR, Phelps ME, Hoffman EJ: Noninvasive assessment of coronary stenoses with myocardial perfusion imaging during pharmacologic coronary vasodilation. V. Detection of 47 percent diameter coronary stenosis with intravenous nitrogen-13 ammonia emisson-computed tomography in intact dogs. Am J Cardiol 47: 200, 1979.
4. Bergmann SR, Fox KAA, Rand AL, McElvany KD, Welch MJ, Markham J, Sobel BE, Quantification of regional myocardial blood flow in vivo with $H_2^{15}O$. Circulation 4:724, 1984.

5. Huang SC, Schwaiger M, Carson RE, Carson J, Hansen H, Selin C, Hoffman EJ, MacDonald N, Schelbert HR, Phelps ME: Quantitative measurement of myocardial blood flow with oxygen-15 water and positron computed tomography: An assessment of potential and problems. J Nucl Med 26:616, 1980.

6. Ruddy TD, Yasuda T, Barlai-Kovach M, Nedelman MA, Moore, RH, Alpert NM, Correia JA, Newell JB, Okada RD, Boucher CA, Strauss HW: Measurement of both left ventricular function and regional myocardial perfusion with ^{133}Xe in dogs. Eur J Nucl Med 12:533, 1987.

7. Korhola O, Valle M, Frick MH et al.: Regional myocardial perfusion abnormalities of xenon-133 imaging in patients with angina pectoris and normal coronary arteries. Am J Cardiol 39:355, 1977.

8. Remme WJ, Krauss XH, Van Hoogenhuyze DCA, Cox PH, Storm CJ, Kruyssen DA: Continuous determination of regional myocardial blood flow with intracoronary krypton-81m in coronary artery disease. Am J Cardiol 56:445, 1985.

9. Kirk GA, Adams R, Jansen C, Judkins MP: Particulate myocardial perfusion scintigraphy: Its clinical usefulness in evaluation of coronary artery disease. Semin Nucl Med 7:67, 1977.

10. Sia STB, Holman BL, McKursick K, Rigo P, Gillis F, Sporn V, Perez-Balino N, Mitta A, Vosberg H, Szabo Z, Schwartzkopff B, Moretti J, Davison A, Lister-James J, Jones A: The utilization of Tc-99m-TBI as a myocardial perfusion agent in exercise studies: Comparison with Tl-201 thallous chloride and examination of its biodistribution in humans. Eur J Nucl Med 12:333, 1986.

MYOCARDIAL PERFUSION ASSESSED BY NUCLEAR MAGNETIC RESONANCE

X.H. Krauss, A. de Roos, S. Postema, J. Doornbos, E.E. van der Wall,
A.E. van Voorthuisen, A.V.G. Bruschke.

In 1946 the groups of Bloch (6) and Purcell (35) described independently
from each other a phenomenon which is known as Nuclear Magnetic Resonance.
It appeared that certain atomic nuclei, when placed in a strong magnetic
field, absorb electromagnetic waves of a particular frequency (radiowaves,
1-100 MegaHerz) and re-emit some of the absorbed energy in the form of
radiosignals with the same frequency. In fact this resembles the
resonance of a tuning fork when the right tone is struck.
Atomic nuclei contain protons and neutrons which possess an intrinsic
momentum (spin), but pairs of these nuclei are aligned in such a way that
their spins will cancel each other out. Therefore only nuclei with an
unpaired proton or neutron will possess a "net spin" and since these
nucleons have an associated electric charge, a magnetic field is
generated. Such a nucleus can be regarded as a small magnet bar or
magnetic dipole, which makes it sensitive to an externally applied
magnetic field (fig. 1).

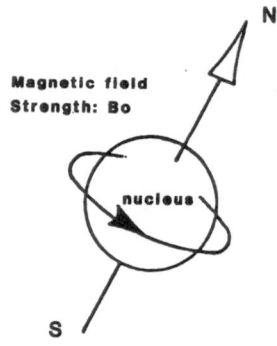

**Magnetic field
Strength: Bo**

*FIGURE 1. The nucleus spins around in a mag-
netic field with a frequency (w) which is
directly proportional to the magnetic field
strength (Bo) as is described in the Larmor
equation: $w = y/2\pi$. Bo*

*$y =$ the gyromagnetic ratio, a speci-
fic constant for each sensitive
nucleus.*

In the absence of a magnetic field these nuclei are randomly oriented and
the sum of their magnetic moments will be zero. However, when a magnetic
field is applied, the nuclei for example protons (^{1}H) will align with or
against this field. There is no intermediate state and more protons are
aligned with the field than against it since their energy state is more
favourable. This results in a nuclear magnetization vector parallel to the
direction of the external magnetic field, like a compass needle that
aligns with the earth's magnetic field.
In this state the protons will be sensitive to electromagnetic waves with
radio-frequency, which must be equal to their own Larmor-frequency.
Such a radio-frequency (RF) pulse will deflect the nuclear magnetization
vector away from the direction of the magnetic field. When this pulse is

switched off the magnetization-vector will return to its original direction and during this process radiowaves with the same frequency are emitted. These radio-signals will diminish in intensity when more nuclei have returned to their equilibrium. This process is called RELAXATION and is characterized by two time constants T1 and T2.

An extensive description of these phenomena is beyond the scope of this article, and the readers are referred to textbooks or articles which are specifically dedicated to this subject.

In table I some atomic nuclei with strong NMR-properties are shown. The most sensitive atom is Hydrogen (^{1}H), which contains only one proton and is the most abundant atom in the human body. Its Larmor frequency in a field-strength of 1 Tesla is 42.58 MegaHerz.

Fluor-19 is less sensitive to NMR, relative sensitivity 83% of ^{1}H, with a Larmor-frequency of 40.05 MHz/T.

Other nuclei like Sodium (^{23}Na), Phosphorus-31 and Carbon-13 have a much lower sensitivity for NMR than protons. Besides the concentrations of these atoms in the tissues are less than that of ^{1}H. For that reason their NMR-properties in living tissues can only be studied if a much stronger magnetic field is applied (12,21,33,36).

Table I: MEDICALLY RELEVANT NUCLEI FOR NMR

nucleus	natural relative abundance	relative sensitivity	Larmor-frequency
Proton (^{1}H)	99.98%	100%	42.58 MHz/T
Fluor-19	100%	83%	40.05 MHz/T
Sodium (^{23}Na)	100%	9.3%	11.26 MHz/T
Phosphorus-31	100%	6.6%	17.24 MHz/T
Carbon-13	1.1%	1.6%	10.71 MHz/T

NMR-SPECTROSCOPY

Chemical Shift:
NMR-sensitive nuclei, placed in a magnetic field, will only respond to RF pulses of their specific Larmor-freqency. This frequency is directly proportional to the external magnetic field-strength experienced by these nuclei. The electrons surrounding the nucleus will slightly alter this magnetic field. For that reason the exact resonance-frequency of the atoms will vary according to the amount and the chemical binding of these electrons. When a chemical compound is irradiated with a RF pulse which contains several frequencies (wide bandwidth) then each nucleus of the compound will re-emit only that RF-signal which fits its Larmor-frequency. These emitted radiowaves form a "Spectrum" of several frequencies as is demonstrated in fig. 2, the proton-NMR-spectrum of alcohol.

Other changes in the environment of the nuclei, like pH or physical state will also lead to variations of the resonance frequency. Protons of water for example show a narrow resonance frequency peak, which widens about 40.000 times when it is frozen to ice.

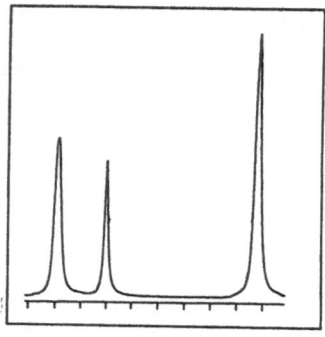

FIGURE 2. ^{1}H-NMR spectrum of C2.H5.OH

The protons bound to different Carbon or Oxygen atoms have a slightly different resonance frequency.

FIGURE 3: PHOSPHORUS-31 NMR SPECTRUM OF THE HEART

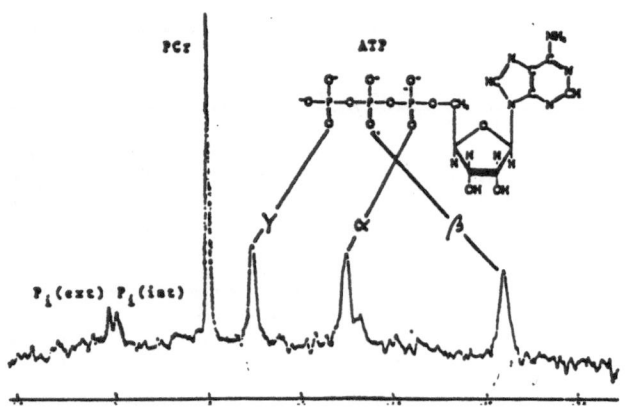

Resonance Frequency
P.i   : 17.237257 MHz/T
PCr : 17.237172 MHz/T
y-ATP: 17.237131 MHz/T
a-ATP: 17.237042 MHz/T
b-ATP: 17.236895 MHz/T

Figure 3 shows the ^{31}P-NMR spectrum of a rat heart in the intact animal. It was obtained via a coil which was applied around the heart surgically (3, 7,11,17,36). These coils can be implanted for several months thus yielding important information on the metabolism of phosphates in the myocardium (24,25), although some signals are derived from the intracardiac bloodpool.

The first peak at the left (Pi) arises from inorganic phosphates. The site of the peaks in the spectrum depends on the pH of the sample, which thus can be measured exactly. (32)

The following large peak of the spectrum is emitted by the ^{31}P-nuclei of Phospho-Creatine (PCr), the most important energy-store of the cell, and which is followed by the three peaks from ATP.

Several authors have used the ratio PCr/Pi as a reliable measure of aerobic metabolism in the heart. Fig. 4, shows the ^{31}P-NMR spectra of a rat's heart, which is made hypoxic by lowering the oxygen content of the inspired air. This leads to an irreversible cardiac failure which is preceded by a fall of the PCr/Pi ratio and severe acidosis.

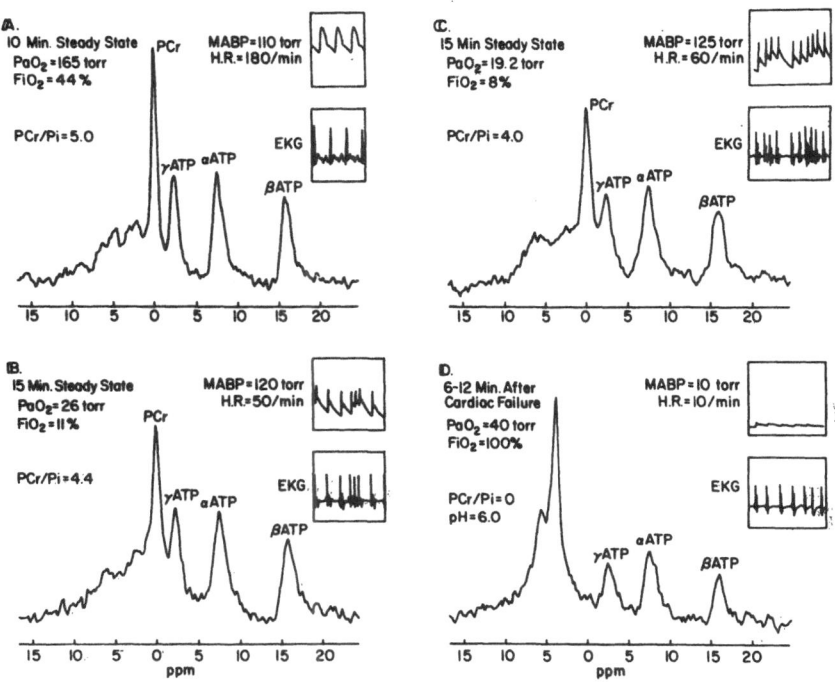

FIGURE 4. 31P-NMR spectra illustrating the PCr/Pi ratio in a rat heart which is made hypoxic by lowering the inspired oxygen content (FiO₂). The inserts show the arterial blood pressure curve and the ECG. Reprinted from Chance, B et al., Circulation 72, Suppl 4: 103, 1985 (by permission of the American Heart Association, Inc.)

In humans ^{31}P-NMR spectroscopy has been performed with the help of a surface coil, which is placed over the sternum (11,48). This coil serves as an antenna which detects the weak signals from the myocardium. Through special localizing techniques (7) the changes in ^{31}P metabolism can be followed, as demonstrated in fig. 5.

These examples show the enormous potential of NMR-spectroscopy in the description of metabolic processes in vivo. Improvements of this technique can be expected in the exact localization of the investigated sample.

Other developments will include the NMR-spectroscopy of other nuclei: Fluor-19 (33), Sodium-23 and Carbon-13.

It is more than likely that NMR-spectroscopy will play a major role in the early detection of metabolic derangements of the myocardium due to perfusion defects.

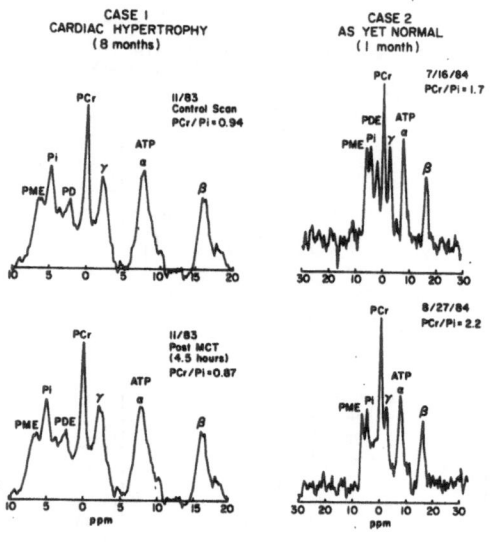

FIGURE 5. Here are shown the ^{31}P-NMR spectra of two baby brothers, case 1 suffering from severe cardiac failure due to congenital cardiomyopathy. Note the very prominent Pi-peak in this infant and the abnormal PCr/Pi ratio. A meal with Medium Chain Triglycerides (MCT) did increase this ratio in case 2 but not in the diseased child. Reprinted from Chance et al. Circulation 72, Suppl 4: 103, 1985 (by permission of the American Heart Association, Inc.)

NUCLEAR MAGNETIC RESONANCE IMAGING (=NMRI)

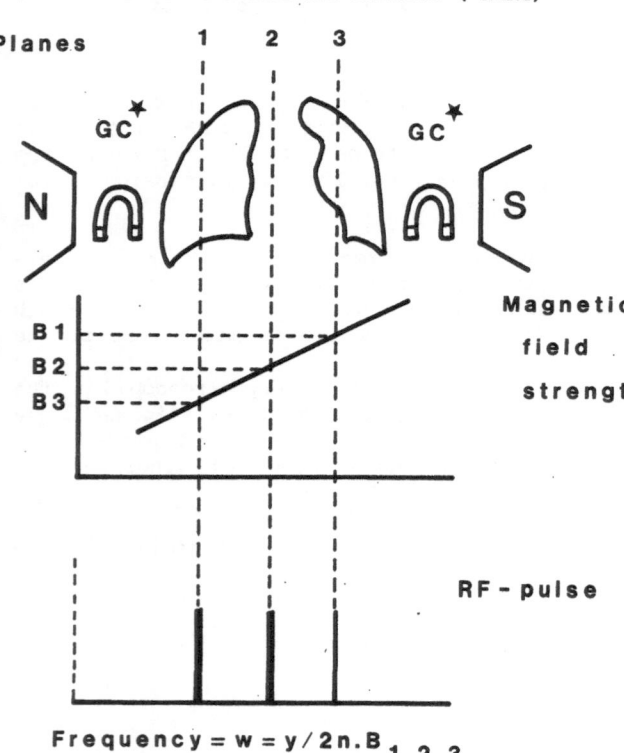

FIGURE 6. PLANE SELECTION IN NMR-IMAGING The principle of selection of the imaging plane is shown. By applying a gradient in the magnetic field (B) it is possible to excite selectively the protons in a certain plane by a "tailored" Radio Frequency (RF) Pulse, with a narrow rectangular frequency distribution. By changing the frequency of this RF-pulse other planes can be excited according to the Larmor-equation

NUCLEAR MAGNETIC RESONANCE IMAGING (=NMRI or MRI)

NMR-imaging is a form of computer-assisted tomography by analysis of emitted radiosignals. In this way it can be compared to X-ray - CT-scanning or Positron-emission tomography. It was first performed by Lauterbur (27) in 1973, almost 30 years after the findings of Bloch and Purcell. Imaging of the structures in the excited planes can be performed by the so-called 2-dimensional Fourier-analysis. This technique employs magnetic field gradients in the direction of the x- and y-axis of the plane (phase- and frequency-encoding gradients). These cause changes in the phase and frequency of the emitted radiosignals. By Fourier-analysis of the radio-signals in both directions, a 2-dimensional tomogram can be constructed. The image quality of these tomograms depends on the contrast in signal intensity between the different tissues. The signal intensity is influenced by the following properties of these tissues:

1. Proton density
   Lungs, for example, contain very few protons, so they appear very dark.
2. Flow
   In rapidly flowing fluids the excited protons will be eliminated from the selected plane before the image is constructed. For that reason large vessels or cardiac cavities with rapid bloodflow will also appear black. On the other hand slowly moving fluids might intensify the emitted signal and appear very bright.
3. Relaxation times, T1 and T2
   The difference in relaxation times is the basis of NMR-imaging. For a detailed descripton the readers are referred to the textbooks. In principle this phenomenon can be compared to the effect of dropping a lump of sugar in a cup of tea. This will induce a wavefront which will extinguish slowly. This "relaxation" of the tea is characterized by a certain time constant.

   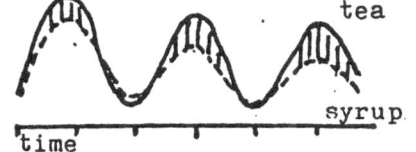

   If we now drop the same lump into a bowl of syrup, it is noticed that the relaxation is much faster. Super-imposing the waves of tea and syrup will show that in the beginning both have almost the same amplitude. Some time later it is seen that the waves are much larger in tea than in syrup. This difference in amplitude can be transformed in contrast in the NMR-image. Fig. 7 shows how this phenomenon is used in NMRI.

CARDIAC NUCLEAR MAGNETIC RESONANCE IMAGING

NMR-tomography of the heart is subject to many more technical problems. The most important are:
MOTION ARTIFACTS: The rapidly moving cardiac structures cannot be imaged through conventional NMR-techniques because of the prolonged acquisition time which is required. This problem has been met by summation of many acquisitions taken at a fixed interval (trigger delay) after the QRS complex of the ECG (44). This technique is also used in the Multiple Gated Acquisition technique used in radionuclide studies. A disadvantage of this method is an important increase of the scanning time which may produce artifacts caused by respiratory or other movements of the patient.

Another problem is the EXCENTRIC LOCATION OF THE HEART (1,13,14,28), which also varies during contraction. This necessitates double angulation of the imaging planes if a tomogram through the long or short axis of the ventricles is required. The imaging planes in fact should be changed during contraction!

Finally the high signal intensity of slowly moving blood will cause many FLOW-ARTIFACTS which disturb the exact delineation of the cardiac chambers and myocardium.

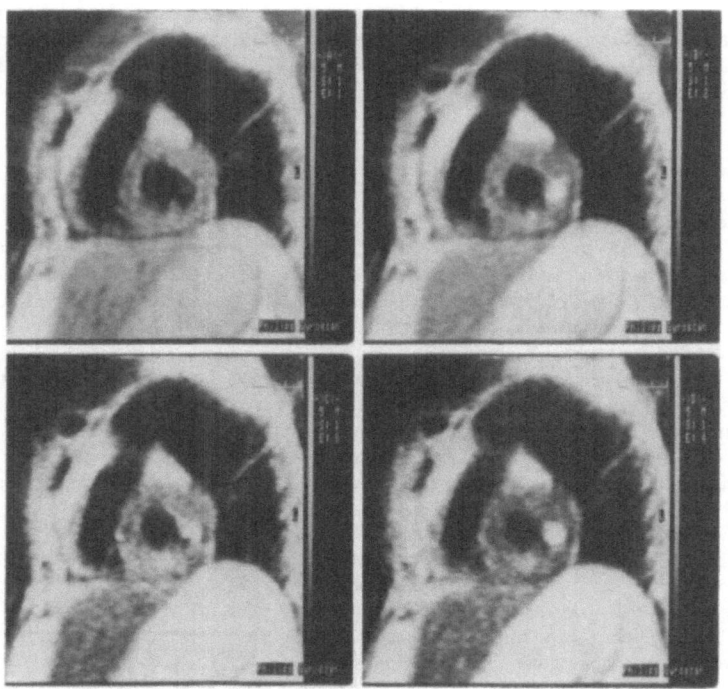

FIGURE 7. Four multi-echo tomograms through the short axis of the left ventricle of the heart. A spin-echo technique was used with a Repetition Time (TR) equal to the RR-interval of the ECG and a Trigger delay of 200 msec. The images were constructed after 30 msec (A); 60 msec (B); 90 msec (C); and 120 msec (D). In the first image (A) the left ventricular myocardium seems to have a uniform signal intensity. The later tomograms show a bright spot in the posterior wall due to prolongation of the relaxation time (T2) in that area. This was caused by a recent myocardial infarction of the posterior wall.

These problems have sofar prevented the widespread use of NMRI in patients with ischemic heart disease. Only recently several authors have tried successfully to describe a serious potential implication of this disease, namely MYOCARDIAL INFARCTION

They found that the most reliable characteristics of infarction in Cardiac-NMR are (2,4,9,10,15,16,18,22,23,29,31,37,43):

1. Regional systolic wall-thinning of the infarcted area.
2. Increased signal intensity of the myocardium, especially when T2-weighted Spin-echo images are constructed as in fig. 7.
3. Increased intra-cavitary signal intensity in the areas adjacent to the infarction (45).

According to these authors criterion No 1 is the most specific and criterion No 2 the most sensitive change in acute myocardial infarction. Criterion No 3 has a very low specificity (45).

These observations have led us to study (26) the diagnostic accuracy of NMRI in the detection and localization of an acute myocardial infarction in man. For that reason the results of NMRI were compared with those of thallium-201 scintigraphy. We evaluated 20 patients with an acute myocardial infarction proven by typical changes of the ECG and an increase of cardiac serum enzyme levels. NMRI was performed 3-14 days after the infarction, but thallium-201 exercise scintigraphy had to be done after 2-6 weeks, which is not appropriate in the acute phase of a myocardial infarction.

Criterion No 1 was tested in a series of T1-weighted Spin-Echo images with a TE of 30 msec through the long and short axis of the left ventricle. This was performed on a 0.5 Tesla Philips Gyroscan employing the Plan-scan technique. Furthermore in selected slices a multi-echo series with a TE of 30-60-90-120 msec was constructed in order to visualize areas with increased T2-relaxation times; criterion No 2. The results are presented below in table 2. The sensitivity of criterion No 1 appeared to be rather low, since only 11 of the 20 patients (55%) showed this phenomenon. In contrast, T2-weighted imaging displayed an increased signal of the infarcted area in 17 of the patients. The sensitivity of this criterion is comparable to that of thallium scintigraphy (85 vs. 90%).

MAGNETIC RESONANCE IMAGING vs THALLIUM 201-PERFUSION STUDIES

20 patients with a recent Myocardial Infarction

Localization:	T1-MRI	T2-MRI	TL201	ECG/Angio
anterior/ septal	6	8	9	9 patients
inferior	4	5	6	7 patients
lateral	1	4	3	4 patients
total	11	17	18	20 patients

TABLE 2
The accuracy of the localization-technique of a patient with Myocardial Infarction by NMRI and Tl-201 scintigraphy in 20 patients compared to ECG-changes and coronary angiography. T1-MRI = T1-weighted spin-echo NMR imaging with a TE of 30 msec. T2-MRI = T2-weighted multi-echo-NMRI with TE of 30-60-90-120 msec.

T2-WEIGHTED MRI vs TL201 PERFUSION IN MYOCARDIAL INFARCTION

Comparison of normal (–) and abnormal (+) Segments

	TL201 (+)	TL201 (–)	
T2-MRI (+)	28	11	39
T2-MRI (–)	9	52	61
	37	63	100

To improve the comparison between T2 NMR-imaging and Tl-201 perfusion we divided the image of the left ventricular wall into 5 segments: 1 = septum; 2 = anterior; 3 = lateral; 4 = inferior; and 5 = apex.
Through a special scoring-system it then was decided whether a segment was abnormal (+) or normal (-). Afterwards the results of NMRI and Tl-201 perfusion were compared as is displayed.

In 80% the findings on T2-NMRI and Tl-201 scans were in accordance with each other. Twenty-eight segments were scored as abnormal and 52 as normal by both methods.
In 9 segments a Tl-201 defect was found while NMRI appeared to be normal. At least 2 patients (with 4 of these segments) suffered a small extension of an old infarction in the same area. This might explain the discrepancy of these findings. The sensitivity of T2-NMR seems to be too low to detect such changes in the borderline area of an old infarction.
In 11 segments T2-weighted NMRI showed an increased signal intensity with normal Tl-201 perfusion. In some patients this might have been caused by high intracavitary flow-signal which easily leads to errors in the delineation between myocardium and blood. In 2 patients with a proven infarction the NMRI was clearly abnormal, but their Tl-201 scintigraphy appeared completely normal. Both suffered a very small infero-posterior infarction.
This finding might be explained by the fact that the NMRI-changes were induced by edema with so little cell-necrosis that it could not be detected on the Tl-201 scan which was performed much later. This is in agreement with several other investigators, who found a linear relation between T1- and T2-relaxation times and tissue water content (9,18,23,43).
The conclusion of our study is that the accuracy of T2-weighted NMRI in detecting and localizing a myocardial infarction is comparable to thallium-201 perfusion scintigraphy. The advantages of NMRI are that it can be repeated harmlessly and can be performed in the early stage of infarction. In that phase Tl-201 scans can only be done at rest which diminishes the diagnostic information.

Other advantages of NMRI are that the anatomical resolution is much better and damage caused by the infarction is displayed exactly. This is especially true for left ventricular aneurysms, pericardial effusions, ventricular or atrial dilatations and even ventricular septal defects. In fig. 8 and 9 several examples are shown.

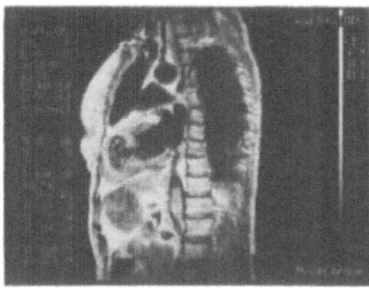
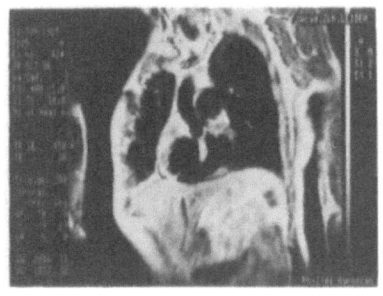

FIGURE 8
A patient with a large LV-aneurysm

FIGURE 9
A ventricular septal defect caused by rupture of the infarcted inferior wall.

FUTURE DEVELOPMENTS OF NMR-IMAGING

New developments which can be expected in NMR-imaging are improvements of image quality through a reduction of the artifacts (14). The exact DETERMINATION OF RELAXATION-TIMES of the different areas of the myocardium will be extremely helpful in detecting changes in tissue water or lipid content (9,18,31,43). The group of Edinburgh (4) proved that it is possible to identify the position and size of myocardial infarctions in man by using calculated T1-images. Another recently developed technique is NMR-ANGIOGRAPHY. Several authors (41) described methods which enable the construction of 16 to 32 ECG-triggered images of the heart and great vessels during the cardiac cycle. When these images are fused into a "movieloop" one gets the impression of a cine-angiogram of the contracting heart. Because this technique is very sensitive to flow, the signal intensity of blood moving in one direction will show a remarkable increase, whereas fluids moving to the opposite side and turbulent blood flow appear dark. This method offers an excellent insight of flow patterns through valves and vessels revealing abnormalities like regurgitations, shunts, and dissections.
Another advantage will be the possibility to assess wall motion of the ventricles, so functional consequences of impaired myocardial perfusion can be detected. Another improvement of the image quality can be obtained by the use of PARAMAGNETIC CONTRAST-AGENTS. These substances reduce the relaxation times T1 and T2 and for that reason contrast in T1-weighted images will increase, while T2-weighted signal intensity diminishes. These qualities can be used to delineate perfusion defects or a delayed washout of underperfused areas. A well-known contrast agent is GADOLINIUM-DTPA, and its pharmacological properties make it clinically very useful (8, 16,

30,37,40,42,46,47).
A promising technique will be NMR-CHEMICAL SHIFT IMAGING. By employing the
small differences in Larmor-frequency due to chemical bindings the signal
intensity of certain substances can be increased or reduced. In this way
it is possible to perform a kind of chemical distribution analysis, which
enhances contrast between, for example, lipids and water (39). Some
authors already speculated on the possibility to display lactate
accumulation or local acidosis! (5)

At last we would like to mention recent progress in NON-PROTON NMR-IMAGING
of Fluor-19 (33) or Sodium-23 (12,21). The use of Fluoro-carbons for NMRI
of reduced coronary flow has been described (34). This opens the possibility to display local metabolism of fluorinated compounds like Fluor-
deoxy-glucose, by superimposing these Fluor-images on conventional Proton-
NMRI. Hilal et al. (21) reported the first clinical NMR-images of sodium
distribution in the human head. They were able to display recent strokes
which were not detectable on X-ray CT-scans. This technique might be extremely useful for the detection of myocardial edema (12), although
technical problems have to be overcome before it will be ready for clinical applications.

In this overview it was attempted to give an impression of the possible
role of Nuclear Magnetic Resonance in the investigation of the coronary
circulation. There is no doubt that at this moment Cardiac-NMR-imaging is
still in the early stage of development. The potentials of this technique
for clinical purposes will become evident in the near future.

RECOMMENDED LITERATURE OF BASIC PRINCIPLES
Cardiovascular Metabolic Imaging. Circulation 72, suppl 4, p. 79-121,
1985.
Gadian DG: Nuclear Magnetic Resonance and its application in living
systems, Oxford University Press, Oxford, 1982.
Higgins CB: Overview of Magnetic Resonance of the Heart, 1986. AJR
146:907-18, 1986.
Koutcher JA: Burt CT: Principles of imaging by Nuclear Magnetic Resonan-
ce. J. Nucl. Med. 25:371-82, 1984.
Kramer DM: Basic Principles of Magnetic Resonance Imaging. Radiol.
Clinics of North America 22:765-78, 1984.
Partain CL, Price RR, Rollo FD, James EA, eds: Nuclear Magnetic Resonan-
ce Imaging, WB Saunders Co., Philadelphia, 1983.
Pykett IL, Newhouse JH, Buonanno FS, Brady TJ, Goldman MR, Kistler JP,
Pohost GM: Principles of Nuclear Magnetic Resonance Imaging, Radiology,
143:157-68, 1982.
Radda GK: Potential and limitations of Nuclear Magnetic Resonance for
the cardiologist, Br. Heart. J. 50:197-201, 1983.
Reeves RC, Evanochko WT, Pohost GM: Potential approaches to evaluating
the Cardiovascular Systems using NMR. Progr. Cardiovasc. Dis. XXIX:53-64,
1986.
Rholl KS, Levitt RG, Glazer HS, Gutterez FR, Murphy WA, Lee JK, Geltman
EM, Peterson RR: Oblique magnetic resonance imaging of the cardiovascular
system. RadioGraphics 6:177-188, 1986.
Young SW: Nuclear Magnetic Resonance Imaging, Basic Principles. Raven
Press, New York, 1984.

REFERENCES

1. Akins EW, Hill JA, Fitzsimmons JR, Pepine CJ, Williams CM: Importance of imaging plane for magnetic resonance imaging of the normal left ventricle. Am. J. Cardiol. 56:366-72, 1985.
2. Akins EW, Hill JA, Sievers KW, Conti CR: Assessment of left ventricular wall thickness in healed myocardial infarction by Magnetic Resonance Imaging, Am. J. Cardiol. 59:24-8, 1987.
3. Barrett EJ, Alger JR, Zaret BL: Nuclear Magnetic Resonance Spectroscopy: Its evolving role in the study of myocardial metabolism. JACC 6:497-501, 1985.
4. Been M, Smith MA, Ridgeway JP, Brydon JW, Douglas RH, Kean DM, Best JJ, Muir AL: Characterization of acute myocardial infarction by gated magnetic resonance imaging. Lancet 2 (8451):348-50, 1985.
5. Behar KL, Roman DL, Shulman RG, Petroff OAC, Prichard JW: Detection of cerebral lactate in vivo during hypoxemia by ^{1}H NMR at relatively low field strength (1.9 T). Proc. Natl. Acad. Sci. USA, 81:2517-9, 1984.
6. Bloch F, Hansen WW, Packard H: The nuclear induction experiment. Physical Rev. 70:474-85, 1946.
7. Bottomley PA: Noninvasive study of high-energy phosphate metabolism in human heart by depth-resolved ^{31}P NMR spectroscpy. Science 229-769-72, 1985.
8. Brasch RC, Weinmann HJ, Wesbey GE: Contrast-enhanced NMR imaging: animal studies using Gadolinium-DTPA complex. AJR 142:625-30, 1984.
9. Brown JJ, Strich G, Higgins CB, Gerbert KH, Slutsky RA: Nuclear magnetic resonance analysis of acute myocardial infarction in dogs, the effect of transient coronary ischemia of varying duration and reperfusion on spin lattice relaxation times. Am. heart J. 109486-90, 1985
10. Buda AJ, Aisen AM, Juni JE, Gallagher KP, Zotz RJ: Detection and sizing of myocardial ischemia and infarction by nuclear magnetic resonance imaging in the canine heart. Am. Heart J. 110:1284-90, 1985.
11. Chance B, Clark BJ, Nioka S, Subramanian H, Maris JM, Argov Z, Bode H: Phosphorus nuclear magnetic resonance spectroscopy in vivo. Circulation 72, suppl. 4:103-10, 1985.
12. Cannon PJ, Maudsley AA, Hilal SK, Simon HE, Cassidy F: Sodium nuclear magnetic resonance imaging of myocardial tissue of dogs after coronary artery occlusion and reperfusion. JACC 7:573-9, 1986.
13. Dinsmore RE, Wismer GL, Levine RA, Okada RD, Brady TJ: Magnetic resonance imaging of the heart: positioning and gradient angle selection for optimal imaging planes. AJR 143:1135-42, 1984.
14. Edelman RE, Thompson R, Kantor H, Brady TJ, Leavitt M, Dinsmore R: Cardiac function: evaluation with fast-echo MR imaging. Radiology 162:611-15, 1987.
15. Flipchuck NG, Peshock RM, Malloy CR, Corbet JR, Rehr RB, Buja LM et al.: Detection and localization of recent myocardial infarction by magnetic resonance imaging. Am. J. Cardiol. 58:214-9, 1986.
16. Goldman MR, Brady TJ, Pykett IL, Burt JT, Buonanno FS, Kistler JP et al.: Quantification of experimental myocardial infarction using nuclear magnetic resonance imaging and paramagnetic ion contrast enhancement in excised canine hearts. Circulation 66:1012-16, 1982.
17. Grove TH, Ackerman JJH, Radda GK, Bore PJ: Analysis of rat heart in vivo by phosphorus nuclear resonance. Proc. Natl. Acad. Sci. USA 80:7491-5, 1980.

18. Higgins CB, Herfkents R, Lipton MJ, Sievers R, Sheldon P, Kaufman L, Crooks LE: Nuclear magnetic resonance imaging of acute myocardial infarction in dogs, alterations in magnetic relaxation times. Am. J. Cardiol. 52:184-8, 1983.

19. Higgins CB, Lanzer P, Stark D, Botvinick E, Schiller NB, Crooks L, Kaufman L, Lipton MJ: Imaging by nuclear magnetic resonance in patients with chronic ischemic heart disease. Circulation 69:523-31, 1984.

20. Higgins CB, Byrd BFD, McNamara MT, Lanzer P, Lipton MJ, Botvinick E, Schiller NB, Crooks LE, Kaufman L: Magnetic resonce imaging of the heart, a review of the experience in 172 subjects. Radiology 155:671-9, 1985.

21. Hilal SK, Maudsley AA, Ra JB, Simon HE, Roschmann P, Wittekoek S, Cho ZH, Mun SK: In vivo NMR imaging of Sodium-23 in the human head. J. Comp. Ass. Tomography 9:1-7, 1985.

22. Johnston DL, Thompson RC, Lui P, Dinsmore RE; Wismer GL, Saini S, Kaul S, Rosen BR, Brady TJ, Okada RD: Magnetic resonance imaging during acute myocardial infarction. Am. J. Cardiol. 57:1059-65, 1986.

23. Johnston DL, Brady TJ, Ratner AV, Rosen BR, Newell JB, Pohost GM, Okada RD: Assessment of myocardial ischemia with proton magnetic resonance: effects of a three hour coronary occlusion with and without reperfusion. Circulation 71:595-601, 1985.

24. Kantor HL, Briggs RW, Balaban RS: In vivo ^{31}P Nuclear magnetic resonance measurements in canine hearts using a catheter-coil. Circ. Res. 55:261-6, 1984.

25. Koretzky AP, Wang S, Murphy-Boesch J, Klein MP, James TL, Weiner MW: ^{31}-P NMR spectroscopy of rat organs in situ, using chronically implanted radiofrequency coils. Proc. Natl. Acad. Sci. USA 80: 7491-5, 1983.

26. Krauss XH, de Roos A, Doornbos J, van der Wall EE, van Voorthuisen A, Bruschke AVG: Magnetic resonance imaging versus thallium-201 myocardial perfusion studies in patients with a recent myocardial infarction (abstr.) JACC 9 (No. 2): 74A, 1987.

27. Lauterbur PC: Image formaton by induced local interactions: examples employing nuclear magnetic resonance. Nature 242:190-1, 1973.

28. Longmore DB, Lipstein RH, Underwood SR, Firmin DN, Houndsfield GN, Watanabe M et al.: Dimensional accuracy of magnetic resonance studies of the heart. Lancet (8442) p. 1360-2, 1985.

29. McNamara MT, Higgins CB: Magnetic resonance imaging of chronic myocardial infarctions in man. AJR 146:315-20, 1986.

30. McNamara MT, Wesbey GE, Brasch RC, Sievers R, Lipton MJ, Higgins CB: Magnetic resonance imaging of acute myocardial infarction using a nitroxyl spin label (PCA). Invest. Radiol. 20:591-5, 1985.

31. McNamara MT, Higgins CB, Schlechtmann N, Botvinick E, Lipton MJ, Chatterjee K, Amparo EG: Detection and characterization of acute myocardial infarctions with the use of aged magnetic resonance. Circulation 71:717-24, 1985.

32. Moon RB, Richard JH: Determination of intracellular pH by ^{31}P magnetic resonance. J. Biol. Chem. 248:7276-8, 1973.

33. Nelson TR, Newman FD, Schiffer LM, Reith JD, Cameron SL: Fluorine nulcear magnetic resonance: calibration and system optimization. Magn. Reson. Imaging 3:267-73, 1985.

34. Nunnally RL, Babcock EE, Horner SD, Peshock RM: Fluorine-19 NMR spectroscopy and imaging investigations of myocardial perfusion and cardiac function. Magn. Reson. Imaging 3:399-405, 1985.

35. Purcell EM, Torrey HC, Pound RV: Resonance absorption by nuclear magnetic moments in a solid. Physical Rev. 69:377, 1946.
36. Radda GK, Bore PJ, Rajagopalan B: Clinical aspects of ^{31}P NMR spectroscopy. Br. Med. Bull. 40:155-9, 1984.
37. Rehr RB, Peshock RM, Malloy CR, Keller AM, Parkey RW, Buja LM, Nunnally RL, Willerson JT: Improved in vivo magnetic resonance imaging of acute myocardial infarction after intravenous paramagnetic contrast agent administration. Am. J. Cardiol. 57:864-8, 1986.
38. Rokey R, Verani MS, Bolli R, Kuo LC, Ford JJ, Wendt RE, Schneiders NJ, Bryan RN, Roberts R: Myocardial infarct size quantification by MR imaging early after coronary occlusion in dogs. Radiology 158:771-4, 1986.
39. Rosen BR, Wedeen VJ, Brady TJ: Selective saturation NMR imaging. J. Comp. Ass. Tomography 8:813-8, 1984.
40. Runge VM, Clanton JA, Wehr CJ, Partain CL, James AE, jr: Gated magnetic resonance imaging of acyte myocardial ischemia in dogs: Application of multi-echo techniques and contrast enhancement with GDDTPA. Magn. Reson. Imaging 3:255-66, 1985.
41. Sechtem U, Pflugelder PW, White RED, Gould RG, Holt W, Lipton M, Higgins CB: Cine MR imaging: potential for the evaluation of cardiovascular function. AJR 148:239-46, 1987.
42. Tscholakoff D, Higgins CB, Sechtem U, McNamara MT: Occlusive and reperfused myocardial infarcts: effect of Gd-DTPA on ECG-gated MR imaging. Radiology 160:515-9, 1986.
43. Tscholakoff D, Higgins CB, Sechtem U, Caputa G, Derugin N: NMR of reperfused myocardial infarct in dogs. AJR 146:925-30, 1986.
44. Van Dijk P: ECG triggered NMR imaging of the heart. Diagn. Imag. Clin. med. 53:29-37, 1984.
45. Von Schulthess GK, Fisher M, Crooks LE, Higgins CB: Gated MR imaging of the heart: Intracardiac signals in patients and healthy subjects. Radiology 156:125-32, 1985.
46. Weinmann HJ, Brasch RC, Press WR, Wesbey GE: Characteristics of Gadolinium-DTPA compex: a potential NMR contrast agent. AJR 142:619-24, 1984.
47. Wesbey GE, Higgins CB, McNamara MT, Engelstadt BL, Lipton MJ, Sievers R, Ehman RL, Lovin J, Brasch RC: Effect of gadolinium-DTPA on the magnetic relaxation times of normal and infarcted myocardium. Radiology 153:165-9, 1984.
48. Whitman GJR, Chance B, Bode H, Maris J, Haselgrove J, Kelly R, Clark BJ, Harken AH: Diagnosis and therapeutic evaluation of a pediatric case of cardiomyopathy using phosphorus-31 Nuclear magnetic resonance spectroscopy. JACC 5:745-9, 1985.

CORONARY ARTERIAL FLOW MEASUREMENTS BY DOPPLER TECHNIQUES

DAVID H. SIBLEY, M.D.

In 1958, Mason Sones first performed selective coronary angiography (1). Since that time, clinical decisions involving ischemic heart disease have been based on the amount of obstruction visually estimated to be present in an epicardial coronary artery. The assumption was made that one could estimate the reduction in myocardial perfusion based on the visual interpretation of the anatomy. Gould found that coronary hyperemia after an intracoronary injection of contrast decreased when there was 30-45% stenosis and disappeared completely when there was 88-93% stenosis. This flow response appeared to be a quantitative measure for physiologically assessing critical coronary stenosis and flow reserve. This study showed that although the coronary arteriogram does provide anatomic definition of coronary lesions, it offers little evaluation of their hemodynamic consequences short of a near total occlusion (2).

The effect of a coronary stenosis on myocardial perfusion is an integrated response of an anatomic-hemodynamic system. The severity of coronary stenosis is one part of the anatomic system and the percent stenosis alone does not describe the supply of blood flow to the myocardium. Coronary perfusion pressure, coronary vascular tone, collateral flow and stenosis configuration all affect myocardial perfusion. Kirkeeide et al. (3) showed that coronary flow reserve is a single functional measure of coronary stenosis severity that is determined by all the hemodynamic variables and geometric characteristics of that stenosis.

Marcus et al developed a Doppler probe which could be coupled to the surface of coronary vessels at the time of cardiac surgery with a small suction cup (4) (Fig.1). They found changes in mean coronary flow velocity were closely correlated to changes in coronary flow over a wide range (15-400 ml/min.). Reactive hyperemia in the coronary circulation of dogs determined with this new Doppler system was similar to that obtained simultaneously with an electromagnetic flow meter. Phasic coronary velocity was measured with a signal-to-noise ratio that exceeded 20:1. After 20 seconds of coronary occlusion, the ratio of peak to resting velocity was 5.8 ± 0.6. This provided the first quantitative measurements of coronary reactive hyperemia in humans.

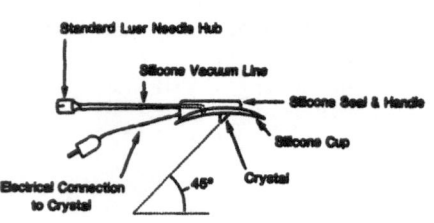

1

White et al. used Marcus' previously validated epicardial Doppler probe to study reactive hyperemic responses at operation after 20 seconds of coronary arterial occlusion. These patients had isolated, discrete coronary lesions usually estimated by cineangiography to have 10-95% stenosis. Coronary flow reserve did not correlate well with percent diameter stenosis as estimated by angiography (R = -0.25) (Fig. 2). This

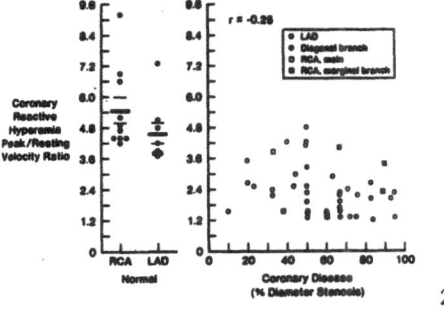

study suggested that the physiological effects of the majority of coronary obstructions cannot be determined accurately by coronary angiography.

Hartley and Cole (6,7) developed the first Doppler coronary catheter capable of on-line continuous measurements of coronary blood flow velocity and coronary flow reserve in humans. A 20 MHz directional pulsed Doppler ultrasonic flow meter was used to drive an annular shaped crystal mounted on the tip of a Sones catheter. This catheter was capable of recording blood velocity from the aorta and coronary arteries of dogs while radiographic contrast was injected. Because of its size (5F), this catheter was too large to be placed subselectively in the coronary circulation.

Wilson (8) validated the ability of a 3F coronary catheter with a side-mounted piezoelectric crystal to provide accurate, continuous on-line measurements of coronary blood flow velocity and vasodilator reserve (Fig. 3). In 10 normal patients, intracoronary meglumine diatrizoate increased coronary blood flow velocity to 3.5 times that at rest (range 2.8 - 5.0). Coronary blood flow velocity rose five fold after an intravenous infusion of Dipyridamole (range 3.8 - 7.0) (Fig. 4, 5).

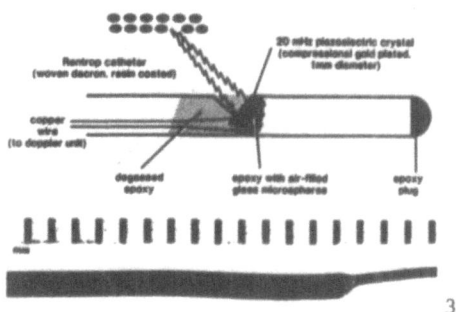

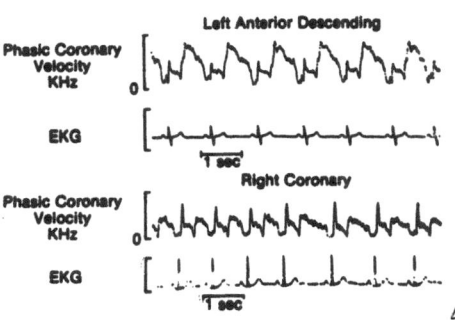

Poor signal quality was obtained in 12 of 70 patients studied with this catheter. The limitation of the system appeared to be the inability to steer the catheter away from small branch vessels in the arterial wall. No catheter lumen was available for guide wire placement; thus it was difficult to control direction of the catheter in the coronary circulation.

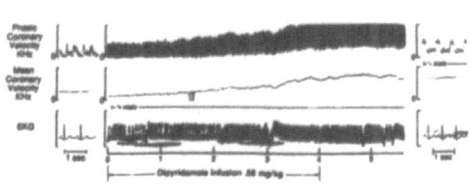

CATHETER WITH DOPPLER PROBE AT TIP

To provide a consistent and clinically safe method of measuring coronary blood flow velocity and coronary flow reserve, we developed a 3F Doppler coronary catheter with an internal lumen that accommodates a standard angioplasty steerable guidewire (9). The guidewire allows precise placement and easy adjustment of the catheter in the coronary circulation. A circular 20 MHz. ceramic crystal capable of both transmitting and receiving acoustic signals is attached to the tip of a USCI Rentrop reperfusion catheter (Millar Instruments). This catheter is 4F in the main body, with a wire weave for torque control, and the distal 20cm tip tapers to 3F (1mm outer diameter). Two wires attached to the crystal pass within the catheter between the outer catheter sheath and an inner lumen tubing traverses the full length of the catheter. The internal lumen is 0.015 inch (0.038cm) and will accommodate a 0.014 inch (0.0356cm) flexible, steerable guidewire (Fig. #6). An electrical leakage test was zero at either polarity, using a device capable of detecting one microamp at 600V.

A range-gated 20MHz pulsed Doppler velocimeter connected to the proximal end of the catheter detects the Doppler shift of the echos from the blood cells within the adjustable sample volume which is 1-12mm distal to the catheter tip. The Doppler frequency is related to the velocity of the reflectors (red blood cells) by the Doppler equation: $\Delta F = 2 \cdot F \cdot V / C \cdot \cos(\Theta)$ where F = the Doppler shift frequency, ΔF = transmitter frequency (20MHz), V = average velocity of the blood cells within the sample volume, C = speed of sound in blood (1500m/s), and Θ = angle between the sound beam and the direction of blood flow. Using an end mounted crystal with the catheter parallel ($\pm$ 20) to the vessel axis, $\cos(\Theta) = 1 \pm 6\%$, and the relation between the Doppler shift and velocity is approximately 3.75 cm/s per kHz. The 20MHz ultrasound frequency and the 62.5 kHz pulse repetition frequency allow the recording of velocities up to 115cm/s at 1-12mm distances from the crystal face.

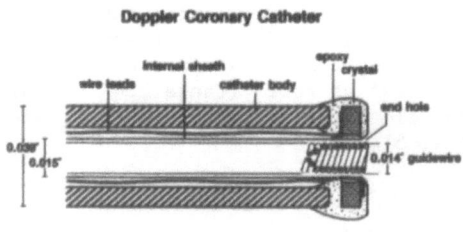

Doppler Coronary Catheter

6

The pulsed Doppler velocimeter provides two simultaneous outputs that represent the spatially averaged velocity within the sample volume. Each is a measure of the frequency of zero crossings of the Doppler audio signal calibrated at 0.25V/kHz, but each has different amounts of filtration. The phasic output displays the pulsatile velocity signal with a band pass from direct current to 15 Hz, and the mean output (which eliminates the pulsations) has a band pass from direct current to 0.25 Hz. Because of the uncertainties in relating the measured frequency shift within the sample volume to the average velocity across the lumen or to volume flow, the data are expressed in terms of the measured frequency shift in kHz.

The relation between the mean Doppler frequency shift measured by the Doppler catheter and timed volume collections was determined by placing the Doppler catheter in a 2.6mm diameter polyethylene tube system filled with whole blood and connected to a roller pump. Flow was altered by adjusting the roller pump and measured with a graduated cylinder and stop watch. Measurements of blood flow calculated from the mean velocity and polyethylene tube cross sectional area were closely correlated with timed collections of blood flow over a broad range (r = 0.96, range = 14-192 ml/min.) (Fig. 7). Animal validation studies were performed using large mongrel dogs. An extra vascular cuff-type Doppler probe was positioned on the surface of the dissected left circumflex coronary artery. An 8F right coronary guiding catheter was then passed through the left carotid artery sheath under fluoroscopy and positioned at the ostium of the left main coronary artery. Reactive hyperemia was induced by a 5 ml injection of meglumine diatrizoate through the guiding

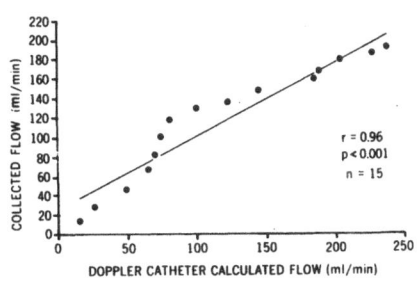

7

catheter into the left circumflex coronary artery. Several measurements of coronary blood flow velocity at rest and after hyperemia with the cuff-type Doppler probe were performed before the Doppler coronary catheter was advanced into the left circumflex coronary artery. The Doppler catheter was preloaded with a 0.014 inch flexible, steerable guidewire. Under fluoroscopic guidance, the guidewire was positioned in the left circumflex coronary artery in a position just proximal to the epicardial Doppler probe. The Doppler coronary catheter was advanced through the guiding catheter over the guidewire into the left circumflex artery and placed in position proximal to the cuff-type Doppler probe. Care was taken not to have arterial branches exiting the left circumflex artery between the extravascular and intracoronary crystals. An optimal signal was obtained by moving the catheter slightly within the arterial lumen, placing torque on the flexible guidewire extending through the tip of the Doppler catheter and adjusting the range-gate control. Sixty-seven measurements of rest and hyperemic coronary blood flow velocity (induced by a 5 ml injection of meglumine diatrizoate) were then performed simultaneously by the cuff-type Doppler probe and the Doppler coronary catheter. The ratio of the peak-to-rest blood flow velocity was used as a measurement of coronary flow reserve (Figs. 8, 9).

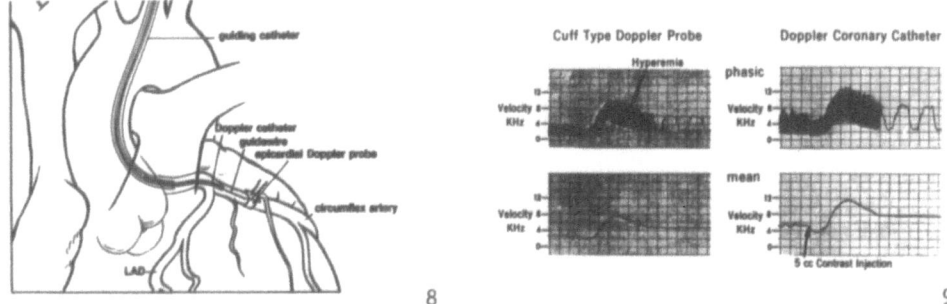

8   9

Measurements with the epicardial cuff-type Doppler probe before the Doppler catheter was placed in the coronary artery were averaged. The mean rest flow velocity was 3.12kHz (SD = 1.62). The same number of epicardial Doppler measurements were averaged immediately after the Doppler catheter was placed in the left circumflex artery and the mean rest flow velocity was 3.19kHz (SD = 1.45). The mean peak/rest velocity ratio was 3.04 (SD = 1.15) without and 3.18 (SD = 1.65) with the Doppler catheter in the left

174

circumflex artery.   The   means   were not significantly different using a
paired t-test.

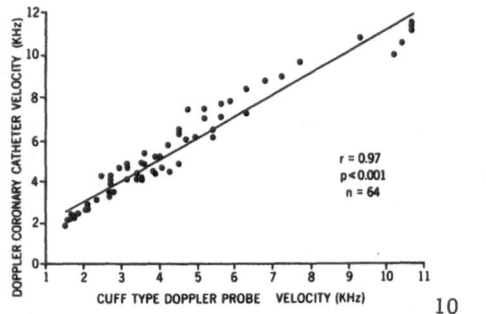

10

Sixty-four simultaneous measurements of coronary blood flow velocity at rest were obtained with the cuff-type Doppler probe placed immediately distal to the intracoronary Doppler catheter position (Fig. 10). Coronary blood flow velocity was altered over a wide range and the paired measurements correlated highly (R = 0.97, range = 1.53 to 10.6kHz, slope = 1.03). Sixty-seven simultaneous measurements of peak/rest velocity ratio were obtained with the cuff-type Doppler probe positioned immediately distal to the intracoronary Doppler catheter (Fig. 11).   The peak/rest velocity ratio values were positively correlated (r = 0.72, range = 1.30 to 8.12, slope = 0.902).

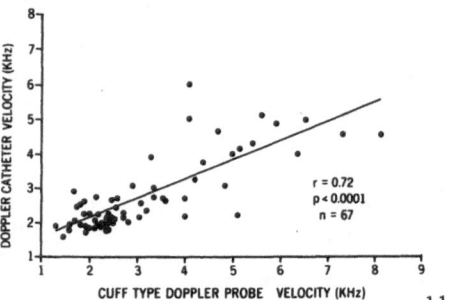

11

In two dogs, the right femoral arteries were dissected and a segment was isolated that was visually estimated to be the size of the left circumflex coronary artery (2-3mm). The branches in the segments were ligated. The distal end of the artery was cannulated with polyethylene tubing and flow through the tubing was controlled with a pinch clamp. The 8F guiding catheter was advanced down the descending aorta into the right femoral artery to a position proximal to the dissected segment of femoral artery. The 0.014 inch steerable guidewire was then placed in the dissected femoral artery segment and the Doppler catheter was advanced to a position proximal to the insertion of the polyethylene tubing. Timed volume collections were made with a graduated cylinder-stopwatch technique while simultaneously measuring mean blood flow velocity with the Doppler catheter. Fifteen volume collections were made from the first dog with a range of 6-266ml/min. (r = 0.98). Eighteen volume collections were made from the second animal with a range of 19-282ml/min. (r = 0.96) (Fig. 12).

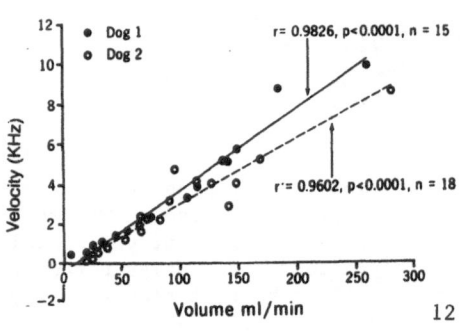

12

In one dog, a right thoracotomy was performed with the animal on its left side. A small incision was made in the right atrial appendage and a 2.5F pediatric Foley catheter was advanced through the right atrium into the coronary sinus. The balloon was inflated with 3ml saline solution. The Doppler coronary catheter was then placed in the left anterior descending artery and an optimal signal obtained. Coronary blood flow velocity was altered over a large range using intravenous Dipyridamole

(0.56mg/kg) and Papaverine (10-20mg). Timed volume collections of coronary sinus flow were made with a graduated cylinder-stopwatch technique. Simultaneous mean coronary blood flow velocity was measured with the Doppler catheter. Twelve timed volume collections of coronary sinus flow were positively correlated with mean rest coronary blood flow velocity measured in the left anterior descending coronary artery (r = 0.78, range = 10.5-19.5ml/min., slope = 1.15) (Fig. 13). In 5 dogs, the left circumflex coronary artery was opened by an incision at autopsy and care- fully inspected. No evidence of trauma or thrombus formation was found.

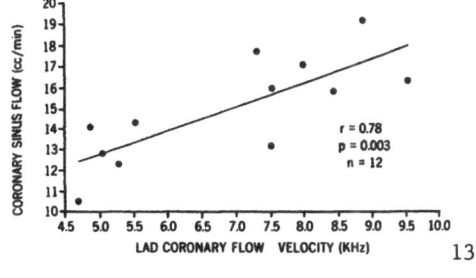

13

HUMAN CATHETERIZATIONS

The Doppler coronary catheter has been used to measure coronary blood flow velocity in patients undergoing diagnostic coronary angiography and percutaneous transluminal coronary angioplasty. The studies have included coronary artery cannulations in the left anterior descending, the left circumflex, the right coronary artery and saphenous vein grafts. Examples of the phasic tracings for the left main, right, left circumflex, and left anterior descending coronary arteries are shown in Figure 14. An example of a hyperemic response in the right coronary artery induced by 5ml injection of meglumine diatrizoate is seen in Figure 15.

Human Catheterization — Phasic Doppler Tracings

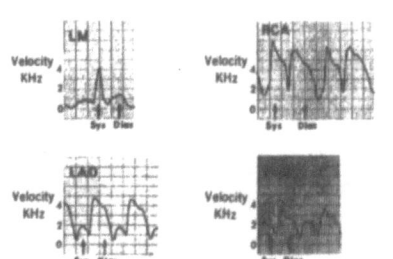

14

Figure 16 demonstrates rest and peak coronary blood flow velocity measured proximal to a 90% stenosis of the mid-left anterior descending coronary artery before and after this vessel was dilated by coronary angioplasty. Stable velocity recordings were obtained in all coronary artery cannulations. There have been no complications during these procedures. There has been no evidence of dissection or thrombus formation or subsequent angiograms.

An important advantage of this steerable catheter is that it can be safely and easily passed in the major arteries of the coronary circulation. The steerable nature of the guidewire catheter system allows precise adjustment and positioning of the Doppler crystal. This was not possible with previous Doppler catheters; consequently, the safety of positioning and stability of signals was not optimal (6,8). The end mounted crystal has advantages over the side mounted crystal. This is most obvious in the Doppler equation itself (Doppler frequency shift = $2 \cdot F \cdot V / C \cdot \cos(\Theta)$). The angle of the side mounted crystal in relation to blood flow is 45°. If this angle were to vary 15° in either direction and blood flow velocity were to remain constant, the Doppler frequency shift could vary as much as 23% from baseline. On the other hand, with an end mounted crystal, the theoretical angle of the acoustic signal to blood flow is 0°. If the angle of the tip of the Doppler catheter were to change by 15° in either

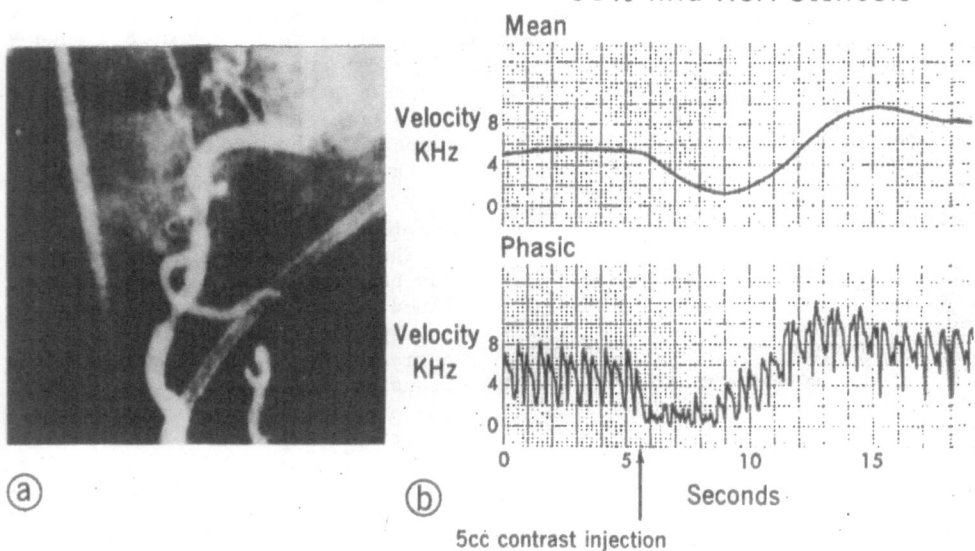

50% Mid RCA Stenosis

Mean

Velocity KHz

Phasic

Velocity KHz

Seconds

5cc contrast injection

15

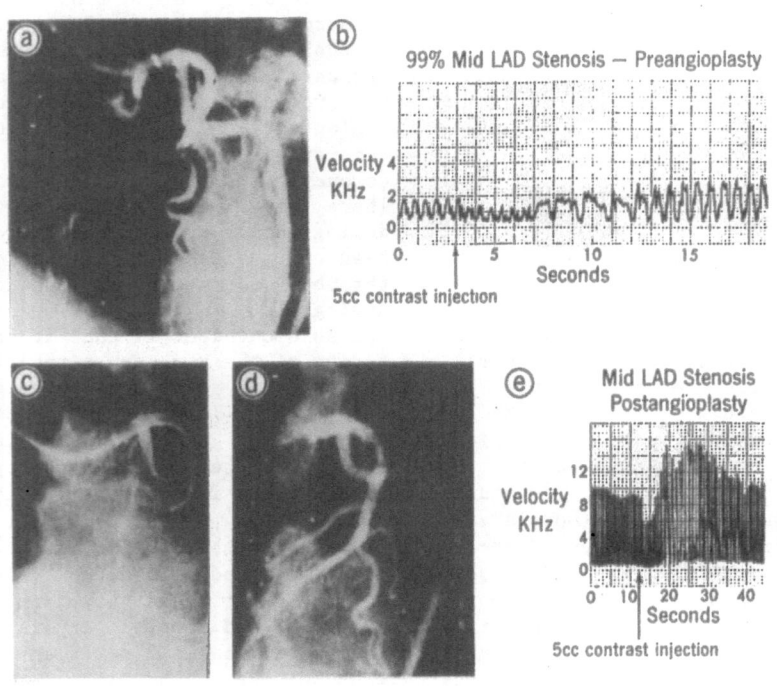

99% Mid LAD Stenosis — Preangioplasty

Velocity KHz

Seconds

5cc contrast injection

Mid LAD Stenosis
Postangioplasty

Velocity KHz

Seconds

5cc contrast injection

16

direction, the change in Doppler frequency shift would be a maximum of 3.5%.

Our measurements with the cuff-type Doppler probe before and after the Doppler catheter was placed in the coronary artery showed no significant change in either rest mean coronary blood flow velocity or coronary vasodilator reserve. This data suggests that this intracoronary Doppler catheter does not obstruct coronary flow.

One potential problem in correlating changes in flow with mean blood flow velocity is a possible change in vessel caliber as the flow is varied. If vessel caliber were to increase after a vasodilating agent was administered, flow could increase while mean blood flow velocity remained constant. If the relation between changes in mean blood flow velocity and flow were to remain linear over a wide range, this would indicate no significant change in the diameter of the vessel being studied. Our data confirmed a very linear correlation over a wide range of flows (6-282 ml/min.) collected from the femoral artery. Previous studies (7,8) also showed excellent linear correlations between maximal flow velocity and flow over a wide range of flow rates. Studies of compliance properties of epicardial coronary arteries in dogs provide further evidence that the caliber of the vessel does not change with increasing flow (11,12).

The cross sectional area of the distal segment of the Doppler catheter is less than 0.8mm2. In a normal left anterior descending coronary artery, this is less than 7% of the cross sectional area of the proximal segment and less than 22% of the area of the middle segment (12). It has previously been shown that maximal coronary blood flow is not affected until at least 36 ± 10% luminal area narrowing is present (13). One must consider the possibility that this small coronary catheter could obstruct flow in arteries that are diffusely diseased.

The success of transluminal coronary angioplasty has been judged by improvement of percent luminal diameter stenosis or a decline in the mean transtenotic pressure gradient after dilatation. Visual estimation of improvement in stenosis during coronary angioplasty is often difficult. Pressure gradients are not consistently useful and frequently difficult to obtain. A decline in the mean transtenotic pressure gradient in a tortuous vessel can be misleading due to changes in the intrinsic catheter gradient (14,15,16). Mean transtenotic pressure gradients have often been useful in predicting myocardial ischemia associated with coronary stenosis of moderate angiographic severity (17). Post dilatation high residual transtenotic pressure gradients may predict exercise induced ischemia (18) and restenosis (19,20). Obtaining pressure gradients during coronary angioplasty is a cumbersome, time consuming effort requiring calibration of two pressure transducers and meticulous flushing of the catheters, Y-connectors and manifolds. All instantaneous pressure gradients must be compared to the intrinsic catheter gradient which may vary by 10-20 mm/Hg between the pre and post dilatation measurements depending on the tortuosity of the vessels studied and kinks or bends in the catheter (21). A transtenotic pressure gradient measured at angioplasty usually overestimates the true resting gradient as a function of the angioplasty catheter diameter (24).

DOPPLER ANGIOPLASTY CATHETER

To provide a new physiological measure of the success of coronary angioplasty, we developed a balloon dilatation catheter with an end mounted Doppler crystal for coronary flow velocity measurement (23). An annular 20mHz ceramic crystal capable of being both a transmitter and receiver of acoustic signals is attached to the tip of a standard, low profile balloon dilatation catheter. Two wires attached to the crystal pass within the catheter between the outer sheath and an inner lumen tubing that traverses the full length of the catheter. The internal lumen will accommodate a 0.014 inch guidewire (Fig. 17). The catheter is connected to a directional 20mHz pulsed Doppler velocimeter. Baseline mean blood flow velocity was measured with the balloon deflated across the area of stenosis. Between each balloon inflation, a new mean coronary blood flow velocity was measured (Fig. 18).

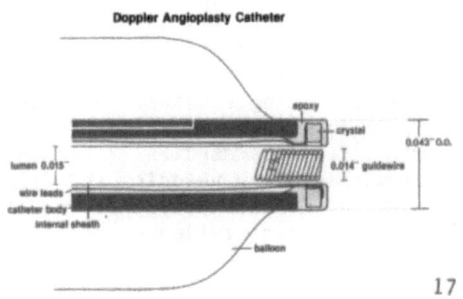

Doppler Angioplasty Catheter

17

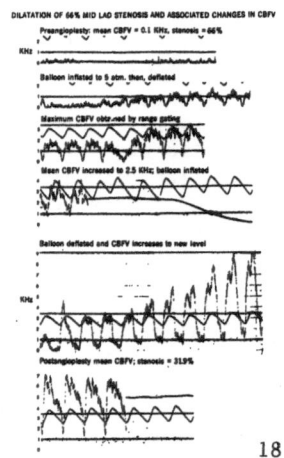

18

We attempted to dilate 18 coronary stenoses in 17 patients. Using the criteria of 20% or greater reduction of luminal diameter stenosis and less than 50% residual stenosis, we successfully dilated 15 stenoses in 17 attempts using the Doppler angioplasty catheter. In one patient with a 95% stenosis of the left circumflex artery, we were unable to pass the angioplasty catheter across the stenosis. Subsequently, a lower profile dilatation catheter was used to cross and successfully dilate the stenosis. This patient was excluded from further statistical analysis.

The coronary artery percent luminal diameter stenosis ranged from 61-95% [(mean 75 $\pm$ 15) (SD)] prior to angioplasty and was reduced to 3-55% (mean 30 $\pm$ 15) after angioplasty. These means were significantly different using a paired t-test (P = 0.0001, N = 16). The percentage improvement in the coronary stenosis varied from 11-96% (mean 57 $\pm$ 24). One angioplasty was unsuccessful by angiographic criteria (Patient #14). A clinically insignificant subintimal nonobstructive dissection was present in the area of dilatation of 5 patients. One of these five patients failed to increase coronary blood flow velocity (30% reduction in flow velocity) despite angiographic success (65% diameter stenosis improved to 40% stenosis). No other complications occurred during angioplasty or the immediate hospital recovery period. Coronary blood flow velocity improved after angioplasty in 15 of the 16 patients in whom these measurements were obtained. Initial blood flow velocity with the deflated balloon catheter positioned across the stenosis ranged from 0.1 to 5.2KHz (mean 0.9 $\pm$ 1.3). The final blood flow velocity after angioplasty with the deflated balloon catheter positioned across the stenosis ranged from 0.7 to 6.2KHz (mean 2.4 $\pm$ 1.5). These means were significantly different using a paired t-test (P = 0.02, N = 16). The percentage improvement in coronary blood flow velocity after each coronary angioplasty varied from -30 to +4300% (mean 732 ± 1125) (Fig. 19). This did not correlate well with the percentage improvement in luminal diameter stenosis (r = 0.51, P = 0.04).

Coronary Blood Flow Velocity (KHz) With Angioplasty # Dilatation

Patient#	Pre	1	2	3	4	5	6	Post	%improvement
1	1.3	3.0	4.9	4.7	4.9	4.6	4.3	4.3	231
2	5.2	4.0	5.2	6.2				6.2	19
3	0.8	1.4	2.4	2.4				2.4	200
4	0.2	0.9	1.8	2.2	2.5			2.5	1150
5	0.4	1.0	1.5					1.5	275
6	0.3	1.0	1.1	*0.5	1.7	3.0		3.0	900
7	0.1	1.9	3.4	4.4				4.4	4300
8	0.1	1.1	1.6	1.9	2.0			2.0	1900
9	0.3	1.6	0.6	1.2	0.8	1.6	0.8	0.8	167
10	0.4	1.2	1.1	1.1	0.9			0.9	125
11	0.4	2.2	2.1	1.9				1.9	375
12	1.9	2.4	1.9	1.9	2.9	3.0		3.0	58
13	0.2	0.3	0.4	0.5				0.8	300
14	1.2	1.6	1.2	1.5	1.7			1.7	42
15	0.1	0.9	1.1	1.2	1.7	1.8		1.8	1700
16	1.0	0.9	0.9	0.7				0.7	-30
17	not recorded								
Mean	0.9	1.6	2.0	2.2	2.1	2.8	2.6	2.4	732 %

* balloon passed across second stenosis

19

The success of coronary angioplasty has been largely judged on the reduction in luminal diameter stenosis estimated by coronary arteriography. Frequently, video monitors and recorders are used in the catheterization laboratory to provide immediate visual assessment of the dilatation; however, the resolution of video images are limited and can be misleading. Reviewing the developed cineangiograms is more reliable but requires time for processing of film. With good cineangiograms, uncertainty of the functional severity of stenosis may still exist. Recent evidence has indicated a poor correlation of the physiological significance of a coronary stenosis with its angiographic appearance (5). Previous studies show that a normalized mean pressure gradient is often a reliable and practical guide to the functional severity of a coronary stenosis. It can be obtained and is useful in documenting the physiological success of coronary angioplasty (21). Unfortunately, tortuous vessels may cause kinking of the fluid filled balloon catheter and spuriously alter pressure measurements. This is frequently the case in the right and in the circumflex coronary arteries.

The new Doppler angioplasty catheter used in this study provides an additional physiological measurement of the success of coronary angioplasty. Data was easily obtained in 16/17 patients attempted. Neither the tortuosity of the vessel nor the position of the stenosis in the vessel affected the Doppler angioplasty catheter measurements. In the human catheterization laboratory, the improvement in coronary blood flow velocity was seen immediately on the oscilloscope. The velocimeter provided a continuous audio signal indicating second-to-second changes in coronary blood flow velocity. Changes in blood flow velocity caused by obstruction from the guiding catheter were readily apparent. Minimal time was required to set up, calibrate and zero the Doppler system.

The coronary blood flow velocity measured with this new Doppler angioplasty catheter is artifactual. The artifact is created by the relationship of the deflated balloon diameter to the stenosis luminal diameter (22). Previous studies have shown that transtenotic pressure gradients measured during coronary angioplasty overestimate the true resting gradient in a predictable manner. This is dependent on the ratio of the catheter diameter to the stenosis diameter (22). One can assume that the coronary blood flow velocity measurements are altered in a similar manner. Despite the artifact, other investigations (24,25) have shown that transtenotic pressure gradients are useful in the assessment of coronary angioplasty. Considering these previous findings, the physiological assessment of coronary angioplasty, although artifactual, acutely gives an online instantaneous measure of success. Theoretically, both coronary blood flow velocity and transtenotic pressure gradients would be useful modalities. Coronary blood flow velocity measurement offers the advantages of an absence of a fluid filled catheter and the inherent miscalculations associated with tortuous vessels. The longterm clinical outcome associated with final transenotic pressure gradients is well known (20). This remains to be elucidated with coronary blood flow velocity measurements.

CONCLUSIONS

The steerable Doppler coronary catheter provides a safe method of determining coronary vasodilator reserve in humans. It has tremendous potential in assessing the physiologic significance of coronary disease in patients with angina but otherwise anatomically insignificant disease. It should be useful in assessing the neurohumoral and pharmacologic control of coronary blood flow. As more experience is gained with the Doppler catheter, coronary hemodynamics will play a larger role in our understanding of ischemic heart disease.

REFERENCES

1. Sones FM Jr, Shirey EK, Prondfit WC, Westcott RN: Cine-coronary arteriography. Circulation 20: 773, 1959 (abstract).

2. Gould KL, Lipscomb K, Hamilton GW: Physiologic basis for assessing critical coronary stenosis. Am J Cardiol 33: 87, 1974.

3. Kirkeeide RL, Gould KL, Parsel L: Assessment of coronary stenoses by myocardial perfusion imaging during pharmacologic coronary vasodilation. VII. Validation of coronary flow reserve as a single integrated functional measure of stenosis severity reflecting all its geometric dimensions. J Am Coll Cardiol 7: 103–113, 1986.

4. Marcus ML, Wright CB, Doty DB, et al: Measurements of coronary velocity and reactive hyperemia in the coronary circulation of humans. Circ Res 49: 877–891, 1981.

5. White CW, Wright CB, Doty DB, et al.: Does visual interpretation of the coronary arteriogram predict the physiologic importance of a coronary stenosis? N Engl J Med 310: 819–824, 1984.

6. Cole JS, Hartley CJ: The pulsed Doppler coronary artery catheter. Preliminary report of a new technique for measuring rapid ranges in coronary artery flow velocity in man. Circulation 56: 18–25, 1977.

7. Hartley CJ, Coles JS: A single-crystal ultrasonic catheter-tip velocity probe. Med Instrum 8: 241–243, 1974.

8. Wilson RF, Laughlin DE, Ackell PH, et al.: Transluminal subselective measurement of coronary artery blood flow velocity and vasodilator reserve in man. Circulation 72: 82–92, 1985.

9. Sibley DH, Millar HD, Hartley CJ, Whitlow PL: Subselective measurement of coronary blood flow velocity using a steerable Doppler catheter. J Am Coll Cardiol 8: 1332–1340, 1986.

REFERENCES (continued)

10. Ishida T, Lewis LM, Hartley CJ, Entman ML, Field JB: Comparison of hepatic extraction of insulin and glucagon in conscious and anesthetized dogs. Endocrinology 112: 1098-1108, 1983.

11. Patel DJ, Janicki JS: Static elastic properties of the left coronary circumflex artery and common carotid artery in dogs. Circ Res 27: 149-158, 1970.

12. Vieweg WVR, Alpert JS, Hagar AD: Caliber and distribution of normal coronary artery anatomy. Cathet Cardiovasc Diagn 2: 269-280, 1976.

13. Folts JD, Gallagher K, Rowe GG: Hemodynamic effects of controlled degrees of coronary artery stenosis in short-term and long-term studies in dogs. J Thorac Cardiovasc Surg 73: 722-777, 1977.

14. Kent KM, Bertivoglio LG, Block PL, Cowley MJ, Dorros G, Gosselin AJ, Gruentzig A, Myler RK, Simpson J, Stertzer SH, Fisher L, Gillespie MJ, Detre KM, Kelsey SF, Mullin SM; Mock MB: Percutaneous transluminal coronary angioplasty - Report from the registry of the National Heart Lung and Blood Institute. Am J Cardiol 49: 2011-2020, 1982.

15. Kent KM, Bonow RO, Rosing DR, Ewels CJ, Lipson LC, McIntosh CL, Bucharach S, Greer M, Epstein SE: Improved myocardial function during exercise after successful percutaneous transluminal coronary angioplasty. N Engl J Med 306: 441-446, 1982.

16. Gruntzig A, Senning A, Siegerthaler WE: Non-operative dilatation of coronary artery stenosis. Percutaneous transluminal coronary angioplasty. N Engl J Med 301: 61-68, 1979.

17. Ganz P, Abben R, Friedman PL, Farnic JD, Barry WH, Zevin DC: Usefulness of transstenotic coronary pressure gradient measurements during diagnostic catheterization. Am J Cardiol 55: 910-914, 1985.

18. Peterson RJ, King SB, Fjaman WA, Douglas JS, Jones RH: Relationship of coronary artery stenosis and gradient to exercise-induced ischemia (abstract). J Am Coll Cardiol 1(2): 673, 1983.

19. Hoffmeister JM, Whitworth HB, Leimgruber PP, Abi-Mansour P, Tate JM, Gruntzig AR: Analysis of anatomic and procedure factors related to restenosis after double lesion coronary angioplasty (abstract). Circulation 72 (Suppl.III): III-398, 1985.

20. Leimgruber PP, Roubin GS, Hollman J, Cotsonis GA, Meier B, Douglas JS, King SB, Gruentzig AR: Restenosis after successful coronary angioplasty in patients with single vessel disease. Circulation 73: 710-717, 1986.

21. Haraphongse M, Tymchak W, Burton JR, Rossall RE: Implication of transstenotic pressure gradient measurement during coronary angioplasty. Cathet Cardiovasc Diagn 12: 80-84, 1986.

REFERENCES (continued)

22. Leiboff R, Bren G, Katz R, Korkes R, Ross A: Determinants of
     transstenotic gradients observed during angioplasty: An experimental
     model. Am J Cardiol 52: 1311-1317, 1983.

23. Sibley DH, Bulle TM, Baxley WA, Dean LS, Whitlow PL: Continuous on-
     line assessment of coronary angioplasty with a Doppler tipped balloon
     dilatation catheter. Circulation 74 (Suppl. II): II-459, 1986.

24. Serruys PW, Wijns W, Reiber JHC, de Feyter P, van der Brand M,
     Piscione F, Hugenholtz PG: Values and limitations of transstenotic
     pressure gradients measured during percutaneous coronary angioplasty.
     Herz 10: 337-342, 1985.

25. Wijns W, Serruys PW, van der Brand M, Zeegers E, Koopman CJ, Reiber
     JHC: Transstenotic pressure gradients obtained during coronary
     angioplasty are useful but artefactual measurements (abstract).
     Circulation 70 (Suppl. II): II-299, 1984.

IV
Myocardial reperfusion

METABOLIC ASPECTS OF MYOCARDIAL REPERFUSION

T.J.C. RUIGROK AND J.H. KIRKELS

INTRODUCTION
The consequences of a severe reduction or total cessation of myocardial blood supply are a reduced availability of oxygen and substrate, a transition from aerobic to anaerobic metabolism, and accumulation of metabolic byproducts. Under these circumstances myocardial high-energy phosphate stores rapidly decrease and cytosolic Na^+ and Ca^{++} concentrations increase. Prolonged ischemia results in disruption of the cell membrane due to changes in tissue osmolarity, and phospholipase-activated degradation and free radical-induced peroxidation of membrane phospholipids.

In the clinical situation a number of interventions is available to induce reperfusion of the ischemic myocardium: thrombolytic therapy, angioplastic techniques and surgical revascularization. However, it is well-established that coronary reperfusion is not always beneficial but may exacerbate the ischemia-induced damage of severely but not irreversibly damaged cells. It is very difficult, particularly in patients, to predict whether reperfusion will be beneficial or deleterious since the condition of the myocardium at the moment of reperfusion is determined by a number of factors, such as the duration of ischemia and the presence of collateral blood flow. The ultimate cause of reperfusion injury is the failure of the tissue to maintain homeostasis with respect to Ca^{++}. The transition of reversible to irreversible damage can be delayed by hypothermia or the administration of Ca^{++} antagonists and beta-adrenergic blocking agents, provided that these interventions are introduced before or early during ischemia.

Tissue that is severely damaged, although not yet irreversibly injured, deserves special attention. Under these circumstances reperfusion may be either beneficial or deleterious, depending on the conditions of reperfusion and the composition of the reperfusion medium. There is increasing experimental evidence that the outcome of an ischemia-reperfusion intervention is not only determined by the extent of damage at the end of the ischemic period, but may be positively influenced by e.g. a temporary reduction of the Ca^{++} concentration in the reperfusion medium. In this way the potentially salvageable tissue would be protected from further damage due to its ability to maintain homeostasis with respect to Ca^{++}.

CALCIUM HOMEOSTASIS DURING NORMAL CORONARY PERFUSION
The sarcolemma maintains a large gradient of Ca^{++} between the extracellular fluid and the cytosol. The extracellular Ca^{++} concentration is approximately 10^{-3} mol/l, whereas the cytosolic Ca^{++} concentration fluctuates between 10^{-7} mol/l during diastole and 10^{-5} mol/l during systole. During the plateau phase of the action potential a small amount of Ca^{++} enters the myocardial cell through the slow channels (Figure 1; mechanism 1). Subsequently, a relatively large amount of Ca^{++} is released from the sarcoplasmic reticulum (SR), according to the 'Ca^{++}-induced Ca^{++} release' theory

186

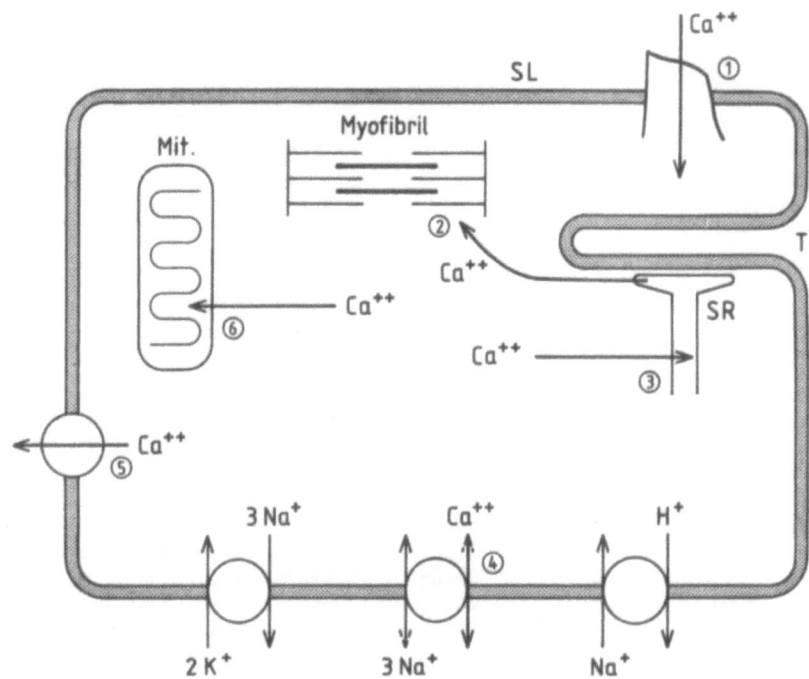

FIGURE 1. Schematic representation of a number of ion fluxes in the myocardium that are responsible for, or influence the cytosolic Ca^{++} concentration. (1) Ca^{++} influx through voltage-operated channels, (2) Ca^{++} release from sarcoplasmic reticulum (SR), (3) ATP-dependent uptake of Ca^{++} by SR, (4) Na^+-Ca^{++} exchange mechanism, (5) Ca^{++} pump of the sarcolemma (SL), (6) Energy-dependent uptake of Ca^{++} by mitochondria (Mit.). In addition, the Na^+-K^+ pump and Na^+-H^+ exchange mechanism are shown. T = transverse tubular system.

(Figure 1; mechanism 2). As the cytosolic Ca^{++} concentration rises from 10^{-7} mol/l to the systolic value of 10^{-5} mol/l, Ca^{++} binds to troponin C, which enables actin and myosin to interact, and contraction occurs. At the beginning of diastole Ca^{++} is pumped back into the SR by a Ca^{++}-dependent ATPase (Figure 1; mechanism 3). The small amount of Ca^{++} entering the cell during each depolarization is extruded by the Na^+-Ca^{++} exchange mechanism and, to a lesser extent, by the sarcolemmal Ca^{++} pump (Figure 1, mechanisms 4 and 5)[1].

METABOLIC CONSEQUENCES OF ISCHEMIA
     A severe reduction or total cessation of coronary perfusion leads to a reduced availability of oxygen and substrate. The reduced availability of oxygen causes a transition from aerobic to anaerobic metabolism, a decrease of myocardial high-energy phosphate stores, accumulation of inorganic phosphate and intracellular acidosis. An important consequence of depletion of the high-energy phosphates is that the ionic homeostasis of the myocardial cells is disturbed. The cells gain Na^+ and lose K^+ [2], due to inhibition of the Na^+-K^+ pump. Intracellular accumulation of Na^+ and other ions (H^+, inorganic phosphate and lactate)leads to an increase of intracellular osmolarity and, because of this, to cell swelling. Although the tissue con-

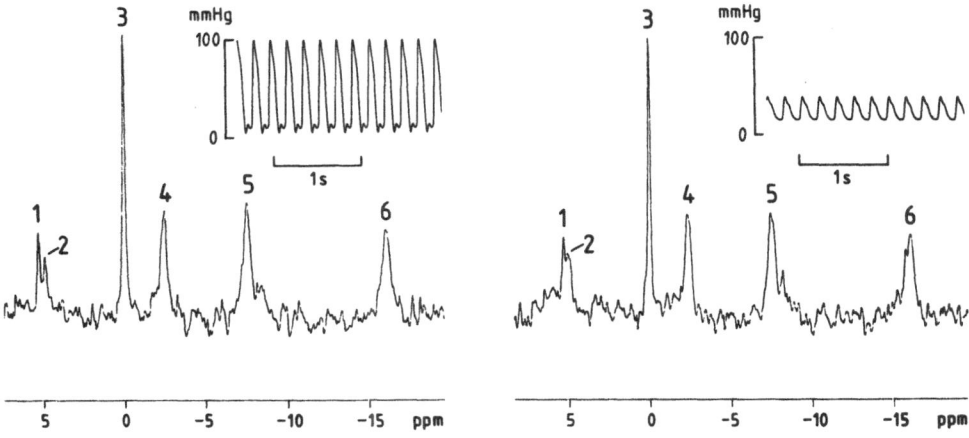

FIGURE 2. ^{31}P NMR spectra and left ventricular pressure recordings obtained between 25 and 30 minutes of control perfusion of an untreated (left) and diltiazem-treated (right) rat heart. Diltiazem (5×10^{-6} mol/l) was added to the perfusate during the last 10 minutes of control perfusion. The spectra were obtained from 128 scans. Numbered peaks are: (1) extracellular Pi, (2) intracellular Pi, (3) CP and (4) the γ-, (5) the α- and (6) the β-phosphate groups of ATP.

tent of Ca^{++} does not significantly increase during ischemia [3], the cytosolic Ca^{++} concentration may rise, due to an impairment of the Ca^{++}-accumulating activity of the SR. Ca^{++}-dependent ATPases will then be activated, causing a further breakdown of high-energy phosphates. Ca^{++} antagonists may reduce the energy requirements of the heart during the early phase of ischemia and, in this way, may delay the transition of nonlethal to lethal cell damage.

^{31}P NMR experiments

We have used phosphorus nuclear magnetic resonance (^{31}P NMR) spectroscopy to illustrate the effects of a temporary cessation of coronary perfusion on the energy metabolism in the isolated perfused rat heart, in the presence or absence of the Ca^{++} antagonist diltiazem. Hearts from male Wistar rats were perfused at 37°C using the Langendorff technique at a constant pressure of 10.0 kPa (75 mm Hg). The perfusate had the following composition (mmol/l): NaCl, 124; KCl, 4.7; $CaCl_2$, 1.3; $MgCl_2$, 1.0; $NaHCO_3$, 24.0; Na_2HPO_4, 0.5; glucose, 11.0. After equilibration with 95% O_2 and 5% CO_2, the pH of the perfusate was 7.35 ± 0.05. The heart rate was maintained at 300 beats/minute by right ventricular pacing with KCl-wick electrodes, connected to a Grass S88 stimulator. Left ventricular pressure was measured according to the method of Neely et al. [4]. The perfusion sequence was: 30 minutes of control perfusion, 30 minutes of total ischemia and 30 minutes of reperfusion. When diltiazem (5×10^{-6} mol/l) was used, the drug was added to the perfusate during the last 10 minutes of control perfusion.

^{31}P NMR spectra were obtained on a Bruker MSL spectrometer equipped with a wide bore (150 mm) 4.7 Tesla superconducting magnet. Spectra were obtained during 5 minutes from 128 scans. Zero ppm was assigned to the resonance position of creatine phosphate (CP). Intracellular and extracellular pH were measured from the chemical shift of the inorganic phosphate (Pi) peaks, using a titration curve obtained from a solution containing ATP (10 mmol/l), CP (10 mmol/l), Pi (10 mmol/l), NADPH (10 mmol/l), glucose-6P (10

188

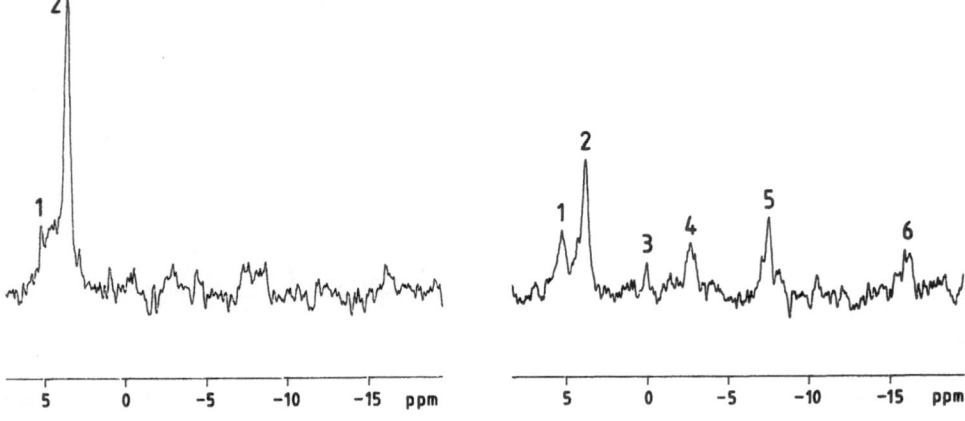

FIGURE 3. ^{31}P NMR spectra obtained between 10 and 15 minutes of total
ischemia of an untreated (left) and diltiazem-treated (right) rat heart.
The spectra were obtained from 128 scans. For identities of numbered peaks
see legend to Figure 2.

mmol/l) and $MgCl_2$ (10 mmol/l).

Figure 2 shows NMR spectra of rat hearts, obtained between 25 and 30
minutes of control perfusion without (left) and with (right) diltiazem.
From the position of the extracellular Pi peak, extracellular pH in both
hearts was calculated to be 7.4, i.e. the pH of the perfusate. Intracellular pH amounted to 7.1 and 7.0, respectively (Table 1). Left ventricular
developed pressure was 90 mm Hg in the untreated heart and 24 mm Hg in the
treated heart, as a result of the negative inotropic effect of diltiazem in
the concentration used.

During ischemia, myocardial high-energy phosphate levels decreased rapidly in the untreated heart. Figure 3 shows that in the spectrum obtained between 10 and 15 minutes of total ischemia, the CP and ATP peaks were no
longer perceptible. The intracellular Pi peak shows a marked increase; the
corresponding intracellular pH value amounted to 5.8. On the other hand, in
the diltiazem-treated heart there was a considerable amount of ATP and also
some CP left between 10 and 15 minutes of ischemia. The intracellular Pi
peak was less pronounced and intracellular pH amounted to 6.2. Between 25
and 30 minutes of ischemia CP and ATP were depleted in both hearts (not
shown). Intracellular pH amounted to 5.8 in the untreated heart and 6.0 in
the diltiazem-treated heart.

These results show that diltiazem added to the perfusate before the onset
of ischemia, protects the heart against some of the consequences of normo-
thermic global ischemia. Intracellular acidosis developed less rapidly and
myocardial CP and ATP contents decreased at lower rates than in the untreated heart.

METABOLIC CONSEQUENCES OF REPERFUSION

Figure 4 shows ^{31}P NMR spectra after reperfusion of the untreated and
diltiazem-treated heart. Between 25 and 30 minutes of reperfusion, there
was no recovery of ATP and some recovery of CP in the untreated heart. In
the Pi region a complex pattern can be seen, consisting of four peaks (1
and 2a-c). Peak 1 corresponds to a pH value of 7.3, i.e. the extracellular
pH. Peaks 2a-c are attributed to different intracellular phosphate pools,

TABLE 1. Intracellular pH values of an untreated and diltiazem-treated (5×10^{-6} mol/l) rat heart.

	Intracellular pH	
	Without diltiazem	With diltiazem
Between 25 and 30 minutes of control perfusion	7.1	7.0
Between 10 and 15 minutes of total ischemia	5.8	6.2
Between 25 and 30 minutes of total ischemia	5.8	6.0
Between 25 and 30 minutes of reperfusion	6.1 - 7.0	7.0

with corresponding pH values ranging from 6.1 - 7.0. A possible interpretation of this result is that the untreated heart was only partially reperfused; the parts that remained ischemic may be responsible for the lower pH values. During reperfusion of the diltiazem-treated heart, intracellular pH returned to its original value of 7.0. There was a good recovery of CP and ATP. Left ventricular pressure recordings show a marked increase in enddiastolic pressure and a poor recovery of developed pressure in the untreated heart and a complete recovery of mechanical activity in the treated heart. Similar results were obtained in earlier studies in which the effects of the Ca^{++} antagonist nifedipine were investigated [5,6].

Reperfusion of myocardial tissue after 30 minutes of ischemia may result in an excessive rise of tissue Ca^{++} [7]. The consequences of such a gain in Ca^{++} include activation of Ca^{++}-dependent phospholipases and proteases, and redistribution of phospholipids, causing sarcolemmal disruption. Ca^{++}-dependent ATPases will be activated, causing a further breakdown of ATP, and mitochondria start accumulating massive amounts of Ca^{++} (Figure 1, mechan-

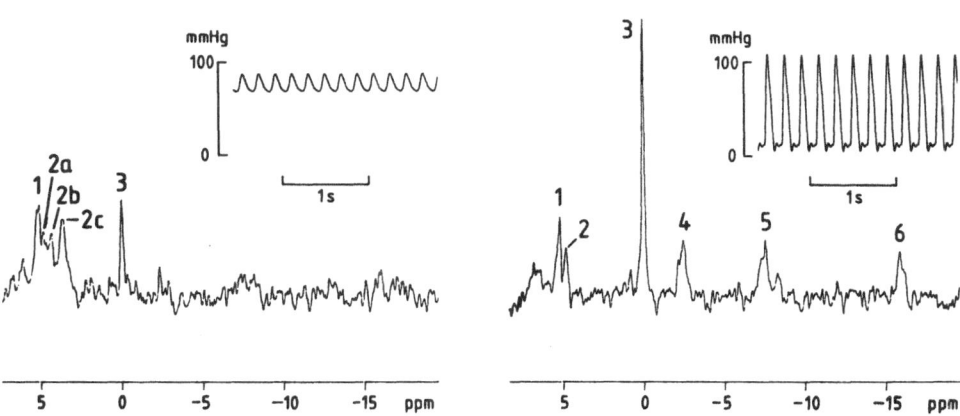

FIGURE 4. ^{31}P NMR spectra and left ventricular pressure recordings obtained between 25 and 30 minutes of reperfusion of an untreated (left) and diltiazem-treated (right) rat heart. The spectra were obtained from 128 scans. Note the complex pattern in the Pi region of the left-hand spectrum. For identities of numbered peaks see legend to Figure 2.

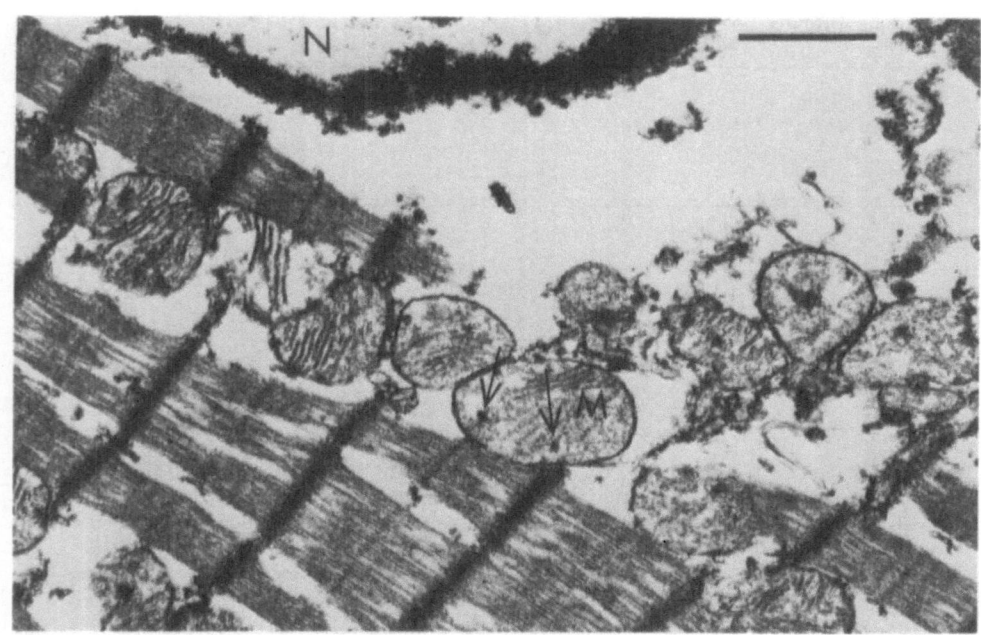

FIGURE 5. Electron micrograph of rat heart muscle after 90 minutes of total ischemia and 30 minutes of reperfusion at 37°C. The ultrastructural
changes include aggregation of chromatin in the nucleus, swelling of mitochondria with formation of electron-dense granules (arrows), contracture of
the myofibrils, and formation of large empty spaces. Marker bar = 1µm.

ism 6), which occurs at the expense of oxydative phosphorylation, thereby
impairing ATP production. Several interventions, such as the use of Ca^{++}
antagonists, are able to prevent ischemia-reperfusion damage, provided that
these interventions are applied prophylactically. There is a number of possible explanations for the recovery of high-energy phosphates and mechanical activity during reperfusion that was observed in our NMR experiments
after diltiazem-pretreatment. Attenuation of intracellular acidosis at the
end of the ischemic period may lead to a reduced exchange of H^+ for Na^+
through the sarcolemmal Na^+-H^+ exchange mechanism (see Figure 1)[8]. Reduced uptake of Na^+ during reperfusion would subsequently diminish uptake
of Ca^{++} by the cells, as a result of the exchange of Na^+ for Ca^{++} through
the Na^+-Ca^{++} exchange mechanism. Another possibility is that the influx of
Ca^{++} through the slow channels was reduced early during reperfusion because
diltiazem was still present in the heart. These two factors could have prevented a severe disturbance of the Ca^{++} homeostasis and a concomitant un-
coupling of the oxidative phosphorylation. A third mechanism may be the
vasodilating properties of the Ca^{++} antagonist, which will improve reperfusion and, in this way, will contribute to a better recovery of metabolism
and function of the heart.
    When the period of ischemia is extended beyond 30 minutes, both biochem-
ical and morphologic changes become irreversible. Phospholipase-activated
degradation and free radical-induced peroxidation of membrane phospholipids, and physical stress due to an increase of tissue osmolarity will ultimately lead to a loss of integrity of the sarcolemma [9]. At this stage,
reperfusion will inevitably exacerbate the ischemic injury. Figure 5 shows

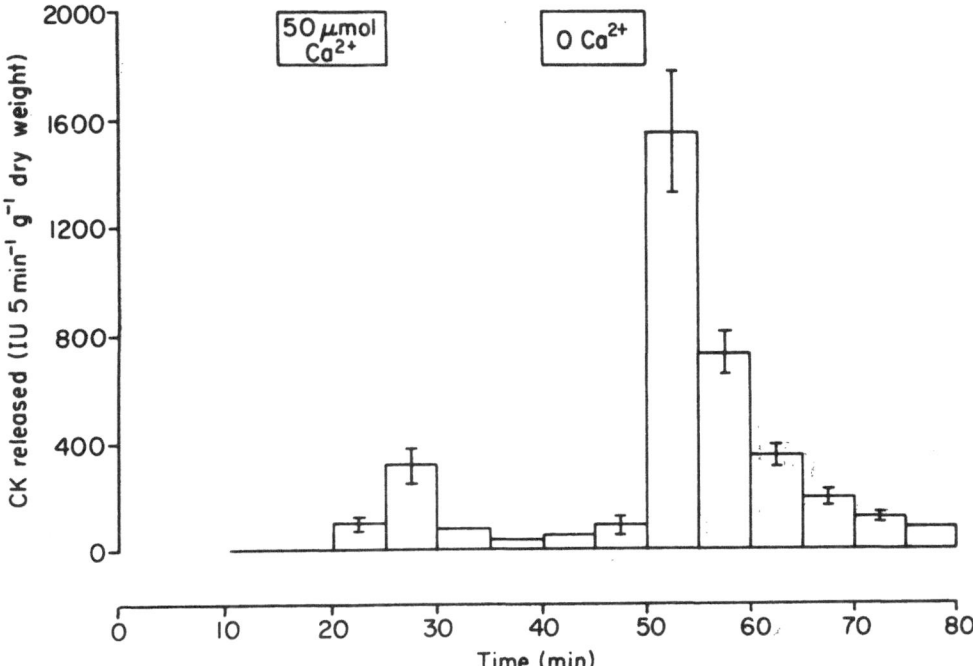

FIGURE 6. Creatine kinase (CK) release from isolated rabbit hearts (n=6). Perfusion sequence was as follows: 15 minutes normal perfusion ([Ca^{++}] = 1.3 mmol/l), 10 minutes low- Ca^{++} (0.05 mmol/l) perfusion, 15 minutes normal perfusion, 10 minutes Ca^{++}-free perfusion, 30 minutes normal perfusion. Note CK release both during and after low-Ca^{++} perfusion, indicating that 0.05 mmol/l Ca^{++} does not entirely protect the rabbit heart against the calcium paradox. From Capucci et al.: Eur. Heart J. 4 (Supplement H), 13-21, 1983. By permission.

the ultrastructure of a rat heart that was reperfused after 90 minutes of total ischemia. The normal architecture of the cell is lost, the myofibrils are contracted and the mitochondria are swollen and contain electron-dense Ca^{++} deposits. It should be noted that these data cannot be directly used to predict whether reperfusion in the clinical situation will be beneficial or deleterious, since collateral flow may delay the transition of nonlethal to lethal injury.

LOW-CALCIUM REPERFUSION

Since uncontrolled Ca^{++} influx constitutes the crucial step in reperfusion damage, a temporary reduction of the Ca^{++} concentration in the reperfusion medium is one of the interventions that may be applied at the time of reperfusion to reduce reperfusion injury [10-16]. In these studies the Ca^{++} concentration during low-Ca^{++} reperfusion varied from 0.75 to 0.05 mmol/l. In three studies the effects of 0.75 mmol/l Ca^{++} were investigated [10,12,14]. Shine and Douglas [12], who studied the isolated vascularly perfused rabbit interventricular septum, observed a significant recovery of ATP and CP contents after 5 minutes of reperfusion with 0.75 mmol/l Ca^{++}. This significantly greater recovery of ATP and CP persisted after an additional reperfusion with 2.5 mmol/l Ca^{++}. Watts et al. [10] and Ferrari et al. [14], who used isolated hearts from rats and rabbits, respectively, were unable to demonstrate a reduction of reperfusion injury during post-ischemic perfusion with 0.75 mmol/l Ca^{++}. It should be noted that, in addition to differences in species, the experimental conditions (e.g. duration of ischemia and heart rate) were different in these three studies. In one of the studies, however, 10 minutes of reperfusion with 0.05 mmol/l Ca^{++}, followed by reperfusion with 1.5 mmol/l Ca^{++}, appeared to be beneficial [14].

A drastic lowering of the Ca^{++} concentration during the early phase of reperfusion will reduce the uptake of Ca^{++} by the cells but may, on the other hand, predispose the cells to the calcium paradox. The term 'calcium paradox' has been introduced by Zimmerman and Hülsmann [17] to illustrate that after Ca^{++}-free perfusion of the rat heart reintroduction of Ca^{++} did not restore function, but resulted in irreversible loss of electrical and mechanical activity, and acute myocardial cell death. The calcium paradox is not limited to isolated hearts of small animals, but has also been demonstrated in the in situ dog heart and in human myocardial tissue [18]. It has been reported that addition of 0.05 mmol/l Ca^{++} to the Ca^{++}-free perfusate protects the perfused interventricular septum of the rabbit against the calcium paradox [19]. However, in another study, in which isolated rabbit hearts were subjected to successive low-Ca^{++} (0.05 mmol/l) and normal-Ca^{++} perfusion, considerable enzyme release was observed during low-Ca^{++} perfusion, as well as during reperfusion (Figure 6)[20]. Furthermore, the sensitivity of the heart to the calcium paradox may be increased under ischemic conditions [21]. As long as the safe lower limit of the Ca^{++} concentration is not established, particularly under ischemic conditions, the possibility of evoking the calcium paradox during low-Ca^{++} reperfusion, should be taken into account. Improvement of reperfusion conditions designed to prevent or reduce reperfusion damage, may turn out to be of great importance to clinical practice, where reperfusion techniques are increasingly used.

REFERENCES

1. Opie LH: The Heart: Physiology, Metabolism, Pharmacology and Therapy. London: Grune & Stratton Ltd, 1984.
2. Reimer KA, Jennings RB & Hill ML: Total ischemia in dog hearts in vitro. II. High energy phosphate depletion and associated defects in energy metabolism, cell volume regulation and sarcolemmal integrity. Circ. Res. **49**, 901–911, 1981.
3. Shen AC & Jennings RB: Myocardial calcium and magnesium in acute ischemic injury. Am. J. Pathol. **67**, 417–440, 1972.
4. Neely JR, Liebermeister H, Battersby EJ & Morgan HE: Effect of pressure development on oxygen consumption by isolated rat heart. Am. J. Physiol. **212**, 804–814, 1967.
5. Ruigrok TJC, Van Echteld CJA, De Kruijff B, Borst C & Meijler FL: Protective effect of nifedipine in myocardial ischemia assessed by phosphorus-31 nuclear magnetic resonance. Eur. Heart J. **4** (Supplement C), 109–113, 1983.
6. Ruigrok TJC, Van Echteld CJA, Borst C & Meijler FL: A phosphorus nuclear magnetic resonance study of the effect of nifedipine on intracellular pH during myocardial ischaemia and reperfusion. In: 6th International Adalat Symposium; New Therapy of Ischaemic Heart Disease and Hypertension (Lichtlen PR, Ed.). Excerpta Medica, Amsterdam, 193–198, 1986.
7. Shen AC & Jennings RB: Kinetics of calcium accumulation in acute myocardial ischemic injury. Am. J. Pathol. **67**, 441–452, 1972.

8. Pierce GN & Philipson KD: Na^+-H^+ exchange in cardiac sarcolemmal vesicles. Biochim. Biophys. Acta **818**, 109–116, 1985.

9. Nayler WG, & Elz JS: Reperfusion injury: laboratory artifact or clinical dilemma? Circulation **74**, 215–221, 1986.

10. Watts JA, Koch CD & LaNoue KF: Effects of Ca^{2+} antagonism on energy metabolism: Ca^{2+} and heart function after ischemia. Am. J. Physiol. **238**, H909–H916, 1980.

11. Koomen JM, Schevers JAM & Noordhoek J: Myocardial recovery from global ischemia and reperfusion: effects of pre- and/or post-ischemic perfusion with low-Ca^{2+}. J. Mol. Cell. Cardiol. **15**, 383–392, 1983.

12. Shine KI & Douglas AM: Low calcium reperfusion of ischemic myocardium. J. Mol. Cell. Cardiol. **15**, 251–260, 1983.

13. Allen BS, Okamoto F, Buckberg GD, Acar C, Partington M, Bugyi H & Leaf J: Studies of controlled reperfusion after ischemia. IX. Reperfusate composition: benefits of marked hypocalcemia and diltiazem on regional recovery. J. Thorac. Cardiovasc. Surg. **92**, 564–572, 1986.

14. Ferrari R, Albertini A, Curello S, Ceconi C, Di Lisa F, Raddino R & Visioli O: Myocardial recovery during post-ischaemic reperfusion: effects of nifedipine, calcium and magnesium. J. Mol. Cell. Cardiol. **18**, 487–498, 1986.

15. Kuroda H, Ishiguro S & Mori T: Optimal calcium concentration in the initial reperfusate for post-ischemic myocardial performance (calcium concentration during reperfusion). J. Mol. Cell. Cardiol. **18**, 625–633, 1986.

16. Kusuoka H, Porterfield JK, Weisman HF, Weisfeldt ML & Marban E: Pathophysiology and pathogenesis of stunned myocardium; depressed Ca^{2+} activation of contraction as a consequence of reperfusion-induced cellular calcium overload in ferret hearts. J. Clin. Invest. **79**, 950–961, 1987.

17. Zimmerman ANE & Hülsmann WC: Paradoxical influence of calcium ions on the permeability of the cell membranes of the isolated rat heart. Nature **211**, 646–647, 1966.

18. Ruigrok TJC & Poole-Wilson PA (Eds): The Calcium Paradox and the Heart: Aspects of Myocardial Integrity and Protection. Eur. Heart J. **4** (Supplement H), 1983.

19. Rich TL & Langer GA: Calcium depletion in rabbit myocardium: calcium paradox protection by hypothermia and cation substitution. Circ. Res. **51**, 131–141, 1982.

20. Capucci A, Janse MJ & Ruigrok TJC: The calcium paradox: an electrophysiological study in the isolated rabbit heart. Eur. Heart J. **4** (Supplement H), 13–21, 1983.

21. Jynge P: Protection of the ischemic myocardium: calcium-free cardioplegic infusates and the additive effects of coronary infusion and ischemia in the induction of the calcium paradox. Thorac. Cardiovasc. Surgeon **28**, 303–309, 1980.

RIGHT VENTRICLE - CORONARY ARTERY FISTULAE AND INTERRUPTION OF
THE LEFT ANTERIOR DESCENDING CORONARY ARTERY IN PATIENTS WITH
PULMONARY ATRESIA AND INTACT VENTRICULAR SEPTUM WITHOUT OPE-
RATION OR SHUNT ONLY

U.SAUER, A.C.GITTENBERGER - DE GROOT, K.BÜHLMEYER, F.SEBENING,
J.APITZ, TÜBINGEN, I.HAMMERER, INNSBRUCK, W.HOFFMANN, HOMBURG,
M.WIMMER, WIEN

INTRODUCTION
    In a recent study (21) we demonstrated by cineangiocardio-
graphy right ventricle (RV) to coronary artery communications
or fistulae (17) as a complicating feature in 26 consecutive
patients (26 of 68 = 38 %) with pulmonary atresia and intact
ventricular septum (PAIVS) which accounts for approximately
1 % of congenital heart anomalies (19). Eighteen of these patients (18 of 26 = 69 %) had interruption of the proximal or
mid left anterior descending coronary artery (LAD), as evidenced by cineangiocardiography and confirmed by histopathological studies in all 7 available heart specimens (12). In these
cases the blood supply of the LAD distal to the interruption
is RV-dependent and occurs during systole through distal, apical fistulae.
    The 2 other conditions in PAIVS with fistulae that have been
shown to require sustained RV blood flow and hypertension to
perfuse part or all of the coronary circulation during systole
are: 1. proximal anatomical discontinuity between the aorta
and the coronary arteries (11,13,21) and 2. co-existing obstructive changes of the wall of the epicardial and intramural
coronary arteries, attributed to the high systolic pressure
perfusion from RV (7,8,12,16,21). In these 3 situations attempts to decompress the hypertensive RV or reduce blood flow
from RV through the fistulae to the coronary circulation may
result in acute myocardial ischemia and death (6,16,21,25).
    In the present study, the anatomy of the coronary arteries
and fistulae, the filling pattern in relation to the extent of
blood supply (regions of perfusion) of the left ventricle (LV)
from the RV through fistulae and evolution, as demonstrated by
biplane RV- and LV-angiography and selective injection in the
ascending aorta, were evaluated. Based on these findings, it
was attempted to delineate risk factors for survival.
    In addition, the angiocardiographic appearance of the ana-
tomy of the RV and the hemodynamics were assessed.
    The study group included only patients with PAIVS with fi-
stulae and interrupted LAD who had either no operation or only
an aorto-pulmonary artery (AO-PA) shunt as the initial operation.

PATIENTS

Between October 1974 and May 1987, 35 patients with PAIVS and RV-coronary artery fistulae were studied. Twenty-three patients (23 of 35 = 66 %) had an interrupted LAD and RV-dependent blood flow and 12 patients (12 of 35 = 34 %) had an uninterrupted LAD. Sixteen patients (16 of 23 = 70 %), all of whom had an interrupted LAD and either no operation - 5 patients (5 of 16) or a shunt operation - 11 patients (11 of 16), form the study group. Ten of these patients were included in the previous study (21). They were initially investigated at a median age of 2 days (1 day - 3 months), with the first shunt operation generally performed within the first week of life (1-34 days, median age 6 days).

All 5 patients without operation and balloon atrial septostomy (BAS) in one, died between 1 day (during cardiac catheterization) and 6.5 months. They include one infant with large AO-PA collaterals who died at 4 months and another with a patent ductus arteriosus (PDA) who died at 46 days after discontinuation of PGE_1 i.v. The possibility of prenatal damage was suggested by the presence of ischemic ST-T changes in the EKG and impaired LV function on angiocardiography at 1 day of age in the latter patient. Extensive fibrosis of the LV- and RV-myocardium was found at autopsy.

In 6 patients (6 of 11), a Waterston anastomosis was performed and in one, initially a BAS - 4 of these infants (4 of 6) died 1 to 100 days postoperatively at 7 to 111 days of age. One of the 2 surviving patients subsequently underwent operative enlargement of the atrial septal defect (ASD) at 1 year of age because of severe narrowing of the ASD. Three patients had an aorto-pulmonary artery Gore-Tex shunt (4-5 mm Ø), in one after a preceding side-to-end anastomosis between the aorta and the pulmonary artery trunk -with 2 intra- and perioperative deaths. Two patients surviving a Blalock-Taussig shunt at 13 days and 1.4 years then underwent a successful modified Fontan operation with direct right atrial-pulmonary artery connection and a modified contralateral Blalock-Taussig shunt at 4.8 and 2.2 years, respectively.

The follow-up in the 5 surviving patients (5 of 16) ranges from 1 to 10 years.

The median age at death of the 11 nonsurviving patients (11 of 16) was 43 days (1 day - 6 months). There were 3 histopathological studies of a total of 5 autopsies.

RESULTS

The results of the 2 groups: nonsurviving and surviving patients are summarized in tables 1.-4. and are also presented individually, including the evolution in the 5 surviving patients in tables 5.-7. For the delineation of risk factors, the comparison of findings of patients with shunt operation who survived (5 of 16) with those who died postoperatively (6 of 16) together with the only infant with pulmonary blood flow through large AO-PA collaterals was considered decisive. This takes into account the difficulty in differentiating the risk for mortality due to the anomalous coronary circulation from that due to the closure of the PDA.

An infundibulum was present in 7 nonsurvivors (7 of 11) and in all 5 survivors as part of a "tripartite" RV in 5 of the former (5 of 7) and in 4 (4 of 5) of the latter group. In 6 patients who did not survive (6 of 11) not all 3 parts of the RV were present: in 4 patients the infundibulum was absent, 2 of these had an inlet portion only. Pulmonary artery trunk atresia in 5 patients was associated with an infundibulum in 3 but with absence of the infundibulum in 2 patients. The tricuspid valve was hypoplastic and restrictive in all patients, and competent in the majority (Table 1.). Pulmonary blood flow depended on the PDA in all but one patient, in whom it occurred through large AO-PA collaterals.

TABLE 1. Right ventricular (RV) anatomy and systolic pressures, pulmonary artery trunk atresia, tricuspid valve (TV) size

	Age at cath/angio median		With RV infundibulum "tripartite"	With RV infundibulum without trabecular portion	Without RV infundibulum trabecular portion with	Without RV infundibulum trabecular portion without
Non-survivors n = 11	2 days (1–3mo)		5	2	2	2
		PA trunk atresia	1	1	1	1
Survivors n = 5	7 mo (1day–8.2yrs)		4	1	0	0
		PA trunk atresia	1	0	0	0
n = 16		5	9	3	2	2

TV ring Ø (mm)	Systolic pressures RV > LV (mmHg)	RV≈LV
7̄ (5–8) 10/11	9̄2̄ (63–115) 8/9	1/9
8̄ (8–15) 5/ 5	1̄2̄2̄ (100–150) 4/ 5	1/ 5
15/16	12/14	2/14

The systolic pressure in the RV was suprasystemic in all but one patient in both groups (Table 1.) which is consistent with a systolic and diastolic pressure difference between the RV and the aorta through the fistulae and the coronary circulation. The negative effect of the blood supply to the subendocardial myocardium of the RV and the coronary arteries was reflected by the pathology of the myocardium and obstructive wall changes of the LAD and intramural coronary arteries in all 3 infants with histopathological studies (10-12, 18). On re-catheterization of 4 surviving patients at 7 months - 8.2 years, the RV hypertension had persisted or further increased (Table 5.).

A "steal" from the aorta into the RV during diastole was documented in 11 infants (11 of 16 = 69 %) (Tables 2. and 7.). It was consistent with a 12-23 % increase of oxygen saturation (O_2 %) in the RV in 7 (7 of 11) and evidenced by a diastolic shunt from the aorta into the RV on aortogram and/or LV angiocardiogram in 8 (8 of 11). Thus, in 4 patients (4 of 11) it was documented by both methods (Fig. 1). Seven of the 11 patients (7 of 11 = 64 %) with "steal" died, 3 after Waterston anastomosis and 4 without operation, including the infant with

TABLE 2. Aorta (AO) → right ventricle (RV) "steal"
+ / or right ventricle → aorta shunt through fistulae

	AO → RV "steal" + RV → AO shunt			AV → RV "steal" ∅ RV → AO shunt			RV → AO shunt only	∅ AO → RV "steal" ∅ RV → AO shunt
	O_2 RV − v̄ = 12-23% +angio	∅ angio	angio only	O_2 RV − v̄ = 13-23% +angio	∅ angio	angio only		
Non-survivors n = 11	1	1	2	2	1	0	1	3
Survivors n = 5	1	1	1	0	0	1	1	0
Total	2	2	3	2	1	1	2	3

v̄, mixed venous blood.

AO-PA collaterals. Four patients (4 of 11) with a "steal" at
the initial investigation and on follow-up angiocardiography
in 2 - are alive.

Seven patients (7 of 16) had a bidirectional shunt (10, 20,
21, 23), that is concurrent with a "steal", a systolic shunt
from the RV into the aorta preferentially through large proximal and mid-fistulae to the LAD and right coronary artery
(RCA), but occasionally, through fistulae at the crux to the
RCA or left circumflex artery (LCX). Three of these patients
(3 of 7) survived and 4 (4 of 7) died without operation, but
AO-PA collaterals in one.

Two patients (2 of 16), one survivor and one nonsurvivor
without operation, had a systolic RV to aorta shunt only.

Further, a higher risk for the coronary artery blood supply
was associated with:
- absent connection between the aorta and a single coronary
  artery in one infant who did not survive
- co-existing interruption of the mid-RCA in 2 patients with
  one survivor who also had a single coronary artery with stenoses in the right coronary arterial branch (Fig.2)
- thus, single coronary artery in 2 patients and

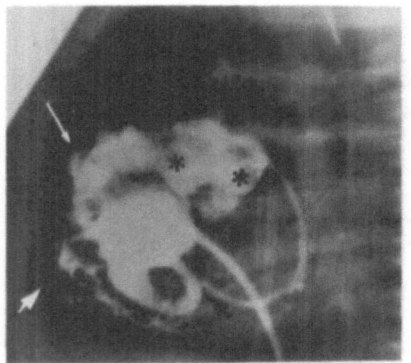 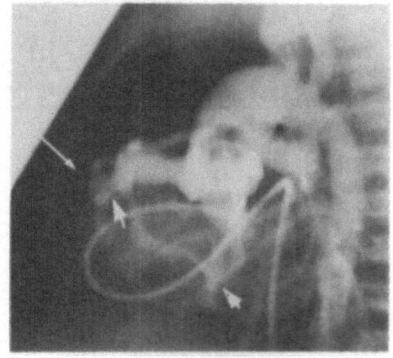

Figure 1. Two-day-old male newborn with PAIVS, RV inlet only
(absent infundibulum and trabecular portion), hypoplastic (Ø
7 mm), competent tricuspid valve, pulmonary artery trunk atresia. No operation. Death at 6.5 months. a) RV cineangiocardiogram, lateral view. Interruption of LAD at fistula to mid LAD
(white arrow). Retrograde filling of distal 2/3 of LAD and collaterals through anterior apical fistula to distal LAD (RV-dependent) (white arrow head). Through fistulae to proximal RCA
and to RCA and LCX at the crux cordis (arrow head) retrograde
opacification of both coronary ostia and aortic sinuses (asterix). b) Aortogram, lateral view. Diastolic aorta - RV "steal"
through fistulae to mid LAD, proximal RCA and to RCA and LCX at
the crux cordis (white arrow heads) consistent with a 13% increase of O_2 in the RV.

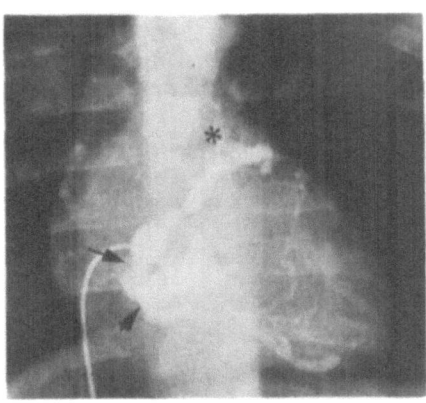 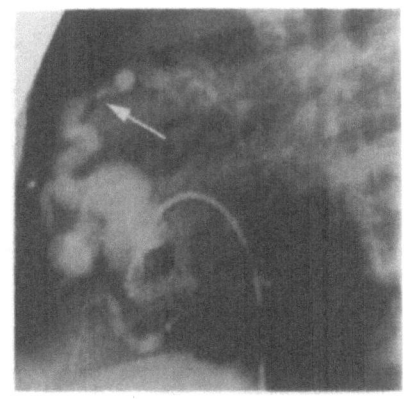

Figure 2. RV cineangiocardiogram of a 8.2 year-old male patient
(no. 1 of the survivors), Waterston anastomosis at 5 days, with
PAIVS, tripartite RV, atresia of distal infundibulum and pulmonary artery trunk, hypoplastic (∅ 15mm), minimally incompetent
tricuspid valve. a) Posteroanterior view. Retrograde filling of
single coronary artery with opacification of left aortic sinus
(asterix) through fistula to mid right coronary arterial branch
(black arrow) which is interrupted and stenosed and of LCX
through fistula at the crux cordis (arrow head). b) Lateral
view. Interruption of the LAD (white arrow) and retrograde filling of distal 2/3 of LAD and collaterals through anterior apical fistula to distal LAD (RV-dependent) (black arrow) and of
LCX through fistula at the crux cordis (arrow head).

- co-existing fistula to coronary vein ("right-sided circular
  shunt" (10)) in one newborn who died
  Right or extreme right dominant type was demonstrated in 9
patients (9 of 16): 8 infants (8 of 9) with right (4 of 8)
and extreme right dominance (4 of 8) died, 3 after shunt
operation and 5 without operation, including the one with AO-
PA collaterals. One patient with extreme right dominance (1
of 9) is alive.
  By contrast, 3 of the remaining surviving patients (3 of 5)
had a left dominant type and in one with a single coronary
artery it was not determined.
  The fistulae were classified according to the location of
their communication with the LCA and RCA as we have described
previously (21) but with the addition of fistulae to the LCX
or its atrio-ventricular and postero-lateral branches (Tables
3. and 6.). Three patients (3 of 16) had LAD-fistulae only,
all died. The remaining patients (13 of 16) had a combination
of proximal +/or mid- and distal fistulae to the LAD and to
the distal RCA at the crux cordis or to the posterior descending artery (RPD). In some of them there were additional fistulae to the apical-distal LAD or to the LCX at the crux as
well as to the proximal +/or mid RCA in various combinations.

TABLE 3. Type of fistulae

Pts. No. (died)	→ LAD prox +/or mid ± dist	→ apex ↓ dist LAD	→ crux ↓ LCX	→ RCA prox +/ or mid	→ crux ↓ RCA + or RPD
(1)	∅	+	∅	∅	∅
(2)	+	+	∅	∅	∅
(1)	+	∅	∅	∅·	+
(1)	+	+	∅	∅	+
3 (1)**	+	+	∅	+	+
4 (3)***	+	∅	+	∅	+
1	+	∅	+	+	+
3* (2)	+	+	+	+	+
Total 16 (11)	15 (10)	10 (7)	8 (5)	7 (3)	13 (8)

*   1 with single coronary artery + RCA – interruption, alive
** 1 with mid RCA–interruption, died
*** 1 with absent connection aorta – single coronary artery, died

The occurrence of fistulae to the LCX in association with fistulae to the proximal +/or mid- and distal LAD and RCA – in 8
patients (8 of 16) with 3 survivors is of special interest.
Six children had no fistulae to the proximal +/or mid RCA, 5
of whom died.
Partition of the LV into regions of perfusion from the RV
through fistulae was based on the observation in each individual patient by whether or not the LAD, particularly the LAD
distal to the interruption, the apical-lateral branches + RPD,
the LCX and the RPD filled through fistulae during systole
from RV on RV angiocardiogram (Tables 4. and 6.). In addition,
it was noted whether or not these arteries were also normally
filled during diastole in an antegrade manner from the aorta
on aortogram and/or LV angiocardiogram or washed out on RV angiocardiogram. In 6 patients (6 of 16), 2 of whom survived,
including one with a single coronary artery and interruption
of both the LAD and main right branch, all regions of the LV
and most of the RV were supplied by the RV. Similarly, LV- and
RV-coronary blood flow was totally RV-dependent in the unique
patient with an absent connection between the aorta and a
single coronary artery. In each of 4 patients most parts of
the LV were supplied by the RV through the fistulae with the
exception of the region in the distribution of the LCX in the
former, and that of the LAD distal to a proximal interruption
in the latter patients. It is suggested that survival in 2 of
these latter patients was enabled by compensatory sustained
right ventricular blood flow and hypertension through the LCX.

In the remaining nonsurviving patient the blood supply from the RV was limited to the capillary bed distal to the inter-rupted LAD and that of the apical-lateral branches.

The coronary arteries to the postero-lateral LV wall, atrio-ventricular branches of the RCA and/or the LCX, exclusively filled retrogradely from RV through fistulae to the RCA or LCX at the crux during systole in 7 patients (7 of 16) with shunt into the aorta in 3 patients (3 of 7). Two patients each had an extreme right and left dominant type, respectively, and in 3 it was undetermined, including one with a single coronary artery. The distribution between the survivors (3 of 7) and the nonsurvivors (4 of 7), one after a Waterston shunt and 3 without operation, including one with AO-PA collaterals, was equal.

However, bidirectional filling (blood supply) of the coro-nary arteries to the postero-lateral LV wall, antegradely du-

TABLE 4. Partition of left ventricle (LV) according to perfusion from right ventricle (RV) through fistulae

	Antero-lateral-septal	Apical-lateral-septal		Postero-lateral-septal		
Fistulae	→ LAD prox +/or mid + distal	→ apex		→ crux		
Coronary arteries	LAD	distal LAD RV-dependent perfusion	apical-lateral branches + RPD	LCX atrio-ventricular + postero-lateral branches	RPD	RCA
All LV n = 6 (4)*	6	5	5	6	1	4
All LAD Ø LCX n = 4 (3)**	4	4	4	0	1	1
Ø dist LAD n = 4 (2)	4	0	2	3	2	4
Fistula → apex only n = (1)	0	1	1	0	0	0
LV + RV RV-dependent; absent connection aorta-single LCA n = (1)	1	0	1	1	1	1
Total n = 16 (11)	15	10	13	10	5	10

() nonsurvivors. LAD, left anterior descending artery. LCX, left circumflex artery. RPD, posterior descending artery. RCA, right coronary artery. *1 with single coronary artery + RCA – interruption, alive. **1 with mid RCA – interruption, died.

TABLE 5. 5 Surviving patients with pulmonary atresia, intact ventricular septum, right ventricle - coronary artery fistulae and interruption of LAD: Follow-up after shunt operation

Pts. No.	Ages at cath/angio 1. +/or 2. last	Operation type age follow-up	RV anatomy with RV infundibulum "tripartite"	without trabecular portion	PA trunk atresia	TV ring Ø (mm)	RV systolic	PA
1 B.S. M	3 d, 5.4 yrs 8.2 yrs	Waterston 5 d 10 yrs	+	Ø	+	– 15	206 (2.) 131	25/13 $\overline{19}$ 16/6 $\overline{9}$
2 R.A. F	1 d 1.3 yrs	1.Waterston ; 2.ASD 1 d, 1 yr 8.8 yrs	+	Ø	Ø	4 9	150 175	– – – –
3 C.P. M	12 d 4 yrs	1.Bl-T R ; 2.Fontan 13 d, 4.8 yrs 4.9 yrs	+	Ø	Ø	8 –	100 –	– – 16/14 $\overline{14}$
4 I.E. F	5 d 1.4 yrs	1.Bl-T L ; 2.Bl-T R 6 d, 2.2 yrs 3.3 yrs	+	Ø	Ø	9 13	75 170	– – – –
5 L.R. M	2 d 7 mo	AO-PA (Ø 4mm) (Gore-Tex) 27 d 1 yr	Ø	+	Ø	– 5	– 108	– – – –

* with single coronary artery + mid RCA interruption. ASD, operative enlargement of atrial septal defect. Bl-T, Blalock-Taussig shunt. PA, pulmonary artery. TV, tricuspid valve. R, right. L, left. – no data, e.g. RV not entered. M, male. F, female.

TABLE 6. Pts. No.	Dominant type	Fistulae → LAD prox +/or mid +dist	Left → apex ↓ dist LAD	→crux ↓ LCX	Right → RCA prox +/or mid	→crux RCA +/or RPD	Perfusion of LV through fistulae antero- lateral- septal	apical- lateral- septal (dist LAD)	postero- lateral- septal
1	?	+ +	+ +	+ +	+ +	+ +	+ +	+ +	+ +
2	R	+ +	+ +	Ø Ø	+ Ø mid RCA	+ +	+ +	+ +	Ø +
3	L	+ –	Ø –	+ +	+ –	+ –	+ –	Ø –	+ +
4	L	+ +	+ +	Ø Ø	+ +	+ +	+ +	+ +	Ø Ø
5	L	+ +	– Ø	– +	– Ø	– Ø	– +	– Ø	– –

TABLE 7. Pts. No.	Shunt through fistulae AO → RV "steal" + RV → AO shunt O_2 RV – $\overline{v}$ = 22; 23 % +angio Øangio angio only	AO → RV "steal" only angio only	RV → AO shunt only	Evolution Progression: "A-V fistulae- like" RV → AO shunt	Regression: closure of fistulae	No change
1	– Ø	– Ø	– +	Ø Ø	Ø Ø	+ Ø	Ø Ø	Ø Ø
2	Ø Ø	Ø Ø	Ø Ø	Ø Ø	+ +	Ø	+ mid RCA	Ø
3	Ø –	+ –	Ø –	Ø Ø	Ø –	–	?	–
4	Ø Ø	+ Ø	Ø +	Ø Ø	Ø Ø	Ø	Ø	+
5	Ø Ø	Ø Ø	Ø Ø	+ +	Ø Ø	Ø	Ø	+

ring diastole from the aorta as well as retrogradely during
systole from RV, appeared to be associated with a more favourable outcome: in all survivors (3 of 7), 2 had a left dominant type and one had a single coronary artery, the filling of
the LCX was bidirectional as well as that of the postero-lateral branches in 2 of them. On the other hand, in each of 2
nonsurviving infants (4 of 7) the LCX and the atrio-ventricular branches of the RCA filled bidirectionally and from RV
only, respectively. One of the former had undergone a Waterston operation, the others had no operation, including the one
with AO-PA collaterals.

Evolution of the coronary circulation (Tables 5.-7.): Rarely
has spontaneous regression of a large fistula in PAIVS been
reported (10,18). We have previously also demonstrated spontaneous closure, or severe narrowing of a large proximal fistula
to the left coronary artery or LAD, with or without simultaneous closure of a co-existing proximal fistula to the RCA, in
each of 4 infants by cineangiocardiography at 1 day to 8
months of age and by corresponding histopathological studies
in one of them. None of these infants had undergone operative
decompression of the RV. In all, spontaneous regression had
resulted in obstruction of the connecting artery with subsequent ischemic changes of the LV myocardium and dyskinesis of
the anterior wall and apex of the LV in 2, respectively (20).
Patient no. 2 of the group of survivors of the present study
was also included in this previously described group with
spontaneous closure of fistulae. Further, patient no. 3 had
multiple large fistulae to all major left and right coronary
arterial branches, excepting the LAD distal to the interruption, and bidirectional shunt at the initial investigation.
But on 2 subsequent studies, the RV could not be probed. The
probability of regression of the fistulae in this child is
suggested by the favourable outcome after a modified Fontan
operation without incorporation of the RV.

The fistulae remained large on follow-up catheterization in
patients no. 4 and 5 at 1.4 years and 7 months respectively,
with persistent bidirectional shunt in the former and a diastolic "steal" from the aorta into the RV on angiocardiography
in the latter.

Progression into an "arterio-venous fistulae-like" systolic
shunt from the RV into the aorta through the proximal as well
as the distal fistulae, preferentially through the LCX was
documented at repeat catheterization at 5.4 and 8.2 years of
age in patient no. 1 with a single coronary artery from the
left aortic sinus and co-existing mid RCA-interruption. The
normal diastolic coronary flow was further impaired by a concurrent diastolic "steal" from the aorta into the RV in this
child. The question is raised as to whether in addition to the
persistence of RV hypertension and multiple stenoses within
the right branch of the single coronary artery, progressive
obstructive changes and increasing resistance in the extra-
and intra-myocardial coronary arteries may have enhanced the
unfavourable development, which accounts for the inoperability
and poor prognosis in this patient.

SUMMARY: findings with relevant effect on the coronary circulation and evolution
- Interruption of the proximal and mid-LAD in all patients, additional interruption of the RCA in 2 and absent connection between the aorta and a single coronary artery in one with the blood supply to the capillary bed distal to the interruption being dependent on sustained RV blood flow and hypertension through the fistulae was a major risk factor for the coronary artery blood supply of the LV myocardium and septum.

In addition to the interruption of the LAD, we had attributed a higher risk for compromise of coronary circulation, and accordingly a major determinate for the choice of surgical procedure, to the "steal" from the aorta into the RV through the fistulae during diastole (21).
- In the selected group of patients in the present study, a "steal" was not a discriminating factor for the outcome: it was distributed equally between the survivors and nonsurvivors with shunt operation or AO-PA collaterals and the patients who died without operation.

Similarly, an incremented risk did not appear to be associated with:
- bidirectional shunt through the fistulae and
- systolic RV to aorta shunt only.
- Right and extreme right dominant type, however, were associated with a higher risk for mortality.
- Fistulae to the LAD only and absence of fistulae to the proximal +/or mid RCA in cases with a combination of fistulae to the left main coronary arterial branches and distal right coronary arteries were associated with an unfavourable outcome.
- Exclusive retrograde filling of the coronary arteries to the postero-lateral LV wall from RV during systole was also equally distributed between the survivors and nonsurvivors with or without shunt operation or AO-PA collaterals.
- However, bidirectional filling of the coronary arteries to the postero-lateral LV wall appeared to be associated with a more favourable outcome.
- The diastolic "steal" from the aorta into the RV and the systolic shunt from RV into the aorta through the fistulae, which may progress into an "arterio-venous fistulae-like" shunt, are the negative effects of the persistence of the suprasystemic systolic pressure in the RV and of the systolic and diastolic pressure difference between RV and the aorta and coronary arteries through the fistulae as well as of the obstructive changes of the extra- and intra-myocardial coronary arteries.

SURGICAL IMPLICATIONS
- Severe hypoplasia of the RV and tricuspid valve in all infants, associated with absent infundibulum in 4 and atresia of the pulmonary artery trunk in 5, but generally with adequate sized pulmonary arteries, - irrespective of the complicating RV - coronary artery fistulae - precluded establishment of RV to pulmonary artery continuity and served as

indication for shunt operation in some infants (1-6, 9,14,15,22). Thus, suggesting a Fontan operation without incorporation of the RV into the right atrial - pulmonary artery anastomosis as the procedure of choice at long term.
- The mortality of the initial shunt operation in these infants with PAIVS, RV-coronary artery fistulae and interrupted LAD (median age 6 days) was 50 %, without operation 100 %.
- Enhancement of the coronary "steal" by the Waterston shunt and large AO-PA collaterals in addition to a diastolic "steal" from the aorta into the RV through fistulae may have played a role in the unfavourable outcome in 3 and one infant, respectively (16). It did, however, not interfere with survival in 4 infants with a Blalock-Taussig shunt in 2 and a Waterston and aorto-pulmonary artery Gore-Tex shunt in one infant each. The "steal" effect of an AO-PA shunt could be avoided by the performance of a Glenn shunt in later infancy.
- Interruption of the LAD ± of the RCA and absent connection between the aorta and a single coronary artery with RV-dependent blood flow preclude decompression of the RV, obliteration of the RV or closure of the fistulae which serve as an outlet for the RV-dependent blood supply distal to the interruption (6,9,10,16,20,21,24).
- However, persistence of the suprasystemic systolic pressure in the RV and of the systolic and diastolic pressure difference between the RV and the coronary circulation through the fistulae after shunt operation alone can result in progression into an "arterio-venous fistulae-like" shunt through the fistulae which further compromises the coronary circulation. Rarely it was associated with spontaneous regression or closure of the fistulae and restoration of normal coronary blood flow.
- To prevent the adverse effects of the RV hypertension on the coronary circulation in infants with PAIVS, fistulae and interruption of the LAD, equilibration of RV and aortic pressures was suggested, but was unsuccessful in 2 patients (9,20,21).

REFERENCES
1. Alboliras ET, Julsrud PR, Danielson GK, Puga FJ, Schaff HV, McGoon DC, Hagler DJ, Edwards WD, Driscoll DJ: Definitive operation for pulmonary atresia with intact ventricular septum. J Thorac Cardiovasc Surg 93: 454-464, 1987.
2. Braunlin EA, Formanek AG, Moller JH, Edwards JE: Angiopathological appearances of pulmonary valve in pulmonary atresia with intact ventricular septum. Interpretation of nature of right ventricle from pulmonary angiography. Br Heart J 47: 281-289, 1982.
3. Bull C, De Leval MR, Mercanti C, Macartney FJ, Anderson RH: Pulmonary atresia and intact ventricular septum: A revised

classification. Circulation 66: 266-272, 1982.

4. Cobanoglu A, Metzdorff MT, Pinson CW, Grunkemeier GL, Sunderland CO, Starr A: Valvotomy for pulmonary atresia with intact ventricular septum. A disciplined approach to achieve a functioning right ventricle. J Thorac Cardiovasc Surg 89: 482-490, 1985.

5. De Leval MR, Bull C, Stark J, Anderson RH, Taylor JFN, Macartney FJ: Pulmonary atresia and intact ventricular septum: Surgical management based on revised classification. Circulation 66: 272-280, 1982.

6. De Leval MR, Bull C, Hopkins R, Rees P, Deanfield J, Taylor JFN, Gersony W, Stark J, Macartney FJ: Decision making in the defintive repair of the heart with a small right ventricle. Circulation 72 (suppl II): 52-60, 1985.

7. Essed CD, Klein HW, Krediet P: Coronary and endocardial fibroelastosis of the ventricles in the hypoplastic left and right heart syndromes. Virchows Arch Path Anat Histol 368: 87-97, 1975.

8. Esterly JR, Oppenheimer EH: Some aspects of cardiac pathology in infancy and childhood. IV Myocardial and coronary lesions and cardiac malformations. Pediatrics 39: 896-903, 1967.

9. Foker JE, Braunlin EA, Cyr JASt, Hunter D, Molina JE, Moller JH, Ring WSt: Management of pulmonary atresia with intact ventricular septum. J Thorac Cardiovasc Surg 92: 706-715, 1986.

10. Freedom RM, Harrington DP: Contribution of intramyocardial sinusoids in pulmonary atresia and intact ventricular septum to a right-sided circular shunt. Br Heart J 36: 1061-1065, 1974.

11. Freedom RM, Wilson G, Trusler GA, Williams WG, Rowe RD: Pulmonary atresia and intact ventricular septum. A review of the anatomy, myocardium and factors influencing right ventricular growth and guidelines for surgical intervention. Scand J Thoracic Cardiovasc Surg 17: 1-28, 1983.

12. Gittenberger-de Groot AC, Sauer U, Bindl L, Babic R, Essed NE, Bühlmeyer K: Competition of coronary arteries and ventriculo-coronary communications in pulmonary atresia with intact ventricular septum. In press.

13. Lenox CC, Briner J: Absent proximal coronary arteries associated with pulmonic atresia. Am J Cardiol 30: 666-669, 1972.

14. Lewis AB, Wells W, Lindesmith GC: Evaluation and surgical treatment of pulmonary atresia and intact ventricular septum in infancy. Circulation 67: 1318-1323, 1983.

15. Milliken JC, Laks H, Hellenbrand W, George B, Chin A, Williams RG: Early and late results in the treatment of patients with pulmonary atresia and intact ventricular septum. Circulation 72 (suppl II): 61-69, 1985.

16. O'Connor WN, Cottrill CM, Johnson GL, Noonan JA, Todd EP: Pulmonary atresia with intact ventricular septum and ventriculocoronary communications: surgical significance. Circulation 65: 805-809, 1982.

17. O'Connor WN, Cash JB, Cottrill CM, Johnson GL, Noonan JA:
    Ventriculocoronary connections in hypoplastic left hearts:
    an autopsy microscopic study. Circulation 66: 1078-1086,
    1982.
18. Patel RG, Freedom RM, Moes CAF, Bloom KR, Olley PM,
    Williams WG, Trusler GA, Rowe RD: Right ventricular volume
    determinations in 18 patients with pulmonary atresia and
    intact ventricular septum. Analysis of factors influencing
    right ventricular growth. Circulation 61: 428-440, 1980.
19. Rowe RD, Freedom RM, Mehrizi A, Bloom KB: The neonate with
    congenital heart disease, 3rd ed. Philadelphia, Saunders
    WB, 1981.
20. Sauer U, Bindl L, Babic R, Gittenberger-de Groot AC, Sink
    JD, De Leval MR, Bühlmeyer K: Communications entre le ven-
    tricule droit et les arteres coronaires chez des nouris-
    sons atteints d'atresie pulmonaire a septum interventricu-
    laire intact. Correlation anatomo-clinique. In: Pathologie
    des Arteres Coronaires 1984, edited by Bex JP, Paris, New
    York, Barcelona, Milan, Mexico, Sao Paulo, Masson 1984:
    60-72.
21. Sauer U, Bindl L, Pilossoff V, Hultzsch W, Bühlmeyer K,
    Gittenberger-de Groot AC, De Leval MR, Sink JD: Pulmonary
    atresia with intact ventricular septum and right ventric-
    le-coronary artery fistulae. Selection of patients for
    surgery. In: Doyle EF, Engle MA, Gersony WM, Rashkind WJ,
    Talner NS (eds) Pediatric Cardiology: Proceedings of the
    second world congress, New York, Springer-Verlag, 1986:
    566-578.
22. Sideris EB, Olley RM, Spooner E, Farina M, Foster E,
    Trusler G, Shaher R: Left ventricular function and compli-
    ance in pulmonary atresia with intact ventricular septum.
    J Thorac Cardiovasc Surg 84: 182, 1982.
23. Sissman NJ, Abrams HL: Bidirectional shunting in a coro-
    nary artery-right ventricular fistula associated with pul-
    monary atresia with intact ventricular septum.
    Circulation 32: 582-588, 1965.
24. Waldman JD, Lamberti JJ, Mathewson JW, George L: Surgical
    closure of the tricuspid valve for pulmonary atresia in-
    tact ventricular septum and right ventricle-to-coronary
    artery communications. Pediatr Cardiol 5:221-224, 1984.
25. Zuberbuhler JR, Anderson RH: Morphological variations in
    pulmonary atresia with intact ventricular septum. Br Heart
    J 41: 281-288, 1979.

Acknowledgements: We wish to thank Miss Yvonne Aeschbach and
Mrs. Joan Deutsch for their help in the preparation of the
manuscript and tables and Mrs. Renate Nowak and Helena Soik
for their secretarial and photographic assistance.

PRESENT PROBLEMS AND NEW ISSUES IN CORONARY ARTERY
SURGERY: AN UPDATE

ROBERT B. KARP, M. D.

Introduction

Coronary artery disease is a multifactorial spectrum and must be approached by definition and analysis of subsets. For the clinician, convenient subsets of coronary artery disease are represented by the following: stable angina, unstable angina, silent ischemia, various combinations of anatomic disease, various derangements of ventricular function, mechanical derangements, electrophysiologic syndromes, congestive heart failure syndrome, associated valvular disease, and various syndromes associated with acute myocardial infarction. These subsets are not necessarily inclusive and not mutually exclusive.

Operations for coronary artery disease were initially designed and found effective for the relief of stable angina pectoris. It was amply demonstrated that a successful coronary artery operation was completely effective in relieving angina in 65 or 70 percent of patients and improving or modifying symptoms in another 20 percent. The surgical result has been found to correlate with the completeness of revascularization and/or freedom from graft occlusion. The relief of angina and, in fact, patency of the aortocoronary conduits is correlated with objective and subjective improvement in treadmill testing. For instance, in 1977, Mathur and Guinn[1] demonstrated in a prospective randomized study that surgical patients had improved exercise performance on treadmill testing on repeated examinations up to three years after operation compared to a similarly matched group of medically treated patients. They demonstrated also that the operated group had a trend toward better survival, less frequent myocardial infarctions, and fewer other major myocardial events. In the CASS study[2], which was primarily designed to evaluate survival in patients having only mild angina, there was, in fact, a significant improvement in freedom from all chest pain in the surgically managed group which differed from that in the medically managed group. In that study also, the use of nitrates and beta blockers was decreased in the surgical group and not changed in the medical group. Exercise performance, as reflected by ST depression, duration of exercise, and freedom from chest pain, was significantly improved in the surgical group and unchanged in the medical group.

The Coronary Artery Surgery Study, CASS

The coronary artery surgery study (CASS)[3] was one of several studies designed to identify whether and in which subsets surgery improved survival. It was assumed for the CASS study that patients with class III or class IV (Canadian Heart Association) angina would benefit from operation. It was also assumed that patients with left main coronary disease, prior coronary artery bypass grafting, overt heart failure, or those aged over 65 should be excluded from randomization because, in many cases, the type of therapy, either medical or surgical, had been well established. In any event, of some 21,000 patients seen at 15 sites in the U.S. and Canada, 16,626 were entered into the registry; 12.7 percent of those were eligible for randomization and 780 were actually randomized. When survival figures for the 390 surgical and 390 medical patients were evaluated at up to six years, there was no difference in survival between medically and surgically assigned patients (Fig. 1). To the surgeon and cardiologist accustomed to the day-to-day evaluation of coronary patients, these data made little sense. For instance, observational studies had shown that retrospective analysis of candidates for operation who had not chosen surgery faired less well than similar patients who had been offered and received operation. Thus, definition of subsets becomes critical when evaluating the universe of coronary artery patients in terms of survival and whether the best treatment is medical or surgical. For instance, when Kaiser(4) and his associates examined patients in the CASS registry who had class III or IV angina and three vessel disease, there was a significant improvement in survival for patients operated upon compared to those not operated upon

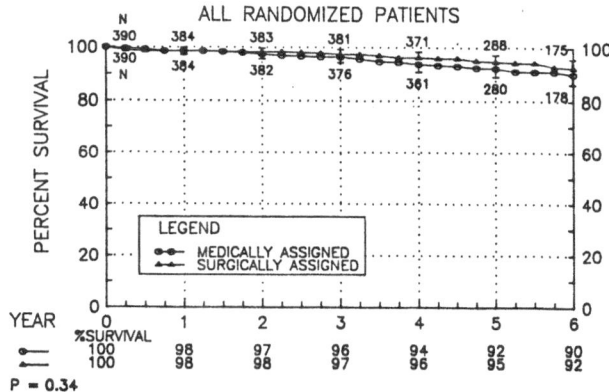

FIGURE 1. Survival Curves of 390 Surgically and 390 Medically Treated Patients Randomized from CASS Database.

(p < 0.001, Fig. 2). As the data accrued from many studies on survival, there occurred a number of persistent factors which predicted an incremental risk with operation. Many of these factors, however, had a greater incremental risk for mortality without operation. For instance, the degree of left ventricular dysfunction, the amount of congestive heart failure, age, smoking history, the urgency or priority of operation, the left ventricular end diastolic pressure, left main coronary artery stenosis, and female gender in multivariate analysis generally are incremental risk factors for mortality in surgically and medically treated patients. Interestingly, recent data suggest that left main stenosis, number of operable vessels, and, to a certain extent, left ventricular dysfunction have been minimized or eliminated as risk factors.

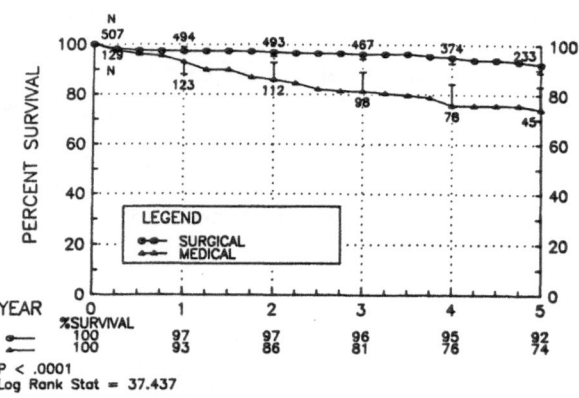

FIGURE 2. Survival Curves of Class III and IV Angina and Three Vessel Disease from the CASS Database.

The European Coronary Surgery Study

The European Coronary Surgery Study[5] is another randomized evaluation of medical and surgical therapy. In this group, however, patients with moderate and severe angina were analyzed. At the end of five years, 94 percent of surgical group and 82 percent of the medical group survived. The difference was significant at p < 0.001. As usual, for left main disease and three vessel disease, the differences were clear and significant between medical and surgical therapy. For two vessel disease, the anatomy was important. In those patients with important left anterior descending stenosis as one of the two vessels involved, surgical survival was significantly better than medical survival. If the left anterior descending was not involved, in those patients with two vessel disease, medical survival was equal to surgical survival.

The first demonstration of the effect of surgery to improve coronary survival was in the left main coronary group in the Veteran's Administration Hospital Study. The only controversy presently existing in patients with left main coronary disease is the priority of their operation. If the patient has unremitting chest pain, arrhythmias, or heart failure, operation is done immediately following catheterization. If the patient is free from these unstable situations, then the operation should be done at the next convenient time on the schedule.

When the patients in the CASS study were evaluated in further subsets, it became apparent that some patients with three vessel disease and minor angina benefited, in terms of survival, from operation. Those patients with ejection fraction less than 0.5 had a significantly improved survival with surgery than with medical therapy. As a corollary, as the ejection fraction diminished from 0.5 to 0.35 to 0.25, the advantage of surgery over medical treatment increased(6).

Coronary Surgery Related to Other Heart Disease

In other areas also, surgery for coronary artery disease has been found to be efficacious. For instance, in those patients having medically intractable ventricular tachyarrhythmias, coronary artery bypass grafting plus a direct approach to endocardial scarring has resulted in freedom from recurrent ventricular tachycardia in the majority of cases and improved survival over medically treated patients. These patients generally have scar or aneurysm formation on the anterior, lateral, or inferior wall of the left ventricle. The aneurysm or scar is resected and the endocardial scar is mapped to find areas of ventricular tachycardia activation, macro-reentry, or early ventricular activation. This area is either resected or encircled by an endocardial and midmyocardial incision. These patients are at higher risk than those for isolated coronary artery bypass grafting and an operative mortality of 10 percent is the norm. Patients are generally restudied in the electrophysiology laboratory seven to ten days postoperatively. Failure to induce ventricular tachycardia predicts excellent survival in this group. If ventricular tachycardia is induced, the patient is placed on one or several antiarrhythmic medications and the EP study repeated.

Unstable angina has also been a controversial area in the spectrum of coronary artery disease as to indication for operation, perhaps not necessarily whether operation ought to be done, but more importantly as to the urgency of operation. Unstable angina, however, is in reality a group of clinical syndromes varying from a slight increase in the intensity of angina to a syndrome characterized by rest pain, ST segment changes, arrhythmias, and pulmonary venous hypertension. There might also be some minor enzyme elaboration. Thus, the clinician must define the degree of instability in each and every patient. In those patients in whom there are arrhythmias, ST segment changes, enzyme enzyme elevations or pulmonary venous hypertension, we have learned that early catheterization and immediate operation result in a satisfactory outcome. In a study by McCormick, et al, of 3,311 patients with unstable angina in the CASS experience, the surgical mortality was 3.9 percent[7]. Determinants of early mortality were age, left ventricular score, and left main disease in a left dominant circulation. Late mortality was predicted by left ventricular score, associated illness, extent of the coronary artery disease, and cardiomegaly. The myocardial infarction rate was low and the relief of angina was excellent. In an earlier study, reported by Conti[8], patients operated upon had a better short and long term survival than those not operated upon. These were patients with preinfarction angina collected from several series. The National Institutes of Health conducted a cooperative study, 1972 to 1976, on unstable angina. In that study, over a four year period, there was no difference in survival between the medical and surgical group. In this writer's opinion, the patients randomized in that group had less severe symptoms and less severe ventricular dysfunction than those usually seen today. Additionally, 40 percent of the patients randomized to medical therapy crossed over to surgery within the duration of the study.

In the early 1980's, one could justify a statement that isolated coronary artery bypass grafting was associated with a 1 percent probability of death. For instance, of 3,608 patients analyzed, 1977 to 1981, at the University of Alabama, there was a 0.72 percent mortality (Fig.3). The mortality, however, increased with age after

Hospital Death after Isolated Coronary Artery Bypass Grafting
and after Left Ventricular Aneurysm
UAB 1977-1981

Category	n	Hospital Death		
		No.	%	CL
Primary Isolated CABPG	3608	26	0.72%	0.58%-0.90%
"LV Aneurysmectomy"	210	11	5.2%	3.7%-7.3%
Isolated with or without CABPG	175	7	4.0%	2.5%-6.2%
With MVR or MVA	8	1	12%	2%-36%
With Surgical Treatment of Ventricular Tachycardia	13	1	8%	1%-24%
With Surgical Treatment of VSD	6	1	17%	2%-46%
Other	8	1	12%	2%-36%

CABPG - coronary artery bypass grafting, CL - 70% confidence limits, LV - left ventricular, MVR - mitral valve replacement, MVA - mitral valve annuloplasty, VSD - ventricular septal defect

FIGURE 3.

the sixth decade. It stands to reason that as the end of the 1980's approaches and we find that more patients are operated upon in the seventh, eighth, and even ninth decade, operative mortality for isolated coronary artery bypass grafting has increased.

Although sometimes controversial, it can be shown that, in general, operation improves survival for patients with coronary artery disease. For instance, five year survival for patients with three vessel coronary artery disease medically treated is estimated to be 65 to 80 percent. A matched population without coronary artery disease has a 95 percent survival, and a population treated with operation has an 88.9 percent survival. It is notable also that operation produces a similarity in survival in patients with two vessel, three vessel, and left main disease, whereas there is a marked dissimilarity among those anatomic groups in their natural history or medically treated follow up. Thus operation neutralizes the effect of severe anatomical disease.

From time to time, patients with carotid stenosis and coronary artery disease are seen. This is particularly true of the coronary artery patient who has a carotid bruit. We have concluded that if the bruit is associated with no symptoms, no further noninvasive or invasive diagnostic test is necessary to define the carotid anatomy. Operation is associated with a low risk and, particularly, a risk which is no different for neurologic complications than in patients without carotid bruit. On the other hand, if the carotid disease is symptomatic, investigation should be done and the more severe lesion approached first. If the carotid disease is of top priority, the carotid operation can be done, followed sequentially by the coronary operation in seven to ten days. Only very infrequently (for instance, left main or unstable angina with a high-grade carotid lesion) should the operation be done simultaneously.

CAD and Valvular Heart Disease

The association of valvular heart disease with coronary artery disease is also an interesting and sometimes controversial surgical problem. There is little question that when important coronary disease is associated with aortic valve disease, the combined operation of coronary artery bypass grafting and aortic valve replacement is necessary. This can be done with a low mortality (5.4% in 220 patients at the University of Alabama), and that mortality is not influenced by the type of valvular lesion or the number of grafts placed. The association of mitral valve disease and coronary artery disease is quite a different story. When mitral incompetence is due to or related to myocardial ischemia, mitral valve replacement and coronary artery bypass grafting have a significantly higher mortality than does the combination when the mitral valve disease is not ischemic. For instance, isolated mitral valve replacement can be said to have a 3 to 5 percent operative mortality. When the mitral valve disease is rheumatic or nonischemic and there is associated, but unrelated, coronary artery bypass grafting, the expected mortality is perhaps 5 to

7 percent.   On the other hand, in the CASS registry, mitral valve replacement associated with ischemic heart disease had a 17 percent mortality and jumped to 40 percent mortality when the operation was performed in an emergent or urgent group of patients.   Thus, we have learned that when coronary artery disease and valvular heart disease are found in the same patient, all coronary disease should be bypassed.   In addition, if one can do a conservative operation or no operation on the mitral valve, the results are likely to be more satisfactory than those when mitral valve replacement is necessary in ischemic heart disease.

Reperfusion

A more controversial discussion centers around early surgical reperfusion for myocardial infarction.   For ten years, the group in Spokane, Washington, has treated many patients with ongoing myocardial infarction by coronary artery bypass grafting.   Their nonrandomized, retrospective study showed superior results in those patients treated surgically compared to those managed medically.   For instance, DeWood[9], in 1979, reported a 5.8 percent 30-day mortality in 187 patients treated surgically compared to an 11.5 percent in 200 patients treated medically in the same hospitals during the same period of time.   The difference, both at 30 days and 56 months, was significant at $p < 0.5$.   Additional studies from that group and others demonstrated that the mortality with surgical reperfusion was less if the patient was operated upon less than six hours from symptom onset compared to greater than six hours from symptom onset.   Phillips and associates[10] from DesMoines, Iowa, had similarly good results in early surgical reperfusion.   Primary surgery in 160 patients was associated with four deaths, two early and two late.   On the other hand, surgery for medical failure, i.e., failure of streptokinase or failure of PTCA, was associated in 21 patients with 6 deaths (29% mortality).   Phillips also showed that surgical reperfusion was associated with a statistically significant improvement in ejection fraction, decrease in left ventricular end diastolic pressure, increase in stroke volume, decrease in end systolic volume, and decrease in end diastolic volume.   Rogers and associates[11] from the University of Alabama suggested that improvement in segmental and global ejection fraction after successful surgical or medical reperfusion was related to the adequacy of preexisting collateral blood flow.   In patients where collateral blood flow had been demonstrated prior to reperfusion, ejection fraction increased; where there was no collateral blood flow, ejection fraction, segmental wall function, and infarct zone ejection fraction showed no change regardless of whether reperfusion was successful or not.

All is not optimistic when one suggests surgery for all patients with myocardial infarction.   For instance, Hochberg[12] demonstrated (Fig. 4) a deleterious effect of early coronary artery bypass grafting on mortality in patients with ejection fraction less than 50 percent. We suggest that if operation can be delayed to three or four weeks postinfarction in those patients with diminished ejection fraction, surgical results and long term outcome will be improved.

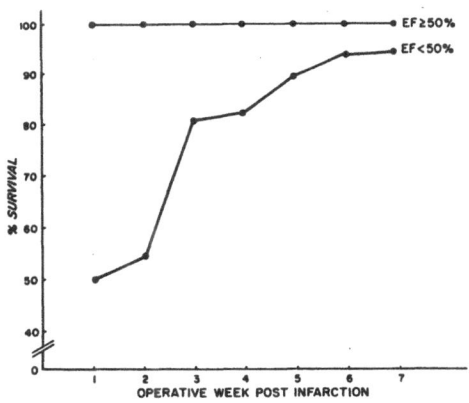

FIGURE 4.   The Effect of Delaying Surgery on Patients with Infarction.

Type of Bypass

The final considerations in this update relate to the type of conduit used to bypass narrowings in the coronary arteries. The two obvious conduits available are the autologous saphenous vein graft and the internal mammary artery graft. The saphenous vein graft can be used as an individual, i.e., end-to-side graft, or a sequential graft basing two or three distal anastomoses of the saphenous vein on one proximal anastomosis to the aorta. There is little to choose in terms of results between the sequential (side-to-side graft) and the end-to-side or individual graft. The former is preferred by some surgeons because of fewer proximal anastomoses, shorter total length of vein necessary, and perhaps, slightly shorter operating time. The obvious disadvantage to the sequential graft is that, if there is a proximal stenosis or occlusion, more myocardium is at risk.

Recently, there has been great enthusiasm for the use of the internal mammary artery, IMA, as one of the primary grafts or as a source of as many grafts as possible. The use of the internal mammary artery was pioneered by Green in New York and by the Cleveland Clinic group, 15 years ago. Many surgeons were reticent to embrace the use of the IMA because of its more tedious operative technique and because of their questions about the adequacy and caliber of the graft to carry adequate blood flow to a large area of the myocardium. Experience has shown, however, that with practice most surgeons can master the use of attached and free internal mammary artery technique and that adequate blood flow can be achieved through the mammary to relieve angina and supply large areas of myocardium. Recently, there have been advocates of sequential internal mammary artery grafting, and there are those who have achieved full and complete revascularization of all three coronary systems using two mammary arteries.

Much of the data generated concerning the internal mammary artery concerned the anastomosis of the left internal mammary to the left anterior descending. For instance, Okies[13] has shown (Fig. 5) that graft patency is significantly improved to the LAD when the mammary is used compared to when the saphenous vein is used. Cosgrove[14] and

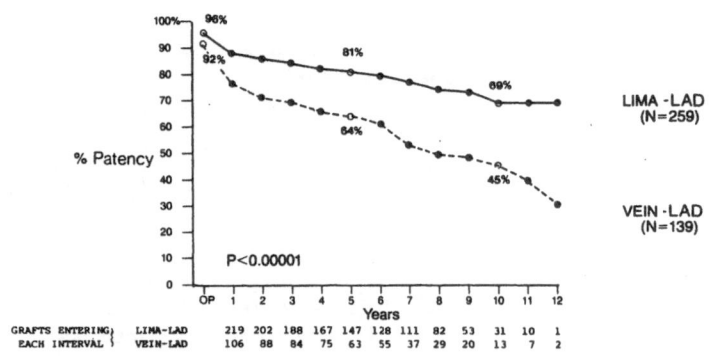

FIGURE 5. Patency in Two Types of Grafts, Internal Mammary Artery (LIMA) and Vein.

others have shown that the incidence of reoperation due to graft failure is decreased when the internal mammary artery is used as one or more of the conduits. Grondin and others have unequivocally demonstrated that there is an inexorable decrease in patency over the years in the saphenous vein. In the first year, this decrease in patency may be due to technical factors, inadequacy of the vein, or to accelerated intimal hyperplasia. The failure rate of the saphenous vein, at one year, is between 7 and 15 percent. Between year two and year five, the failure rate is about 1.5 percent per year in the saphenous vein. After the fifth year, saphenous vein atherosclerosis occurs, and a conservative estimate suggests that, at seven to ten years, only 60 percent of vein grafts will be patent. On the other hand, the patency of the internal mammary artery at seven to ten years may be 85 to 90 percent. Recently, it has been shown that patients having the internal mammary artery operation compared to those having all grafts done with saphenous vein experience equal relief of angina. Thus, the ability of the internal mammary artery to carry sufficient blood was demonstrated.

The final answer to our questions regarding the internal mammary artery was provided by the Cleveland Clinic in a study extending over ten years comparing survival in patients with one or more grafts done with the internal mammary artery to those with all grafts done using saphenous vein[15]. At ten years, the survival in the IMA group was 82.6 percent compared to 71 percent in patients with saphenous vein graft ($p < 0.0001$). Thus, in patients with three vessel disease, the use of the internal mammary artery gives equal relief of angina, longer patency, greater freedom from reoperation, and better survival than does revascularization with only saphenous vein grafting (Fig. 6).

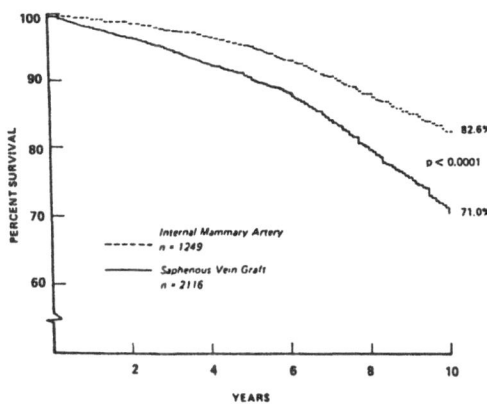

FIGURE 6.   The Effects of Graft Choice on Survival Curves.

Conclusions

The future for coronary artery bypass grafting lies the prospect of more redo operations, the use of additional conduits (such as allograft saphenous vein and allograft internal mammary artery), the use of laser and operative balloon angioplasty, and the greater use of extended endarterectomy.

Better myocardial protection has allowed effective operation in older patients, more severely diseased ventricles, and complex associated malformations.

The one sobering note to this generally optimistic picture is the fact that, in 1986, the mortality for isolated coronary artery bypass grafting and the morbidity associated with it has increased over a period five to ten years ago. The cause of this is not hard to see, in that surgeons have extended the operation to older patients and to sicker patients, many of whom would not have been considered for operation five to ten years ago.

Thus, age, heart failure score, and surgical priority again remain predictors of operative mortality.

REFERENCES

1. Mathur VS and Guinn GA: Prospective randomized study of coronary artery bypass in stable angina: the first 100 patients. Circ 51,52:1-133, 1975.

2. CASS principal investigators and their associates: Coronary artery surgery study (CASS): a randomized trial of coronary artery bypass surgery: quality of life in patients randomly assigned to treatment groups. Circ 68:951-960, 1983.

3. CASS principal investigators and their associates: Coronary artery surgery study (CASS): a randomized trial of coronary artery bypass surgery: survival data. Circ 68:939-950, 1983.

4. Kaiser GC, David KB, et al: Survival following coronary artery bypass grafting in patients with severe angina pectoris (CASS): an observational study. J Thorac Cardiovasc Surg 89:513-524.

5. European Coronary Surgery Study group: Prospective randomized study of coronary artery bypass surgery in stable angina pectoris: a progress report on survival. Circ 65(Suppl. II): II67-II71, 1982.

6. Alderman EL, Fisher L, et al: Results of coronary artery surgery in patients with poor left ventricular function (CASS). Circ 68: 785-795, 1983.

7. McCormick JR, Schick EC, et al: Determinants of operative mortality and long term survival in patients with unstable angina: the CASS experience. J Thorac Cardiovasc Surg 89: 683-688, 1985.

8. Conti CR II, Gilbert JB, et al: Unstable angina pectoris: randomized study of surgical versus medical therapy. Am J Cardiol 35:129, 1975.

9. DeWood MA, Spores J, et al: Medical and surgical management of myocardial infarction. Am J Cardiol 44:1356-1364, 1979.

10. Phillips SJ, Kontahworn C, et al: Emergency coronary artery reperfusion: a choice therapy for evolving myocardial infarction. J Thorac Cardiovasc Surg 86:679-688, 1983.

11. Rogers WJ, Hood WP, et al: Return of left ventricular function after reperfusion in patients with myocardial infarction: importance of subtotal stenoses or intact collaterals. Circ 69:338-349, 1984.

12. Hochberg MS, Parsonnet V, et al: Timing of coronary revascularization after acute myocardial infarction: early and late results in patients revascularized within seven weeks. J Thorac Cardiovasc Surg 88:914-921, 1984.

13. Okies JE, Page US, et al: The left internal mammary artery: the graft of choice. Circ 70:213-221, 1984.

14. Cosgrove DM, Loop FD, et al: Predictors of reoperation after myocardial revascularization. J Thorac Cardiovasc Surg 92:811-821, 1986.

15. Loop FD, Lytle BW, et al: Influence of the internal mammary artery graft on the ten year survival and other cardiac events. N Engl J Med 314:1-6, 1986.

THROMBOLYSIS WITH AND WITHOUT PTCA IN ACUTE MYOCARDIAL INFARCTION

Maarten L. Simoons, M.D., Thoraxcenter, University Hospital Dijkzigt and
Erasmus University Rotterdam, the Netherlands.

Thrombolytic therapy in patients with acute myocardial infarction has been
developed in order to salvage myocardial cells through restoration of
coronary blood flow. The clinical value of various methods for thrombolytic
therapy can be judged by (a) patency of the infarct related vessel after
the intervention, (b) limitation of infarct size, (c) preservation of
global and regional left ventricular function, (d) clinical course in
hospital and after hospital discharge and (e) long term survival. This
sequence of salutary effects of thrombolytic therapy has been shown by the
trial conducted by the Interuniversity Cardiology Institute in the
Netherlands in 533 patients, randomly allocated to conventional treatment
and intracoronary administration of streptokinase (1-6). The improved
survival after intravenous administration of streptokinase has been
documented by the Italian GISSI trial (7) and the ISIS study (8), while
limitation of infarct size and preservation of left ventricular function
after intravenous streptokinase was shown by the ISAM study (9). In this
review the effects of thrombolytic therapy will be described.

Patency of the infarct related vessel

Early angiography, within a few hours after the onset of myocardial
infarction has shown complete occlusion of the infarct related vessel in
approximately 80% of patients. After intravenous administration of
streptokinase approximately half the patients have a patent vessel while
75 - 85% patency can be achieved by intracoronary administration of
streptokinase (2). Newly developed drugs such as recombinant tissue
plasminogen activator (rtPA) have an intermediary effect, leading to
approximately 60 - 70% patency. The fraction of patients with a patent
infarct related vessel is also dependent upon the time interval between
thrombolytic therapy and angiography. The numbers mentioned above have been
obtained by angiography after approximately 1 - 2 hours. If the angiogram
is made at a later stage, for example after one or several days, more
patent vessels are found. In a small number of patients with
persistant occlusion in spite of thrombolytic therapy, patency can be
achieved by immediate perforation of the thrombus and angioplasty
(PTCA)(10). Furthermore immediate PTCA can be applied in order to reduce
the residual stenosis after thrombolysis. This might further improve flow
to the infarcted tissue.

Limitation of infarct size

In the study conducted by the Interuniversity Cardiology Institute of the
Netherlands infarct size was estimated from release of the enzyme alpha
HBDH. In average a 30% reduction of infarct size was observed after
intracoronary streptokinase. In patients treated within one hour after the
onset of symptoms, infarct size was halved, while little effect was
observed in patients treated after four hours (4). In addition myocardial
perfusion was measured by thallium scintigraphy 3 months after the
infarction. Quantitative analysis of thallium scintigrams from 118 patients
admitted to the Thoraxcenter revealed a 13% reduction of scintigraphic
infarct size after thrombolysis. In the same group of patients a 21%
limitation of enzymatic infarct size was observed. Qualitative analysis of
thallium scintigrams from 236 patients with a first myocardial infarction
from the 5 participating centers supported these observations (5). Finally
infarct size can be estimated by the length of the akinetic segement on
contrast angiography. In patients who underwent thrombolytic therapy, the
length of the akinetic segment was considerably shorter than in patients
after conventional treatment (2).
In the ISAM study, infarct size was estimated from serial CK-release. In
patients admitted within 3 hours after the onset of symptoms a 15%
reduction of enzymatic infarct size was observed after intravenous
administration of streptokinase (9). Thus, intravenous streptokinase seems
to be half as effective as intracoronary treatment in terms of infarct size
limitation. This is in agreement with the rate of reperfusion which is also
twice as high after intracoronary streptokinase compared with intravenous
administration.

Global left ventricular ejection fraction was measured by radionuclide
angiography and by contrast angiography in the study conducted by the
Interuniversity Cardiology Institute of the Netherlands. Both showed a
higher global ejection fraction after thrombolytic therapy. The 6%
difference in global ejection fraction was due to smaller end diastolic and
smaller end systolic volumes in the thrombolysis group (2,3,6). Again
differences in global ejection fraction measured by the ISAM study after
intravenous streptokinase were half of those observed after intracoronary
streptokinase (9).

Clinical course after thrombolytic therapy

Patients allocated to thrombolytic therapy in the Netherlands trial had a
more favorable clinical course than the control group. In particular the
incidence of ventricular fibrillation, shock and heart failure during
convalenscence as well as post infarction pericarditis were lower in the
thrombolysis group (table 1). On the other hand thrombolysis resulted in a
number of bleeding complicaions, which were usually limited to arterial and
venous puncture sites. Also recurrent infarction was more prominent after
thrombolytic therapy, while hospital mortality was almost halved (3,5).
Again these data are in agreement with those in the two larger studies on
intravenous streptokinase (7,8).

Table 1 : Clinical Course in Hospital

	Control group	Thrombolysis group	p Value
No. of patients	264	269	
Hospital mortality (14 days)	26	14	0.05
Recurrent infarction (14 days)	9	12	
Angina pectoris	55	57	
Heart failure (coronary care unit)			
Mild	55	54	
Severe	12	10	
Shock	24	13	
Dopamine/dobutamine treatment	42	26	0.03
Respiratory support	11	6	
Intraaortic balloon pump	10	16	
Heart failure during convalescence	53	37	0.05
Ventricular fibrillation	61	38	0.01
Pericarditis	46	19	0.0004
Bleeding	7	53	0.0001
Coronary angioplasty	9	59*	
Bypass surgery	16	29	

Percutaneous transluminal angioplasty was performed more frequently in the thrombolysis group when the 46 patients with angioplasty immediately after thrombolysis are included (*). Only p values of 0.05 or less are reported.

Long term survival

One year survival improved from 84% in conventional treated patients to 90% in patients allocated to the thrombolytic therapy in the Netherlands trial. The greatest improvement of survival was observed in patients with anterior wall infarction (table 2), while only a small difference was observed in patients with inferior wall infarction. Reduction of hospital mortality was also reported by the GISSI study, particularly in patients treated within 3 hours after the onset of symptoms (7). The reported, but not yet published, one year follow up data from that study show consistent reduction of mortality, particularly in patients with anterior wall infarction.

The value of PTCA after thrombolytic therapy

In the Netherlands' trial, immediate PTCA was attempted in 46 patients, and successful in 44 patients. Matched pair analysis of 36 patients who underwent immediate PTCA, compared with patients with similar coronary who were treated in hospitals without PTCA facilities, shows that immediate PTCA lead to a reduction of reinfarction angina. Also Erbel et al. observed a more favorable clinical course in patients who underwent PTCA immediately after intracoronary streptokinase treatment (10). On the other hand, PTCA did not improve the clinical course in patients in whom thrombolysis was achieved with rtPA as reported by the TAMI study.

Table 2

	Inferior infarction			Anterior infarction		
	C	T	p	C	T	p
n	148	139		116	130	
Acute PTCA	–	17 (12%)	–	–	29 (22%)	–
Late PTCA/CABG	28 (19%)	31 (22%)	–	17 (15%)	36 (28%)	0.03
Recurrent MI	9 (6%)	26 (19%)	0.001	5 (4%)	10 (8%)	–
Mortality	17 (11%)	12 (9%)	–	26 (22%)	14 (11%)	0.01

Results of the study conducted by the Netherlands Interuniversity
Cardiology Institute, one year follow-up.
n = number of patients
C = control group
T = thrombolysis group
p = Mann-Whitney rank-sum test (two sided)
PTCA = percutaneous transluminal coronary angioplasty
CABG = coronary artery bypass grafting
MI = myocardial infarction

Conclusion

It is now well established that thrombolytic therapy does improve survival,
and quality of life in patients with acute myocardial infarction. The
treatment is particularly indicated in patients with large anterior
infarction who are admitted within 4-6 hours after the onset of symptoms.
The benefits of thrombolytic therapy in patients with inferior infarction
are less clear, since a high incidence of reinfarction is apparent in this
group (5). At this time it is uncertain which method for thrombolytic
therapy is most cost effective. Intravenous streptokinase is least
effective, but cheep and readily available. The newer agents for
intravenous administration such as rtPA and APSAC are more effective, but
also more expensive (11). The most effective procedure is intracoronary
administration of a thrombolytic agent such as streptokinase,followed in
part of the patients by PTCA. This procedure however requires facilities
for acute angiography and PTCA, and this is thus relative costly. Methods
should be developed for early recognition and immediate treatment of
patients with acute myocardial infarction, preferably before hospital
admission, e.g. by the ambulance service. Comparative studies of various
approaches to thrombolytic therapy are urgently needed.

REFERENCES

1. Simoons ML, Serruys PW, Brand M vd, et al. Improved survival after early thrombolysis in acute myocardial infarction. Lancet, 1985; II : 578-582.
2. Serruys PW, Simoons ML, Suryapranata H et al. Preservation of global and regional left ventricular function after early thrombolysis in acute myocardial infarction. J Am Coll Cardiol 1986; 7 : 729-742.
3. Simoons ML, Serruys PW, Brand M vd, et al. Early thrombolysis in acute myocardial infarction : limitation of infarct size and improved survival. J Am Coll Cardiol, 1986; 7 : 717-728.
4. Vermeer F, Simoons ML, Baer FW, et al. Which patients benefit most from early thrombolytic therapy with intracoronary streptokinase ? Circulation, 1986; 74 : 1379-1389.
5. Vermeer F. Thrombolysis in acute myocardial infarction. Thesis, May 20, 1987. Res JCJ, Simoons ML, Wall EE van der, et al. Long term improvement
6. in global left ventricular function after early thrombolytic treatment in acute myocardial infarction. Br Heart J, 1986; 56 : 414-421.
7. Gruppo Italiano per lo studio della streptochinasi nell'infarto miocardico (GISSI). Effectiveness of intravenous thrombolytic treatment in acute myocardial infarction. Lancet, 1986; I : 397-401.
8. ISIS Steering Committee : Intravenous streptokinase given within 0-4 hours of onset of myocardial infarction reduced mortality in ISIS-2. Lancet, 1987; I: 502.
9. The ISAM Study group. A prospective trial of intravenous streptokinase in acute myocardial infarction mortality, morbidity, and infarct size at 21 days. N Engl J Med, 1986; 314: 1465-1470.
10. Erbel R, Pop T, Henrichs KJ, et al. Percutaneous transluminal coronary angioplasty after thrombolytic therapy : a prospective controlled randomized trial. J Am Coll Cardiol, 1986; 8 : 485-495.
11. Simoons ML, Lubsen J, Serruys PW, Hugenholtz PG. Thrombolytic therapy for acute coronary thrombosis. Eur Heart J, 1987 (in press).

LASER ANGIOSURGERY:
A Brief Overview of Tissue
Micromachining with Spectral Diagnostics.

J.R. Kramer*, S. Strikwerda+, C. Kittrell#, M.S. Feld#

INTRODUCTION

The introduction of percutaneous transluminal balloon angioplasty by Dr. Andreas Gruntzig in 1977 revolutionized the care of many patients with coronary atherosclerosis.[1] Selected individuals with coronary artery disease could be treated in the catheterization laboratory less invasively, at a lower cost and with less hospitalization than would have been required for an open heart operation.[2] Early reports showed that in-hospital mortality (1.1%) was similar to that of open heart surgery.[3] Subsequent improvements in equipment and operator skill led to higher primary success rates[4] and, eventually, to a wider application of the technique.[5-6]

Enthusiasm for percutaneous transluminal angioplasty, however, has been dampened somewhat by the significant incidence of restenosis (up to 49%).[7] Restenosis occurs early (within three to six months) and appears to be the result of intimal proliferation of smooth muscle cells in response to the arterial injury induced by balloon expansion.[8-9] Unfortunately, the likelihood of this response appears to be greatest in the left anterior descending coronary artery.[10] When restenosis occurs, initial gains, in terms of patient comfort and reduced cost, are eroded by the need for follow-up stress tests, repeat catheterizations, repeat balloon angioplasties or open heart surgery.

In an effort to overcome the problem of restenosis, many investigators have begun to explore the use of laser light.[11-13] Because some forms of laser light can be transmitted through optical fibers, a percutaneous approach to plaque ablation seems technically feasible. Conceptually, laser light could vaporize obstructive lesions rather than rip or tear them and, at the same time, cauterize the residual arterial surface reducing the likelihood of a proliferative healing response.[14]

Choy and colleagues were the first to attempt the in vivo removal of atherosclerotic obstructions from human coronary arteries using a laser catheter.[15-16] Figure 1 schematically represents the delivery system used. Coherent blue-green light from an argon ion laser was emitted into a fiberoptic coupler and transmitted to the coronary obstruction via a single, bare, silica fiber with an 85 micron core.

*Cleveland Clinic Foundation. Cleveland, Ohio 44106 USA
+State University of Leiden. Leiden, The Netherlands
#Massachusetts Institute of Technology. Cambridge, Massachusetts 02139 USA

STANDARD LASER LABORATORY

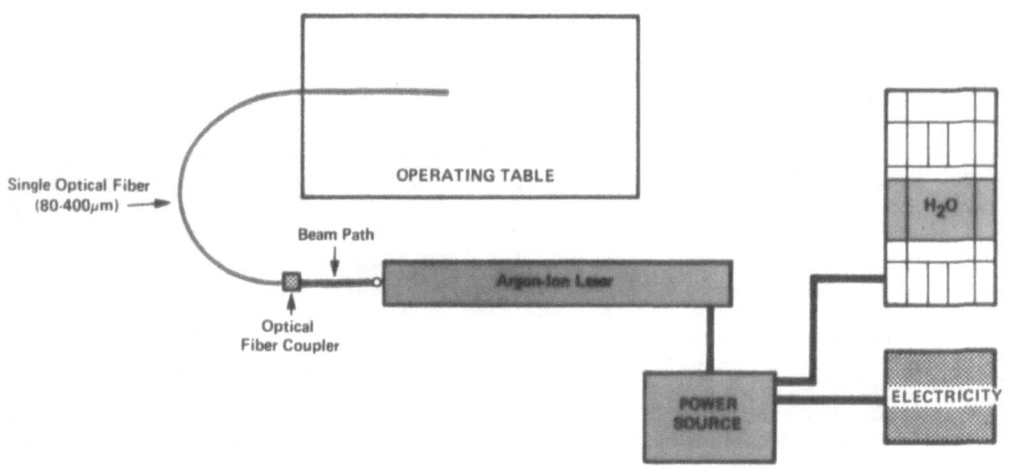

Figure 1. Layout of a standard laser laboratory

During open heart surgery, five arteries, later to be bypassed, were treated with 60 to 1231 joules of blue-green argon ion laser light. Following the laser treatment, each artery received an aorto-coronary saphenous vein graft.[16-17] Problems encountered included perforation, thermal injury to the media, inability to create a large new lumen, and early reocclusion. In a larger sense, these problems related to the simplicity of the delivery system and to:

(1) The inability to precisely control fluence,
(2) an inadequate understanding of dosimetry, and
(3) an inability to aim within the arterial lumen.

In order to study these problems in more detail, physicians at the Cleveland Clinic Foundation and scientists and engineers at the Massachusetts Institute of Technology have established a cooperative research program under the name of "The Lester Wolfe Laser Angiosurgery Research Group" in honor of a visionary and early benefactor. While the research goals of this group are broad, some specific goals include:[18]

(1) Build systems and catheters that will allow precise control of fluence,
(2) describe dosimetry in terms of fluence,
(3) and develop an intra-arterial spectral guidance system.

CONTROL OF FLUENCE

In a certain range of operating parameters, a single relationship exists between the amount of arterial tissue removed and a laser parameter, the fluence. Fluence is described as follows:

$$\text{Fluence} \; \left(\frac{\text{joules}}{\text{millimeter}^2}\right) = \frac{\text{Power (watts) x Time (seconds)}}{\text{Area (millimeters}^2)}$$

Fluence can be controlled by determining laser power, exposure time and spot size. Power (milliwatts to 30 watts) can be controlled by laser beam attenuation or by computer control of the laser output. Time of exposure, when using a continuous wave beam, can be accurately determined by using a shutter, under computer control, to intermittently interrupt the beam. Exposures as short as 5 milliseconds can be obtained using this technique.[19] In the Cleveland Clinic interventional operating room (figure 2-3), energy dosage is under computer control, and can be defined in millijoules.

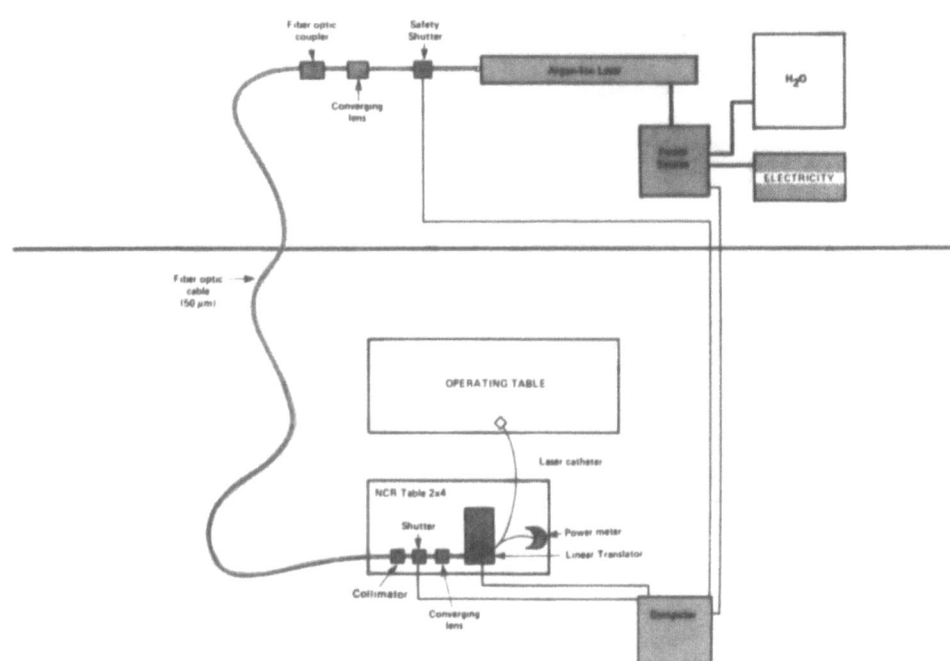

Figure 2. Schematic representation of a laser angiosurgery operating room specifically designed to control energy delivery.

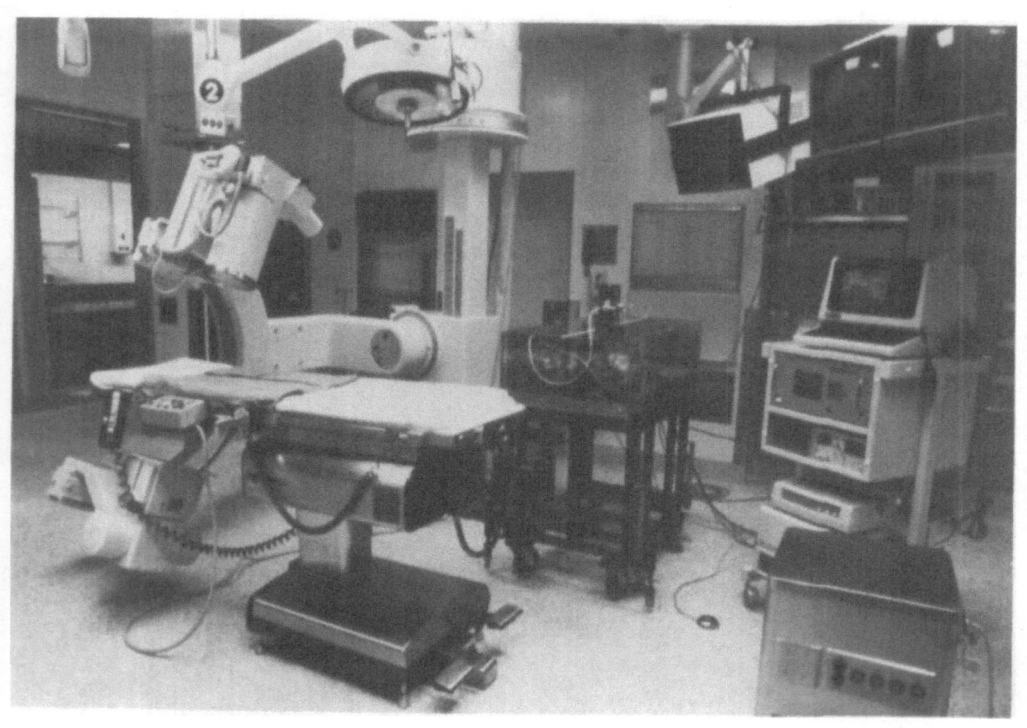

Figure 3. Cleveland Clinic laser angiosurgery operating room. The laser
is housed in a closet outside the operating room (left). A cart carrying
the alignment optics and a shutter and the control computer are in the
operating room (right). The laser is connected to the operating room
cart by a fiberoptic cable running through the ceiling.

In order to completely define fluence, one must know over what area
(spot size) the measured energy is delivered. This can be accomplished
by knowing and controlling the distance between the tip of the optical
fiber and the target.[19-20] An interposing optical shield allows the
fiber tip to target distance to be predetermined (figure 4). Because the
shield is placed in contact with the tissue to be removed, spot size is
known and intervening blood, which would otherwise absorb laser light, is
displaced from the field insuring correct dosimetry.

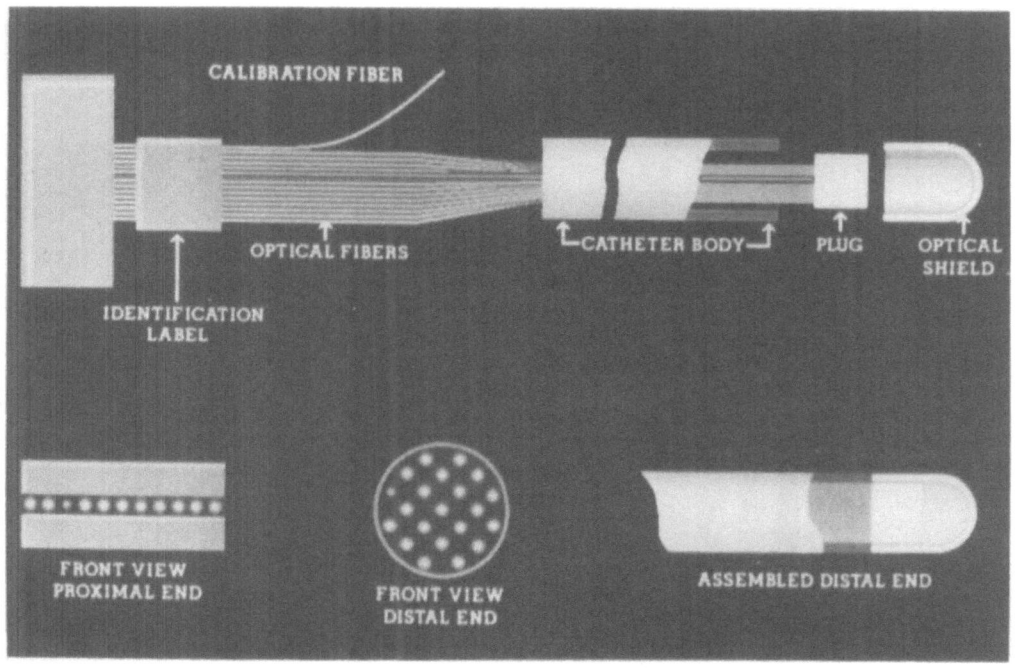

Figure 4. Laser angiosurgery catheter. A preset fiber to shield distance determines spot size and allows the calculation of laser beam intensity.

DOSIMETRY

The difference between successful plaque removal and arterial perforation can be measured in microns. Because tolerances are so tight, an understanding of what happens when light impinges on tissue (ie, dosimetry) is essential. Dr. Strickwerda and colleagues,[21] using atherosclerotic aortic segments obtained at autopsy, blue-green argon ion laser light, and a delivery system to control fluence, have shown that it is possible to remove discrete portions of tissue while leaving the perimeter intact. Time, energy, intensity and fluence thresholds can be defined, ablation efficiencies described, and certain "workable" fluence regions identified[22] (figure 5).

230

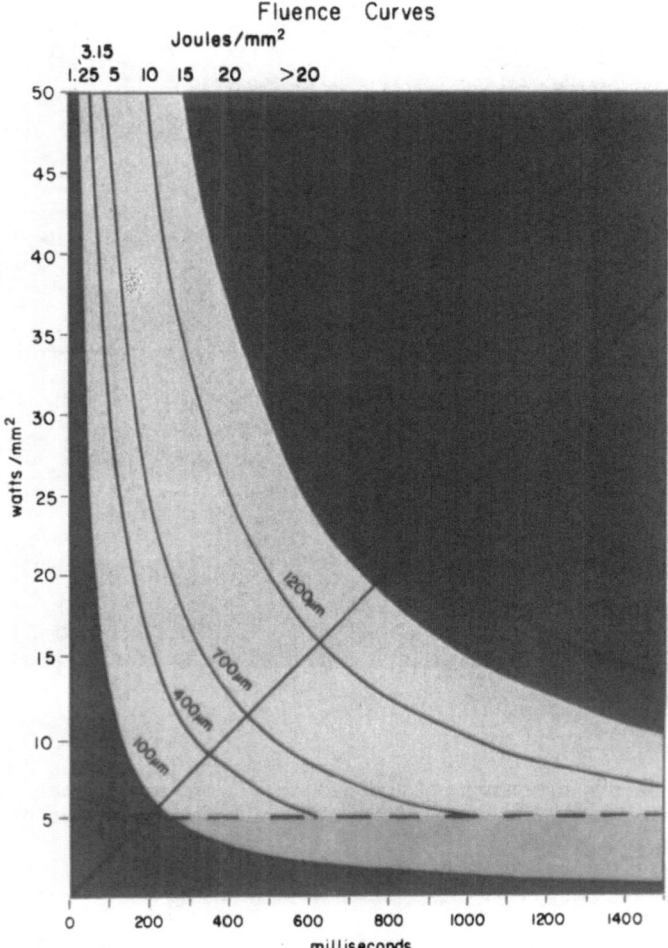

Figure 5. Fluence curves for a spot size of 500 microns. There is a fluence threshold at approximately 1.25 joules/mm^2 and an intensity threshold at approximately 5 watts/mm^2. Once over threshold, depth of penetration and degree of peripheral heat damage are proportional to the fluence delivered. By working near the fluence threshold with adequate intensity, it is possible to ablate tissue while avoiding deep tissue penetration and excessive peripheral thermal damage.

INTRA-ARTERIAL GUIDANCE

Even with precise dosimetry, an aiming method more sensitive than fluoroscopy and angiography will be needed for laser angiosurgery. Dr. Kittrell and colleagues[23] have shown that blood, normal artery, and atherosclerotic plaque can be recognized and differentiated by using the fluorescence induced by exposure to low levels of blue-green laser light. Spectral information from the artery can be collected, analyzed, and displayed before a decision to use high laser power within the arterial lumen is made. Because the laser angiosurgery catheter contains an array of fibers oriented to form a series of overlapping spots, a multipixel image of the arterial lumen can be created, permitting tissue removal with resolution. Computer controlled feedback loops that deliver the correct photon dose to clearly identified targets in the artery can be envisioned[24] (figure 6).

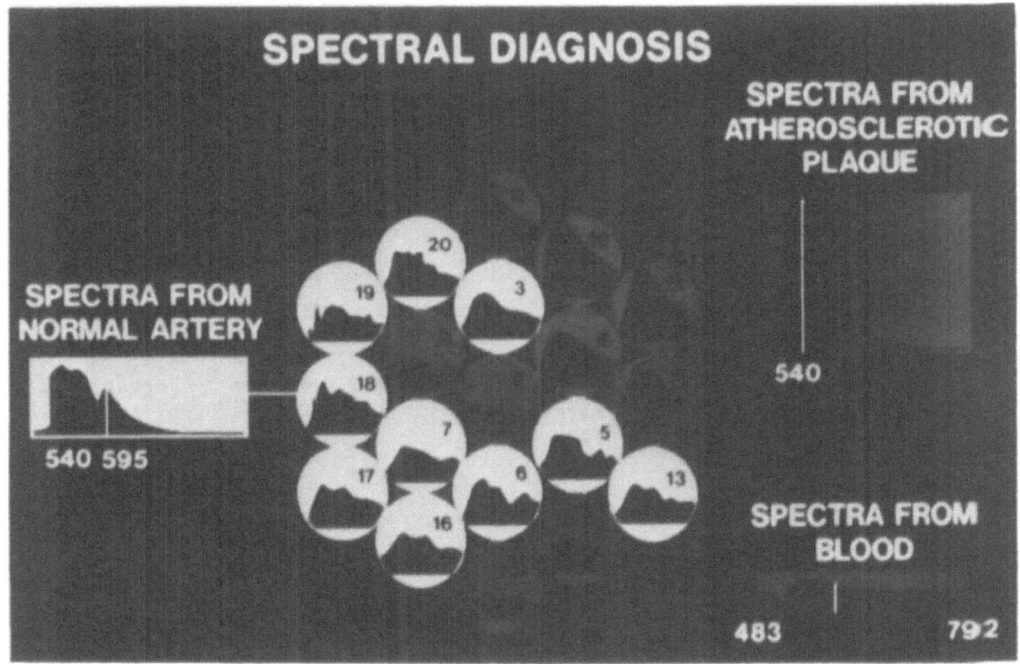

Figure 6. Spectral map obtained from a 19 fiber laser angiosurgery catheter in contact with blood, normal artery and atherosclerotic plaque. Only fibers in contact with plaque would be fired.

SUMMARY

It is technically possible to control the physical factors that define fluence. While the delivery systems and catheters are complex, they are part of todays' technology. With control of fluence, it is possible to describe a dosimetry for precise, controlled tissue removal. The development of intra-arterial aiming systems that ensure the appropriate aiming of a defined photon dose are on the horizon as are clinical protocols for testing these concepts in the operating room environment.

ACKNOWLEDGEMENTS

The authors recognize and appreciate the support of the Lester Wolfe Laser Angiosurgery Research Group at Massachusetts Institute of Technology, the Cleveland Clinic Foundation and American Edwards Laboratories. We thank Ms. Nancy Boyko for preparation of the manuscript.

REFERENCES

1. Gruntzig AR, Senning A, Siegenthaler WE: Non-operative dilatation of coronary artery stenosis. Percutaneous transluminal coronary angioplasty. New England Journal of Medicine 301: 61, 1979.

2. Jang GC, Block PC; Cowley MJ, Gruntzig AR, Dorros G, Holmes DR, Kent KM, Letherman LL, Myler RK, Sjolander SME, Stertzer SH, Vetrovec GW, Willis WH, Williams DO: Relative cost of coronary angioplasty and bypass surgery in a one-vessel model. American Journal of Cardiology 53: 52C, 1984.

3. Dorros G, Cowley MJ, Simpson J, Bentivoglio LG, Block PC, Bourassa M, Detre K, Gosselin AJ, Gruntzig AR, Kelsey SF, Kent KM, Mock MB, Mullin SM, Myler RK, Passamani ER, Stertzer SH, Williams DO: Percutaneous transluminal coronary angioplasty: Report of complications from the National Heart, Lung and Blood Institute PTCA Registry. Circulation 67: 723, 1983.

4. Meier B, Gruntzig AR: Learning curve for percutaneous transluminal coronary angioplasty: Skill, technology or patient selection. American Journal of Cardiology 53: 65C, 1984.

5. Hartzler GO, Rutherford BD, McConahay DR, McCallister SH: Simultaneous multiple lesion coronary angioplasty-a preferred therapy for patients with multiple vessel disease (abstract). Circulation 66: II-5, 1982.

6. Dorros G, Stertzer SH, Cowley MJ, Myler RK: Complex coronary angioplasty: Multiple coronary dilatations. American Journal of Cardiology 53: 126C, 1984.

7. Zaidi AR, Hollman J, Galan K, Belardi J, Franco I, Simpfendorfer CC, Klein MI: Predictive value of chest discomfort for restenosis following successful coronary angioplasty (abstract). Circulation 72: III-456, 1985.

8. Essed CE, Van Den Brand M, Becker AE: Transluminal coronary angioplasty and early restenosis. Fibrocellular occlusion after wall laceration. British Heart Journal 49: 393, 1983.

9. Austin GE, Ratliff NB, Hollman J, Tabei S, Phillips DF: Intimal proliferation of smooth muscle cells as an explanation for recurrent coronary artery stenosis after percutaneous transluminal coronary angioplasty. Journal of the American College of Cardiology 6: 369, 1985.

10. Leimgruber PP, Roubin GS, Hollman J, Cotsonis GA, Meier B, Douglas JS, King SB, Gruntzig AR: Restenosis after successful coronary angioplasty in patients with single vessel disease. Circulation 73: 710, 1986.

11. Lee G, Ikeda RM, Dwyer RM, Hussein H, Dietrich P, Mason DT: Feasibility of intravascular laser irradiation for in vivo visualization and therapy of cardiocirculatory diseases. American Heart Journal 103: 1076, 1982.

12. Abela GS, Normann S, Cohen D, Feldman RL, Geiser EA, Conti CR: Effects of carbon dioxide, Nd-YAG, and argon laser radiation on coronary atheromatous plaques. American Journal of Cardiology 50: 1199, 1982.

13. Choy DSJ, Stertzer SH, Rotterdam HZ, Bruno MS: Laser coronary angioplasty: Experience with nine cadaver hearts. American Journal of Cardiology 50: 1209, 1982.

14. Gerrity RG, Loop FD, Golding LAR, Ehrhart LA, Argenyi ZB: Arterial response to laser operation for removal of atherosclerotic plaques. Journal of Thoracic and Cardiovascular Surgery 85: 409, 1983.

15. Choy DSJ, Stertzer SH, Rotterdam HZ, Sharrock N, Kaminow IP: Transluminal laser catheter angioplasty. American Journal of Cardiology 50: 1206, 1982.

16. Choy DSJ, Stertzer SH, Myler RK, Marco J, Fournial G: Human coronary laser recanalization. Clinical Cardiology 7: 377, 1984.

17. Choy DSJ: Vascular recanalization with the laser catheter. IEEE Journal of Quantum Electronics. QE-20: 1420, 1984.

18. Kittrell C: Strategic plaque initiative. The Spectrograph 6: 1, 1987.

19. Cothern RM, Kittrell C, Hayes GB, Willett RL, Sacks B, Malk EG, Ehmsen RJ, Bott-Silverman C, Kramer JR, Feld MS: Controlled light delivery for laser angiosurgery. IEEE Journal of Quantum Electronics. QE-22: 4, 1986.

20. Cothern RM, Hayes GB, Kramer JR, Sacks B, Kittrell C, Feld MS: A multifiber catheter with an optical shield for laser angiosurgery. Lasers in the Life Sciences 1: 1, 1986.

21. Strikwerda S, Bott-Silverman C, Ratliff NB, Goormastic M, Cothern RM, Costello B, Kittrell C, Feld MS, Kramer JR: The effects of varying argon laser intensity and exposure time on ablation of atherosclerotic plaque. Lasers in Surgery and Medicine, submitted for publication.

22. Partovi F, Izatt JA, Cothern MS, Kittrell C, Thomas JE, Strikwerda S, Kramer JR, Feld MS: A model for thermal ablation of biological tissue using laser radiation. Lasers in Surgery and Medicine, in press.

23. Kittrell C, Willett RL, delos Santos-Pacheo C, Ratliff NB, Kramer JR, Malk EG, Feld MS: Diagnosis of fibrous arterial atherosclerosis using fluorescence. Applied Optics 24: 2280, 1985.

24. Mehta A, Richards-Kortum RR, Ratliff NB, Kittrell C, Feld MS: Real time determination of artery wall composition and control of laser ablation using laser-induced fluorescence. Conference on Lasers and Electro-optics, Baltimore, Maryland, 1987, p. 39.

INDEX